Emergency Medicine Certifying Exam

The Complete Review

Daniel G. Ostermayer, MD
MCGOVERN MEDICAL SCHOOL
THE UNIVERSITY OF OF TEXAS HEALTH SCIENCE CENTER
UT HEALTH
DEPARTMENT OF EMERGENCY MEDICINE

Editors

Brandon R. O'Keefe, MD

MCGOVERN MEDICAL SCHOOL
THE UNIVERSITY OF OF TEXAS HEALTH SCIENCE CENTER
UT HEALTH
DEPARTMENT OF EMERGENCY MEDICINE

Carra G. Banda, MD

MCGOVERN MEDICAL SCHOOL
THE UNIVERSITY OF OF TEXAS HEALTH SCIENCE CENTER
UT HEALTH
DEPARTMENT OF EMERGENCY MEDICINE

Kenneth Paul, MD

MCGOVERN MEDICAL SCHOOL
THE UNIVERSITY OF OF TEXAS HEALTH SCIENCE CENTER
UT HEALTH
DEPARTMENT OF EMERGENCY MEDICINE

Lorenzo Baeza, MD

MCGOVERN MEDICAL SCHOOL
THE UNIVERSITY OF OF TEXAS HEALTH SCIENCE CENTER
UT HEALTH
DEPARTMENT OF EMERGENCY MEDICINE

Cade A. Johnson, MD, MBA, MPH

MCGOVERN MEDICAL SCHOOL
THE UNIVERSITY OF OF TEXAS HEALTH SCIENCE CENTER
UT HEALTH
DEPARTMENT OF EMERGENCY MEDICINE

Jessica Dunn, MD

MCGOVERN MEDICAL SCHOOL
THE UNIVERSITY OF OF TEXAS HEALTH SCIENCE CENTER
UT HEALTH
DEPARTMENT OF EMERGENCY MEDICINE

SPECIAL THANKS TO ECG STAMPEDE FOR THEIR GENEROUS DONATION OF ECGS USED THROUGHOUT THIS BOOK.

Null Publishing

Null Publishing, an independent publisher, provides tools, resources, and expertise to authors publishing educational texts. Authors retain ownership, control, and copyright of their published works and gain the flexibility and power of digital publishing.

For more information visit http://nullpublishing.com or email info@nullpublishing.com.

Preparing for the Certifying Exam

Exam Format

The ABEM Certifying Examination consists of two testing sessions. Each session contains 4 Clinical Decision-Making (CDM) cases at 15 minutes each and 6 Communication/Procedural cases at 10 minutes each. You will manage a simulated trackboard throughout the CDM cases, requiring you to prioritize and multitask across patients just as you would in a real emergency department.

The 8 ABEM Case Types

Clinical Decision-Making (CDM): The core of the exam. You receive a chief complaint, obtain history and physical findings, order and interpret studies, manage the patient, and disposition appropriately. These cases test your ability to recognize emergencies, manage evolving clinical scenarios, and reassess after interventions. Each CDM case includes a trackboard with other patients requiring attention.

Difficult Conversations: You must deliver bad news, discuss goals of care, navigate end-of-life decisions, or address sensitive topics such as substance use, abuse, or unexpected diagnoses. The examiner evaluates your empathy, clarity, and ability to maintain a therapeutic relationship under emotionally charged circumstances.

Managing Conflict: These cases present interpersonal friction with consultants, nursing staff, patients, or families. You must de-escalate, negotiate, and advocate for your patient while maintaining professionalism and collaborative relationships.

Patient-Centered Communication (PCC): You must elicit the patient's perspective, address their concerns and health literacy, provide clear discharge instructions, and ensure shared decision-making. The focus is on whether you communicate in a way the patient can understand and act on.

Prioritization: You manage a busy trackboard with multiple patients at various acuity levels. The examiner evaluates your ability to triage, delegate, and identify which patient needs you most urgently while ensuring no patient is neglected.

Procedures: Using task trainers or simulation equipment, you demonstrate procedural competency. You must verbalize indications, consent, preparation, technique, and post-procedure assessment. Common procedures include airway management, chest tubes, central lines, abscess drainage, and nerve blocks.

Ultrasound: You interpret point-of-care ultrasound images in the context of a clinical scenario. You must identify normal and abnormal findings and integrate them into your clinical decision-making. Common applications include FAST, cardiac, aortic, biliary, renal, and soft tissue ultrasound.

Reassessment/Troubleshooting: After an initial intervention or stabilization, the patient changes. You must recognize clinical deterioration, identify the cause, and adjust your management. These cases test whether you follow up on results, reassess vital signs, and modify your plan when things do not go as expected.

How to Use This Book

The Clinical Care Cases section provides comprehensive CDM-format cases with opening scenarios, diagnostics, management, reassessment, and critical actions. Many cases also include embedded communication challenges (difficult conversations, conflict management, patient-centered communication) identified by their own subheadings within the case. The Prioritization cases toward the end of this section simulate multi-patient trackboard scenarios.

The Procedures section lists critical steps for each procedure to refresh and organize your approach. The Ultrasound section provides anatomic images and interpretation guidance for the point-of-care applications tested on the exam.

For the best simulation of exam conditions, practice with a partner who reads the case and presents clinical information as you request it. Verbalize your actions, thought process, and communication with patients and families rather than silently reading through cases.

Tips for the Exam

Trackboard management: During CDM cases, you will have a trackboard with other patients. Check it at natural transition points (after ordering studies, while waiting for results). Delegate appropriately (nursing reassessments, social work consults). Do not ignore the trackboard, but do not let it distract you from a critically ill patient in front of you.

Time management: You have 15 minutes per CDM case and 10 minutes per communication/procedural case. Move through your assessment efficiently. State your differential early. Do not perseverate on a single aspect of the case. If you are stuck, verbalize your thought process and move forward. The examiner may redirect you if you are spending too long on one area.

Communicate constantly: Narrate everything. Tell the examiner what you are thinking, what you are looking for, what you are ordering, and why. If you are unsure, say so and describe your approach to resolving the uncertainty.

Disposition is part of the case: Every case requires a disposition decision. State your admission or discharge plan, the appropriate level of care, necessary follow-up, and return precautions. Incomplete dispositions lose points.

We also offer an interactive companion course at emcertifyingexam.com

CLINICAL CARE CASES

Fussy Toddler

Opening Scenario

A 3-year-old male is brought in by his parents. The mother is carrying the child, who is crying inconsolably. The father states, "He keeps grabbing his stomach and screaming. This isn't like him."

Initial Assessment

Vitals: BP 89/61, HR 126, RR 24, SpO_2 100% RA, T 36.9°C. Weight: 15 kg

Crying, kicking legs intermittently, inconsolable, making tears.

History

- HPI: Constant crying for 3 hours. Colicky and restless for 12 hours prior with decreased feeding. One episode nonbilious, nonbloody emesis 2 hours ago. No fever. Normal urine output and stool earlier today. Mother noticed a "new diaper rash" on the left side.
- PMHx: Full-term, uncomplicated delivery, immunizations up-to-date
- PSH: None
- Meds/Allergies: None
- Social: Lives with parents and 8-year-old brother

Physical Examination

- General: Crying, inconsolable, moderate pain distress
- HEENT: Normal, making tears, moist mucous membranes
- Chest/Cardiac: Clear bilaterally, normal S1/S2, no murmur
- Abdomen: Soft, nondistended, active bowel sounds, non-tender (no guarding or rebound when distracted), no masses
- GU Exam (CRITICAL — must specifically request): Normal circumcised phallus. Right testicle normal size, position, lie; cremasteric reflex present. Left hemiscrotum erythematous and edematous. Left testicle enlarged, exquisitely tender, high-riding with transverse lie. Cremasteric reflex absent on left.
- Skin: Erythema to left hemiscrotum
- Extremities/Back/Neuro: Normal

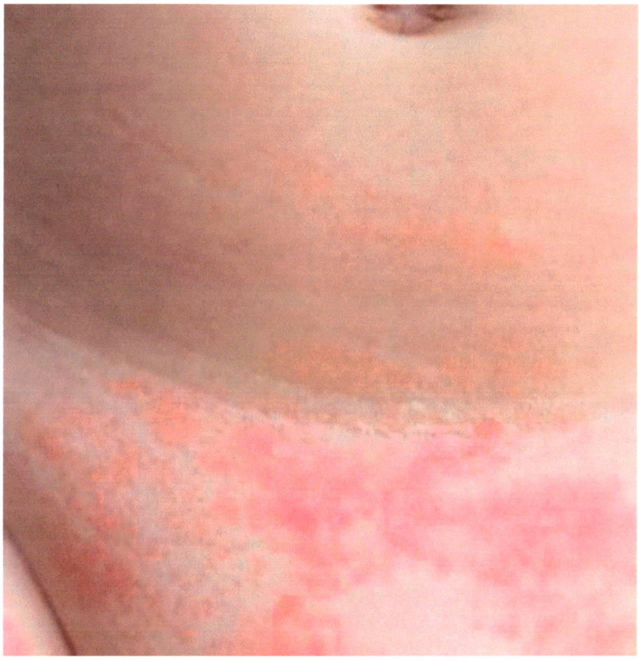

Diagnostic Studies

- CBC: WBC 11.0, Hct 38.1%, Plt 350. BMP and UA normal.
- Testicular US with color flow: Absent arterial flow to enlarged, hypoechoic left testicle; normal flow to right testicle

Management

- IV access (22g or larger), make NPO
- Morphine IV 0.1 mg/kg – do not delay analgesia for imaging or consult
- Order bedside testicular US with color flow Doppler
- Immediate page to Urology or Pediatric Surgery (do not wait for imaging)

Patient Communication

The US tech is at home (45-60 min ETA). Urology has not responded to page. Parents are increasingly distressed: "Why isn't anyone doing anything?"

- Acknowledge the delay; empathetically explain the diagnosis (testicular torsion) and urgency (time-critical to save the testicle)
- Escalate: charge nurse, hospital supervisor, or administrator to expedite tech or arrange transfer
- Communicate urgency directly to consultant: "Surgical emergency with threatened testicle; need immediate response"

Reassessment

After initial morphine: HR increases to 148, crying resumes, grabbing groin saying "Owie, owie."

- Recognize return of pain/tachycardia indicates ongoing ischemia
- With surgical delay >30 minutes and persistent symptoms, attempt manual detorsion
- Explain risks/benefits to parents, obtain consent, provide additional analgesia/sedation
- Technique: Elevate testicle toward inguinal ring and rotate medial-to-lateral ("opening a book") 1.5 rotations (540 degrees). If pain worsens, try opposite direction.

Manual detorsion provides temporary relief (HR 106, consolable), but pain recurs after 30 minutes. Urology arrives and takes patient to OR for scrotal exploration, detorsion, and bilateral orchiopexy.

Critical Actions

- Perform testicular/groin examination on any male child with acute abdominal pain
- Recognize testicular torsion (high-riding, transverse lie, absent cremasteric reflex)
- Order emergent testicular Doppler ultrasound
- Call Urology/Pediatric Surgery immediately (do not wait for imaging)
- Administer opioid analgesia promptly – do not delay for imaging or consult
- Attempt manual detorsion

Found Unresponsive

Opening Scenario

EMS arrives with a 28-year-old female nurse student found unresponsive in the bathroom of an inpatient hospice facility where she works. Last seen normal 90 minutes ago. Hospice staff found her slumped against the wall with an empty pill bottle labeled "Morphine Sulfate ER 30mg". Snoring respirations on scene; supplemental oxygen placed by EMS. No signs of trauma.

Initial Assessment

Vitals: BP 88/54, HR 56, RR 6, SpO_2 88% RA (96% on 15L NRB), T 36.4°C

- Airway: Patent with snoring respirations, no gag reflex
- Breathing: Shallow, irregular, visible respiratory depression
- Circulation: Warm, dry skin; weak pulses; cap refill 2 seconds
- Disability: Unresponsive to verbal stimuli; withdraws to pain; GCS 7 (E2, V1, M4)
- Exposure: No track marks, rashes, or trauma

Immediate actions: Continuous monitoring, two large-bore IVs, NRB mask, fingerstick glucose (94), prepare naloxone, order ECG/CBC/BMP/acetaminophen/salicylate levels/urine tox screen.

History

- HPI: Second-year nursing student volunteering at hospice. Found by aide 15 minutes prior to EMS. No witnessed seizure or vomiting.
- PMHx/Meds/Allergies: Unknown (patient unresponsive)
- Social: Lives with roommate; no known substance use per staff

Physical Examination

- General: Young female, obtunded, minimally responsive to sternal rub
- HEENT: Pupils pinpoint (2 mm bilaterally), reactive; no head trauma; oropharynx clear
- Neck: Supple, no JVD, no meningismus
- Cardiovascular: Bradycardic, regular rhythm, no murmurs
- Pulmonary: Shallow respirations, clear bilaterally
- Abdomen: Soft, nondistended
- Extremities: No edema, no track marks
- Neurological: Withdraws all extremities to pain; no focal deficits

Diagnostic Studies

- CBC: WBC 7.2, Hgb 13.5, Plt 245
- BMP: Na 139, K 4.3, Cl 104, HCO_3 24, BUN 14, Cr 0.9, Glucose 94
- ABG: pH 7.28, pCO_2 72, pO_2 78, HCO_3 25 (acute respiratory acidosis)
- Acetaminophen <10, Salicylates <5, Ethanol undetectable
- ECG: Sinus bradycardia at 54 bpm, normal intervals, no QT prolongation
- CXR: Clear, no aspiration infiltrates, no radio-opaque pills

Management

- Administer naloxone 0.4 mg IV push
- Patient becomes arousable within 2-3 minutes; RR improves to 14, BP 98/64, HR 72, SpO_2 96% on 2L NC

Reassessment

30 minutes later: Patient becomes increasingly somnolent, RR drops to 10. Administer second naloxone 0.4 mg IV and initiate continuous infusion at 0.5 mg/hour. Extended observation required (12-24 hours) due to extended-release morphine formulation outlasting naloxone duration.

Patient Communication

Once awake and alert after naloxone: - Non-judgmental assessment of suicide risk and psychosocial stressors - Explore triggers: academic pressure, hospice-related grief, prior undisclosed substance use - Frame substance use disorder as a medical condition; offer opioid cessation referral and counseling resources

Difficult Conversations

- Discuss opioid use disorder with the patient and also the potential impact on her work due to nature of the use that occurred while she was at work.

Managing Conflict

Patient becomes agitated upon learning of mandatory reporting, demands to leave AMA. Acknowledge fear and anger. Explain medical necessity of 12-hour observation (extended-release formulation risk). Negotiate: expedited social work consult, confidentiality assurances where possible, voluntary substance abuse treatment referral.

Disposition

- ED observation 12-24 hours with continuous pulse oximetry
- Naloxone infusion titrated to RR >12
- Psychiatry consult for suicide risk assessment
- Social work for substance use disorder resources
- Poison Control notification

Critical Actions

- Recognize opioid toxidrome (respiratory depression, pinpoint pupils, AMS) and treat without waiting for tox confirmation
- Incremental naloxone (0.4 mg IV) to avoid precipitating severe withdrawal
- Recognize naloxone duration (20-60 min) is shorter than ER morphine — anticipate re-narcotization and start infusion
- Immediate glucose check
- Screen for co-ingestants (acetaminophen, salicylates)
- Non-judgmental communication about substance use; suicide risk assessment
- Navigate mandatory reporting conversation and AMA conflict
- Extended observation for long-acting opioid with appropriate disposition planning

Abdominal Pain After Travel

Opening Scenario

A 28-year-old woman presents with worsening abdominal bloating and frequent loose stools. She appears tired but walks unaided.

Initial Assessment

Vitals: BP 118/76, HR 98, RR 16, SpO_2 98% RA, T 37.2°C

Tired but no acute distress. Airway patent, lungs clear, warm dry skin, cap refill <2 seconds.

History

- HPI: 28-year-old woman with 3-week history of watery, foul-smelling diarrhea (5-8 episodes daily) following return from Southeast Asia. Associated with significant bloating, early satiety, and mild diffuse abdominal cramping. Denies fever, hematochezia, or melena. Reports approximately 8 lb unintentional weight loss. Symptoms initially improved briefly after return but have persisted and worsened over the past week.
- PMHx: Hypothyroidism
- PSHx: Appendectomy (age 12)
- Medications: Levothyroxine
- Allergies: NKDA
- Social: Graphic designer, lives with partner, occasional alcohol use, denies tobacco or illicit drug use
- FHx: Mother with irritable bowel syndrome; father with type 2 diabetes
- Travel History: Returned 3 weeks ago from a 2-week trip to Cambodia and Vietnam. Consumed street food, fresh vegetables, and untreated well water while trekking in rural areas. Denies recent camping or freshwater swimming in the US.

Physical Examination

- General: Alert, oriented, mild fatigue noted
- HEENT: Mucous membranes slightly dry, oropharynx clear
- Neck: Supple, no lymphadenopathy
- Cardiovascular: Borderline tachycardic, regular rhythm, no murmurs
- Abdomen: Soft, mildly distended with increased tympany to percussion, hyperactive bowel sounds, minimal diffuse tenderness without guarding or rebound, no hepatosplenomegaly
- Rectal: Hemoccult negative brown stool, no masses
- Skin: Warm, dry, no rashes or edema
- Remainder of physical examination normal

Diagnostic Studies

- CBC: WBC 8.2, Hgb 12.8, Hct 41%, Plt 245
- BMP: Na 134, K 3.1, Cl 102, HCO_3 20, BUN 32, Cr 1.0, Glucose 88
- LFTs: AST 28, ALT 24, Alk Phos 95, Albumin 3.8
- Stool: Fecal leukocytes negative, C. difficile toxin negative, O&P sent and pending, Giardia antigen positive

Management

- Peripheral IV access, initiate IV rehydration
- Ondansetron PRN for nausea
- Order CBC, BMP, LFTs, stool for O&P, Giardia antigen, fecal leukocytes, stool culture, C. difficile toxin

Reassessment

After 3 hours: improving nausea, vomited twice, but eager to try and PO. Repeat vitals: BP 110/72, HR 108, RR 18, T 37.4°C.

- Transition to IV NS with 20 KCl at 125 mL/hr
- Metronidazole 500 mg PO (or IV if vomiting persists); prescribe tinidazole as alternative

Patient Communication

- Explain Giardia is a protozoan parasite, not bacterial – typical traveler's diarrhea antibiotics (ciprofloxacin, azithromycin) are ineffective
- 5-7 day treatment course; symptom resolution expected within 2-3 days; complete full course
- Not typically contagious with standard hygiene after treatment initiation; avoid food preparation for 24 hours if in food service
- Screen and treat symptomatic household contacts
- Discuss water purification for future travel

Critical Actions

- Elicit detailed travel history with specific exposures and timing
- Recognize diarrhea >14 days suggests protozoal etiology (Giardia, Entamoeba) rather than bacterial
- Order Giardia antigen and O&P rather than relying solely on bacterial culture
- Identify dehydration on reassessment and transition to IV rehydration
- Replete potassium (K 3.1) with IV fluids
- Select metronidazole or tinidazole for protozoal infection (not fluoroquinolones)
- Arrange outpatient follow-up with repeat stool studies if symptoms persist

Facial Trauma

Opening Scenario

EMS arrives with a 24-year-old male assaulted outside a bar 15 minutes ago, struck multiple times in the face with a baseball bat. Intoxicated but verbal at scene with questionable LOC; increasingly somnolent en route.

Initial Assessment

Vitals: BP 143/83, HR 106, RR 20, SpO_2 95% RA, T 36.2°C, FS 110

Obvious facial deformity with significant active bleeding from nose and mouth. Gurgling respirations. Supine on backboard with C-collar.

- Airway: Compromised – gurgling, blood in oropharynx, significant epistaxis
- Breathing: Tachypneic, SpO_2 declining
- Circulation: Hypertensive, tachycardic

Immediate actions: Chin lift/jaw thrust with C-spine precautions, oropharyngeal suctioning, manual tongue traction. After basic maneuvers, gurgling persists with SpO_2 declining to 90% on 15L NRB mask.

Critical Decision – Airway Management:

This is a difficult airway due to midface trauma. Do NOT proceed with standard RSI (risk of cannot-intubate-cannot-ventilate). Prepare for awake intubation with topical anesthesia and ketamine while maintaining spontaneous respirations. Have cricothyrotomy set at bedside. If awake intubation fails, proceed directly to surgical airway.

After successful awake intubation: SpO_2 improves to 100%.

History

- HPI: Assault with baseball bat to face. Questionable LOC at scene. Intoxicated.
- PMHx/Meds/Allergies: Unknown
- Social: Intoxicated

Physical Examination

After airway secured and hemorrhage control initiated (direct pressure to nares, anterior nasal packing if needed – do not clamp vessels blindly). Two large-bore IVs, T&C for 2 units PRBCs, 1L NS bolus, tetanus prophylaxis, trauma team activation.

After stabilization (BP 128/79, HR 99, SpO_2 100% on ventilator):

- HEENT: Laceration under right zygoma, moderate epistaxis, depressed midface, craniofacial dislocation (maxillary arch moves independently when rocked), nasal deformity, blood in oropharynx
- C-spine: No step-offs or tenderness (collar remains)
- Chest/Abdomen: Normal
- FAST: Negative
- Neuro: Intubated; no focal deficits

Diagnostic Studies

- CT Head: No intracranial hemorrhage or skull fracture
- CT C-spine: Normal
- CT Face: Le Fort II fracture (pyramidal – nasal bridge, maxilla, medial orbital rims)
- CXR: ETT in good position, no aspirated teeth

- CBC: Hct 41.5%, WBC 5.3; INR 1.0; EtOH 340

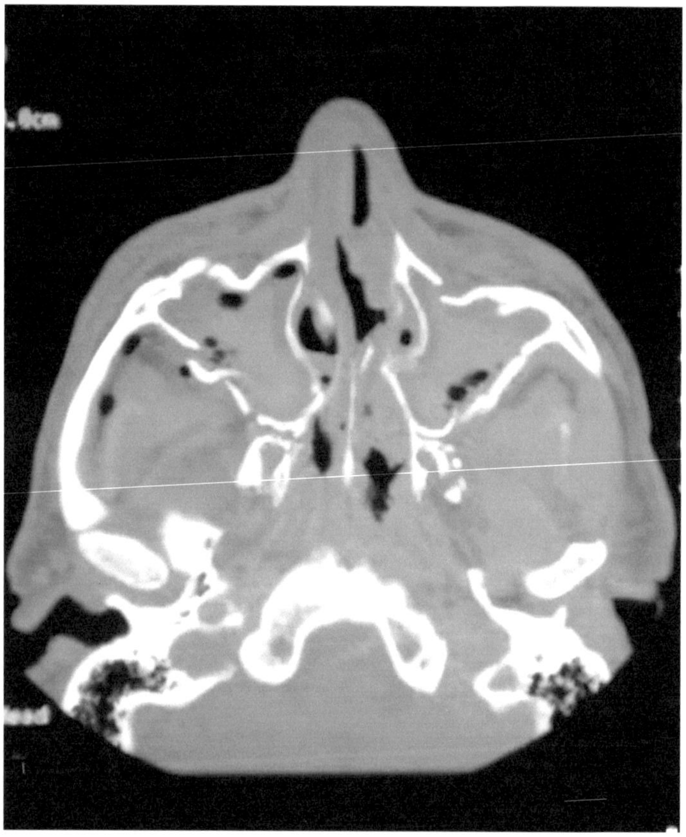

Management

- Consult OMFS and Trauma Surgery immediately
- Maintain C-spine precautions until cleared (blunt facial injury has higher C-spine injury incidence)

Disposition

Admission to trauma service for operative repair of Le Fort II fracture.

Critical Actions

- Recognize difficult airway before giving any paralytic; prepare for awake intubation or surgical airway with cricothyrotomy equipment at bedside
- If failed airway occurs, immediately pivot to cricothyrotomy – do not persist with failed orotracheal attempts
- Control hemorrhage with direct pressure and nasal packing (not blind clamping)
- Maintain C-spine immobilization throughout
- Activate trauma team; complete full secondary survey (do not be distracted by facial injuries)
- Order CT head, C-spine, and facial bones; CXR to rule out aspirated teeth
- Consult OMFS early; admit to trauma service

Toxic Ingestion

Opening Scenario

A 17-year-old female is brought in by her mother with nausea, tremors, and "ringing in her ears" since this morning. She developed a headache last night and took "some pills" before bed. She denies fever, cough, or sick contacts.

Initial Assessment

Vitals: BP 107/56, HR 117, RR 22, SpO_2 98% RA, T 37.2°C

Alert and oriented, mildly tremulous, visible tachypnea/hyperpnea. No acute respiratory distress.

Immediate actions: Large-bore IV, continuous cardiac monitoring, focused medication history, pregnancy test.

History

- HPI: Took six 325-mg aspirin tablets last night for headache. This morning developed nausea, tremors, tinnitus. No fever, cough, or sick contacts.
- Key exam findings: Tachypnea with deep respirations, tinnitus, tremors, diaphoresis, warm flushed skin, dry mucous membranes

Diagnostic Studies

- VBG: pH 7.54, pCO_2 21, HCO_3 17 (mixed respiratory alkalosis and anion gap metabolic acidosis – pathognomonic for salicylate toxicity)
- Salicylate level: 60 (severe toxicity)
- BMP: Na 146, K 3.1, Cl 117, HCO_3 17
- ECG: Sinus tachycardia, no ischemic changes
- Pregnancy: Negative
- Also order: Acetaminophen level (co-ingestion screen), CBC, coagulation studies, LFTs, UA

The pH >7.40 indicates the patient is maintaining respiratory compensation. If pH were <7.35, this would indicate impending respiratory failure and require emergent hemodialysis.

Management

- Urinary alkalinization with sodium bicarbonate drip (goal urine pH 7.5-8.5)
- Aggressively replete potassium (hypokalemia prevents effective alkalinization)
- Contact Poison Control
- Antiemetic (ondansetron)
- Repeat salicylate levels q2h until declining and <20

Hemodialysis Indications:

- Salicylate level >100 (>90 with renal insufficiency)
- Altered mental status, seizures, or cerebral edema
- Refractory acidemia (pH <7.20 despite resuscitation)
- Acute kidney injury or fluid overload
- Respiratory failure requiring intubation

Disposition

ICU admission for serial salicylate levels, continuous monitoring, urinary alkalinization management, and respiratory monitoring.

Critical Actions

- Recognize salicylate toxicity (classic triad: tinnitus, tachypnea, nausea)
- Recognize the danger of intubation: loss of compensatory hyperventilation causes rapid acidemia and cardiovascular collapse; if intubation required, match pre-intubation minute ventilation with bicarbonate bolus ready
- Initiate urinary alkalinization and aggressively replete potassium
- Know hemodialysis indications (level >100, AMS, refractory acidemia, renal failure)
- Screen for co-ingestants (acetaminophen level)
- Contact Poison Control and arrange ICU admission

Severe Respiratory Distress

Opening Scenario

A 37-year-old male is brought to the resuscitation bay by EMS with shortness of breath. He is obese, sitting upright, using accessory muscles, and unable to speak in full sentences.

Initial Assessment

Vitals: BP 156/60, HR 116, RR 28, SpO_2 90% RA, T 36.8°C

- Airway: Patent, no stridor
- Breathing: Diffuse bilateral wheezing, prolonged expiration, poor air movement, decreased breath sounds at bases
- Circulation: Warm skin, normal cap refill, pulses intact

Immediate actions: High-flow O_2 via NRB, two large-bore IVs, continuous monitoring, ECG, portable CXR. Start continuous albuterol nebulizer, ipratropium q20min x 3, methylprednisolone 125 mg IV, consider magnesium sulfate 1-2 g IV over 15 minutes.

History

- HPI: Progressive dyspnea and dry cough over 2 hours. URI symptoms earlier this week. Used albuterol inhaler "several times" at home without relief. Denies fever, chest pain, recent travel/surgery.
- PMHx: Asthma (two prior intubations, two ICU admissions in last 5 years), hypertension, type 2 DM
- Meds: Albuterol and fluticasone inhalers (compliance uncertain), prednisone ("a few days ago")
- Allergies: NKDA
- Social: Denies tobacco, alcohol, drug use

Physical Examination

- General: Moderate respiratory distress, unable to speak in full sentences
- HEENT: Cyanotic lips
- Neck: No JVD
- Chest: Diffuse inspiratory and expiratory wheezing, prolonged expiratory phase, poor air movement, no rales
- Cardiovascular: Tachycardic, regular, no murmurs
- Extremities: No edema
- Peak Expiratory Flow: 180 L/min (severely reduced)

Diagnostic Studies

- ABG: pH 7.45, pCO_2 24, pO_2 62, HCO_3 20
- CBC: WBC 12.0, Hct 36%, Plt 288
- BMP: Na 134, K 4.2, Cl 102, HCO_3 21, BUN 11, Cr 1.0, Glucose 210
- Coags: Normal
- ECG: Sinus tachycardia, no ischemic changes
- CXR: Hyperinflation, no pneumothorax, no infiltrates

Reassessment

Thirty minutes after initial bronchodilator therapy: no improvement. SpO_2 remains 90% on high-flow O_2, RR 28-30, increased work of breathing, peak flow unchanged. Status asthmaticus refractory to initial therapy.

- Escalate: Terbutaline 0.25 mg SC or epinephrine 0.3 mg SC
- Initiate BiPAP with inline continuous nebulized albuterol (trial NIV before intubation in hemodynamically stable patient)
- If no escalation: patient will deteriorate with decreased mental status and rising pCO_2 to 55, requiring emergent intubation

Patient Communication

After stabilization on BiPAP (RR 24, SpO_2 96%), patient begins to speak clearly: "Am I going to be okay? I can't go to the ICU – I have to work tomorrow."

- Explain status asthmaticus in plain terms
- Acknowledge work/financial concerns without dismissing them
- State necessity of ICU monitoring given prior intubations and current severity
- Discuss potential need for intubation if deterioration occurs
- Check understanding and obtain consent for ICU transfer

Disposition

ICU admission for status asthmaticus management.

Critical Actions

- Recognize severe asthma exacerbation and initiate bronchodilators and systemic steroids immediately
- Trial BiPAP before intubation in the hemodynamically stable patient
- Recognize refractory status asthmaticus and escalate therapy (SC terbutaline/epinephrine)
- Recognize impending respiratory failure: normalizing or rising pCO_2 in an asthmatic is a danger sign
- Arrange ICU admission (not general floor due to BiPaP needs)
- Communicate clearly with patient about severity and ICU necessity

Weakness and Lethargy

Opening Scenario

EMS arrives with a 68-year-old female found by her son lying on the couch, too weak to stand. EMS reports she is alert but lethargic with stable vitals; placed on 2L NC for pallor. Son is in the waiting room.

Initial Assessment

Vitals: BP 136/89, HR 79, RR 18, SpO_2 98% on 2L NC, T 36.5°C

- Airway: Speaking in full sentences
- Breathing: No distress, lungs clear
- Circulation: Warm skin, normal cap refill, regular pulse
- Fingerstick glucose: 200
- ECG: Normal sinus rhythm, no ischemic changes

Immediate actions: IV access, fingerstick glucose, order CBC/BMP/LFTs/coagulation studies/lactate, ECG.

History

- HPI: "Extremely weak and lethargic" since waking. Cat died last night. Feels depressed and "not right." Mild headache, generalized malaise. Denies chest pain, dyspnea, syncope, seizure, nausea, vomiting.
- PMHx: Hypertension, hypercholesterolemia
- Meds: Hydrochlorothiazide, simvastatin
- Social: Lives alone. No alcohol, tobacco, or drug use.
- From son: "She seemed confused when I got there. I had to turn off the stove – she left the oven on with the door open. Even the cat… we found it dead this morning."

Physical Examination

- General: Lethargic but arousable, oriented to self and place, pale
- Neuro: Follows commands. Generalized weakness without focal motor deficits. Unsteady gait, dysmetria on finger-to-nose, poor concentration
- Remainder: Normal

Key findings: Environmental exposure (gas stove with door open), dead pet, and cerebellar signs should trigger concern for carbon monoxide poisoning. Place on 100% O_2 via NRB immediately.

Diagnostic Studies

- COHb: 23 (critical; normal <3 in nonsmokers)
- ABG: pH 7.31, PaO_2 399 (on 100% NRB), pCO_2 40, HCO_3 20, calculated O_2 sat 72% (pulse ox cannot distinguish COHb from oxyhemoglobin – falsely normal SpO_2)
- Lactate: 2.2 (mildly elevated)
- Head CT: No acute bleed or mass
- CXR: Normal
- CBC, BMP, LFTs: Unremarkable

Reassessment

After 100% O_2: mild improvement in headache but remains ataxic and lethargic. Persistent neurologic deficits despite oxygen therapy indicate need for escalation.

Management

- Continue 100% oxygen
- Consult hyperbaric medicine center
- Arrange transfer for hyperbaric oxygen therapy (neurologic symptoms with elevated COHb are indications)

Managing Conflict

Son expresses concern: "Can't she just stay here on oxygen? I don't want her transported to another hospital."

- Explain diagnosis in plain terms: carbon monoxide poisoning from the gas stove preventing her blood from carrying oxygen
- Explain that neurologic symptoms (unsteadiness, confusion) and high COHb level require hyperbaric oxygen to prevent permanent brain injury
- Address barriers (cost, distance, inconvenience) and problem-solve
- Maintain firm recommendation while respecting autonomy

Disposition

Transfer to nearest hyperbaric oxygen facility with 100% O_2 maintained during transport.

Critical Actions

- Obtain fingerstick glucose immediately in any weak/altered patient
- Elicit environmental exposure history (stove, combustion source, dead pet)
- Recognize that SpO_2 is falsely normal in CO poisoning; order COHb level specifically
- Place on 100% O_2 via NRB immediately, do not wait for COHb result
- Perform thorough neurologic exam documenting cerebellar signs
- Recognize persistent neurologic deficits as indication for hyperbaric therapy (not just normobaric O_2)
- Consult hyperbaric medicine and arrange transfer
- Address family concerns about transfer empathetically while maintaining firm recommendation

Vision Loss

Opening Scenario

A 70-year-old female presents with vision loss. She is stable, alert, and oriented, sitting comfortably. IV placed by nurse.

Initial Assessment

Vitals: BP 146/74, HR 84, RR 20, SpO_2 98% RA, T 36.9°C

Well-appearing, comfortable, no acute distress. Neurologic exam normal except for vision (see below).

History

- HPI: Progressive, painless vision loss in the right eye starting yesterday, worsened today. Denies "curtain" sensation, photopsias, floaters, eye pain, redness, or tearing. Mild dizziness. Denies headache, jaw claudication, scalp tenderness, fever. Denies weakness, numbness, speech difficulty, facial asymmetry.
- PMHx: Hypertension, type 2 DM, asthma, hypercholesterolemia
- PSHx: Cataract extraction (right eye, 6 months ago)
- Meds: Metformin, hydrochlorothiazide, albuterol, simvastatin
- Allergies: None
- Social: No tobacco, alcohol, or drugs. Lives independently.

Physical Examination

- Visual Acuity: Left eye 20/30; Right eye count fingers at 2 feet (severe loss)
- Pupils: Left reactive, 3 mm. Right sluggish; positive RAPD (right pupil dilates on direct light, constricts with consensual from left – Marcus Gunn positive)
- Confrontational Fields: Unable to assess right eye; left full
- Slit Lamp: Unremarkable bilaterally, no hyphema
- IOP: 14 right, 15 left (normal)
- Fluorescein: No abrasions or ulcerations
- Fundoscopy: Left eye normal. Right eye: optic disc edema with blurred margins, tortuous dilated retinal veins, diffuse intraretinal hemorrhages in all quadrants ("blood and thunder" appearance), macular edema. No cherry-red spot.
- Ocular US: Normal lens, clear anechoic posterior chamber, no membranes or tethering

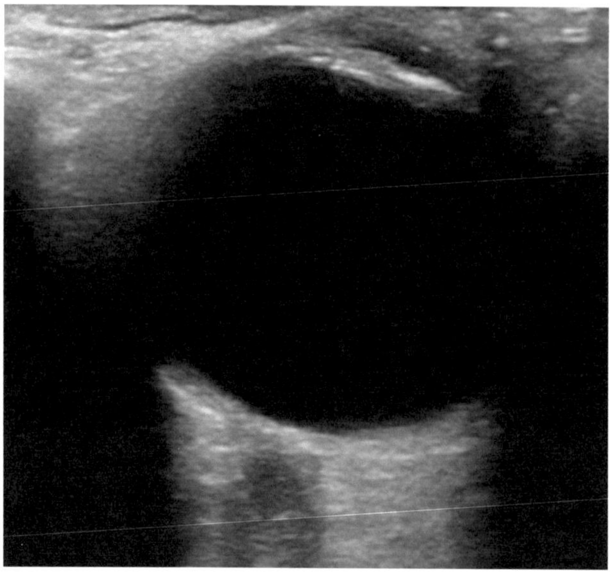

Diagnostic Studies

- CBC: WBC 5.3, Hct 35.1%, Plt 265
- BMP: Na 136, K 3.9, Cl 99, HCO_3 33, BUN 26, Cr 1.3, Glucose 146
- Coags: PT 14, PTT 26, INR 1.1
- ESR 28, CRP 1.2 (not consistent with active GCA)
- ECG: NSR at 84, no ST-T changes
- Head CT: No intracranial hemorrhage, mass, or acute findings

Management

Diagnosis: Central Retinal Vein Occlusion (CRVO). Differential excluded: CRAO (no cherry-red spot), retinal detachment (no curtain/photopsias), vitreous hemorrhage (fundus visible), optic neuritis (painless, older), acute angle-closure glaucoma (normal IOP, painless), GCA (normal inflammatory markers).

- Urgent (same-day) ophthalmology consultation for fluorescein angiography and treatment planning
- Aspirin 325 mg daily (atherosclerotic risk factors)
- Address cardiovascular risk factors (strict glucose and BP control)
- Arrange urgent ophthalmology follow-up for possible anti-VEGF injections or photocoagulation

Disposition

Discharge if ophthalmology can see within 24 hours and safe transport available. Instruct patient not to drive (monocular vision). Return precautions for worsening vision, new headache, or neurologic symptoms. If ophthalmology available then ask for them to see in ED.

Critical Actions

- Obtain focused history asking specifically about curtain sensation, eye pain, jaw claudication/scalp tenderness (GCA screen)
- Perform complete ocular exam: visual acuity in each eye separately, swinging flashlight test for RAPD, fundoscopy, IOP measurement
- Utilize ultrasound to evaluate for other painless causes of visual loss (retinal detachment, vitreous hemorrhage)
- Recognize "blood and thunder" fundoscopic appearance as CRVO

- Order ESR/CRP to exclude GCA in any patient >50 with vision loss
- Order head CT to rule out intracranial pathology
- Urgent ophthalmology consultation
- Initiate antiplatelet therapy and address modifiable cardiovascular risk factors
- Advise patient not to drive; arrange appropriate follow-up

Lower Extremity Weakness

Opening Scenario

A 38-year-old male presents via EMS with severe lower back pain and left lower extremity weakness. He is anxious and asking if he can go home with pain medication.

Initial Assessment

Vitals: BP 142/88, HR 96, RR 16, SpO_2 98% RA, T 37.1°C

Uncomfortable, diaphoretic, lying supine with left leg elevated. Alert and conversant but grimacing with movement. No rashes, deformities, or trauma.

Immediate actions: Two large-bore IVs, analgesia (ketorolac 15 mg IV + morphine 4 mg IV), Foley catheter for post-void residual, continuous monitoring, labs (CBC, BMP, coagulation, T&S).

History

- HPI: Severe lumbar pain began 3 weeks ago after lifting a heavy box at work, initially improved with NSAIDs. Three days ago, pain recurred with increased severity radiating down left posterior thigh to lateral foot. Today noticed "dragging" his left foot, difficulty initiating urination, and new perineal numbness.
- PMHx: Hypertension, hyperlipidemia
- PSHx: Laparoscopic cholecystectomy (2019)
- Meds: Lisinopril, atorvastatin, ibuprofen PRN
- Allergies: NKDA
- Social: Former smoker, occasional alcohol, warehouse supervisor

Physical Examination

- General: Alert, moderate distress, diaphoretic
- Back: Paraspinal spasm, marked tenderness over L4-L5 and L5-S1, limited forward flexion
- Neurologic: Left ankle dorsiflexion 3/5, plantar flexion 4/5. Decreased sensation left lateral foot/sole (S1). Decreased perianal/perineal sensation. Positive SLR at 30 degrees left. Patellar reflexes 2+ bilaterally; Achilles 1+ left, 2+ right.

Patient Communication

Patient expresses fear about surgery, asks to go home with pain medication to "wait and see." Counsel regarding urgency: risk of permanent paralysis and bowel/bladder dysfunction without intervention. Obtain informed consent.

Diagnostic Studies

- CBC: WBC 10.2, Hgb 14.1, Hct 42.3%, Plt 278
- BMP: Na 138, K 4.2, Cl 102, HCO_3 22, BUN 18, Cr 1.1, Glucose 112
- Coags: PT 12.8, PTT 28, INR 1.0
- UA: Normal
- Bladder Ultrasound: distended full bladder
- MRI Lumbar Spine: Large L4-L5 disc herniation with severe central canal stenosis, bilateral neural foraminal compromise, and cauda equina nerve root compression

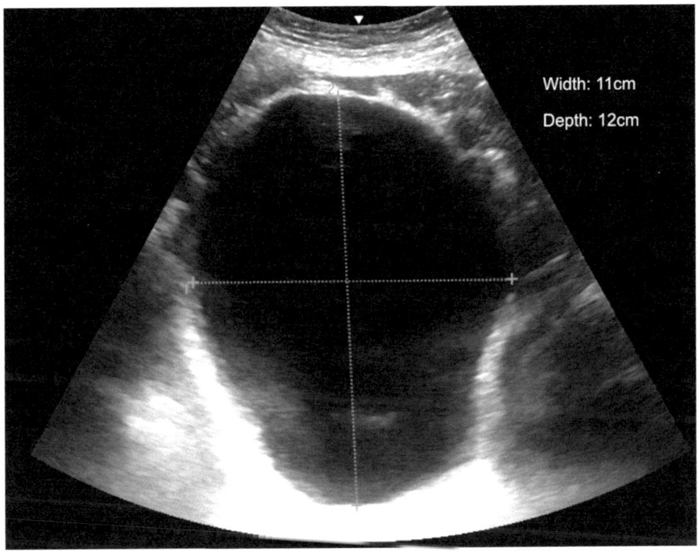

Reassessment

While awaiting MRI: patient reports increasing right leg numbness, unable to dorsiflex right ankle. Repeat vitals stable.

- New right foot drop (dorsiflexion 3/5)
- Bilateral saddle anesthesia
- Post-void residual: 850 mL
- Rectal exam: decreased sphincter tone, no voluntary contraction

Management

- Emergent neurosurgery consultation for operative decompression
- Urgent L4-L5 discectomy and decompression
- Continue IV analgesia and Foley drainage

Critical Actions

- Recognize cauda equina syndrome: urinary retention (PVR >200 mL), saddle anesthesia, progressive lower extremity weakness
- Perform complete neurologic exam including rectal tone, perineal sensation, and specific motor testing
- Identify progressive bilateral deficits on reassessment as indication for emergent intervention
- Order emergent MRI lumbar spine (gold standard) – do not await lab results
- Emergent neurosurgical consultation (surgical emergency)
- Communicate urgency to patient, addressing fears while explaining risks of permanent paralysis/ incontinence
- Do not discharge or delay imaging with classic presentation and progressive symptoms

Upper Abdominal Pain

Opening Scenario

A 58-year-old male with type 2 DM and hypertension presents with epigastric and right upper quadrant pain. He appears uncomfortable. His spouse expresses frustration about the wait time and asks when he can go home.

Initial Assessment

Vitals: BP 156/92, HR 108, RR 18, SpO_2 96% RA, T 38.4°C

Obese, mildly diaphoretic, sitting upright holding RUQ. Alert, speaking in full sentences, grimacing with movement.

Immediate actions: Two large-bore IVs, 1L NS bolus, continuous monitoring, ECG, morphine 4 mg IV, ondansetron 4 mg IV, acetaminophen 1000 mg PO.

History

- HPI: 18 hours of constant, sharp epigastric pain radiating to RUQ and right scapula. Began 2 hours after a large fatty meal. Two similar but milder episodes over 6 months that resolved spontaneously. Persistent nausea with two non-bloody emesis episodes. Subjective fever/chills. Denies diarrhea, chest pain, SOB, dark urine, or pale stools.
- PMHx: Type 2 DM (HbA1c 8.2), hypertension, hyperlipidemia, obesity
- PSHx: No prior abdominal surgeries
- Meds: Metformin, lisinopril, atorvastatin
- Allergies: NKDA
- Social: Long-haul truck driver, former smoker (20 pack-years, quit 5 years ago), occasional alcohol
- FHx: Mother with DM and gallstones; father with CAD

Physical Examination

- General: Moderate distress, reluctant to lie flat
- HEENT: Anicteric sclerae, moist mucous membranes
- Cardiovascular: Tachycardic, regular, no murmurs, no edema
- Pulmonary: Clear bilaterally
- Abdomen: Soft, non-distended, severe tenderness in epigastrium and RUQ, positive Murphy sign, negative McBurney, no rebound or guarding, no masses or hepatosplenomegaly
- GU: No suprapubic or CVA tenderness
- Skin: No jaundice

Diagnostic Studies

- CBC: WBC 17.2, Hgb 14.1, Hct 42.3%, Plt 285
- BMP: Na 140, K 3.8, Cl 104, HCO_3 24, BUN 22, Cr 1.1, Glucose 186
- LFTs: AST 28, ALT 24, Alk Phos 298 (elevated), Total Bili 4.2 (elevated), Direct Bili 3.1 (elevated), Albumin 4.1
- Lipase 45 (normal), Amylase 62 (normal)
- Coags: PT 12.8, PTT 32, INR 0.9
- UA: Bilirubin positive, urobilinogen elevated, otherwise normal
- ECG: Sinus tachycardia at 108, no ST changes

- CXR: No free air, no infiltrates
- RUQ US: GB wall 5 mm (thickened), pericholecystic fluid, gallstone impacted in GB neck, positive sonographic Murphy sign, CBD 4 mm

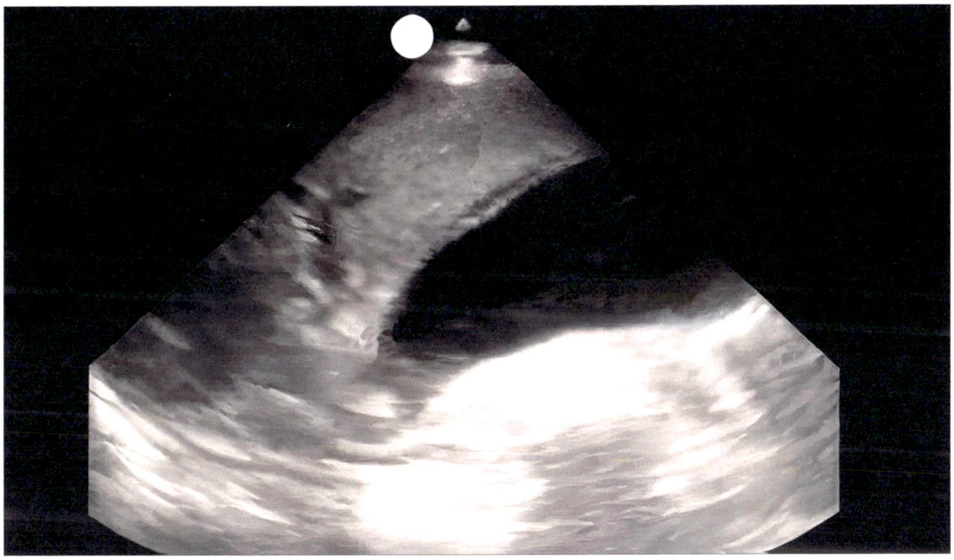

Reassessment

15 minutes post-intervention: Pain improved 8/10 to 5/10. Vitals: BP 148/88, HR 98, T 38.1°C. Patient feels "somewhat better" and asks to go home – has a cross-country delivery tomorrow. Spouse says, "If he says he's better, maybe we should just go."

Partial pain relief with analgesics does not indicate resolution of the underlying surgical condition. Persistent tachycardia and fever despite treatment.

Patient Communication

Patient asks: "Can't you just give me antibiotics and let me follow up next week?"

- Explain acute cholecystitis with cystic duct obstruction in plain language
- Discuss risks of leaving: perforation, peritonitis, sepsis
- Address increased risk of emphysematous cholecystitis and gangrene in diabetics
- Validate employment and financial concerns empathetically
- Explain necessity of admission, IV antibiotics, and surgical intervention
- Assess decision-making capacity; obtain informed consent

Management

- General surgery consultation
- Ampicillin-sulbactam 3 g IV q6h (or ceftriaxone + metronidazole, or piperacillin-tazobactam)
- NPO, IV fluids at maintenance
- Blood cultures (two sets)
- Planned laparoscopic cholecystectomy within 24 hours

Critical Actions

- Recognize acute cholecystitis (post-prandial RUQ pain, fever, leukocytosis, positive Murphy sign)
- Order fractionated bilirubin and alk phos to evaluate for cholestasis
- Identify diagnostic US findings: wall thickening >3 mm, pericholecystic fluid, impacted stone, sonographic Murphy sign

- Initiate empiric IV antibiotics covering biliary flora
- Recognize DM as risk factor for complicated gallbladder disease (emphysematous cholecystitis, gangrene)
- Differentiate from ACS (atypical in diabetics), pancreatitis (normal lipase), cholangitis (no Charcot triad), hepatitis (normal transaminases)
- Address patient's desire for AMA discharge with empathetic but firm communication about surgical necessity
- Consult surgery, make NPO, admit for cholecystectomy

Abdominal Pain and Groin Mass

Opening Scenario

A 55-year-old male is brought in by his wife with severe abdominal pain and vomiting. The nurse reports he appears uncomfortable and hypotensive.

Initial Assessment

Vitals: BP 86/57, HR 89, RR 20, SpO_2 99% on 2L NC, T 37.1°C

Pale, diaphoretic, moderate distress. Alert, speaking in full sentences. Dry oral mucosa. Note: BP 86/57 represents relative hypotension in a patient with known hypertension.

Immediate actions: Two large-bore IVs, aggressive NS bolus (1-2L), supplemental O_2, continuous monitoring.

History

- HPI: 24 hours of progressively worsening abdominal distension and crampy pain. Two episodes bilious vomiting. Swollen, tender right groin that has become "hard" – intermittent groin swelling for years that previously reduced when lying down, but now persistently swollen and more painful than ever. No BM today. Denies fever, chills, chest pain, or SOB.
- PMHx: Hypertension, type 2 DM, asthma, prior cholecystectomy
- Meds: Metformin
- Allergies: Penicillins
- Social: Lives with wife; no tobacco, alcohol, or drugs

Physical Examination

- General: Alert, moderate distress, tachycardic
- Abdomen: Markedly distended, diffusely tender with rebound and guarding, absent bowel sounds, no pulsatile masses
- GU: Large right-sided inguinal hernia – firm, tender, non-reducible, overlying skin dusky/discolored. No scrotal swelling or testicular tenderness.
- Rectal: Normal tone, hemoccult negative
- Skin: Pale, warm

Diagnostic Studies

- ECG: NSR, no acute ST changes

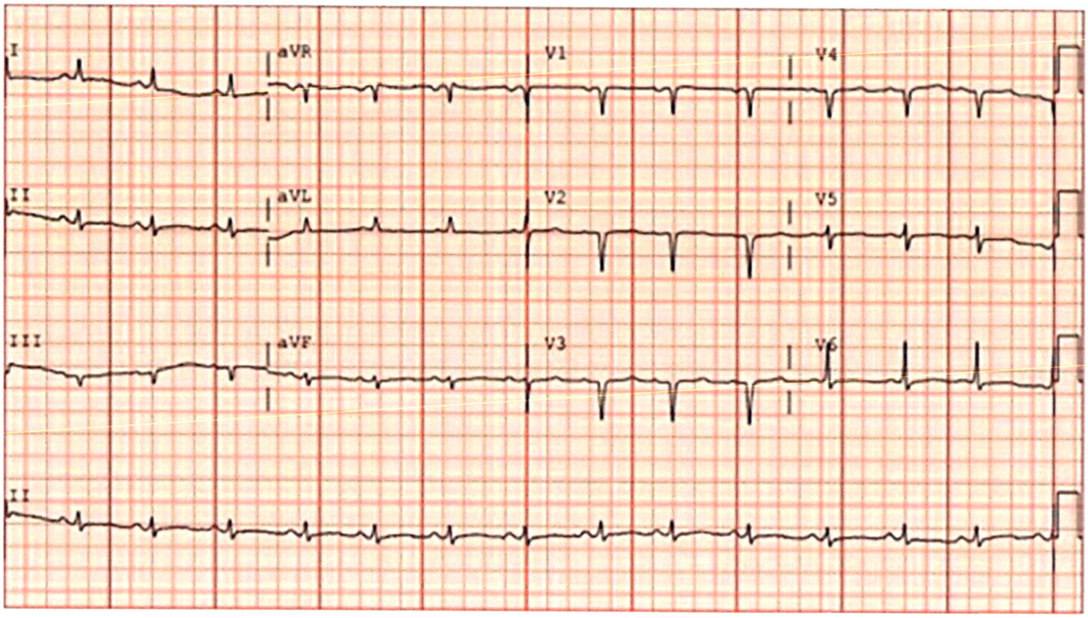

- CBC: WBC 18.4, Hct 52.0% (hemoconcentration), Plt 288
- BMP: Na 139, K 4.6, Cl 92, HCO_3 31, BUN 18, Cr 1.2, Glucose 160
- LFTs: AST 40, ALT 23, Alk Phos 107, T Bili 1.6, D Bili 0.5
- Amylase 123, Lipase 140, Lactate 3.9
- Coags: PT 12.9, PTT 31.2, INR 1.1; UA normal (SG 1.030)
- CXR: No free air
- Abdominal XR: Dilated small bowel loops with multiple air-fluid levels, no pneumatosis

Management

- Do NOT attempt to reduce the hernia given dusky skin changes (strangulation) – reduction could precipitate bowel perforation or release ischemic toxins
- NGT placement for decompression
- Communicate elevated lactate as a sign of ischemia and communicate with surgery before ordering any additional imaging.
- Broad-spectrum IV antibiotics covering gram-negatives and anaerobes (penicillin-allergic: ciprofloxacin + metronidazole, or aztreonam + metronidazole)
- IV opioid analgesia
- NPO
- Emergent general surgery consultation for operative management

Reassessment

After 2L NS and NGT: pain modestly improved (6/10 from 10/10), BP improves to 92/64, but abdominal distension persists and hernia remains non-reducible with dusky skin.

Leukocytosis (WBC 18.4) and hemoconcentration (Hct 52%) raise concern for bowel ischemia/gangrene. Despite normal lactate, clinical picture (peritoneal signs + strangulated hernia) mandates emergent surgical intervention.

Critical Actions

- Recognize hemodynamic instability (relative hypotension in hypertensive patient) and initiate aggressive resuscitation
- Perform thorough exam including GU to discover incarcerated/strangulated inguinal hernia
- Recognize bowel obstruction from imaging (dilated bowel, air-fluid levels)
- Do NOT attempt reduction of hernia with dusky skin changes (strangulation)
- Place NGT for decompression
- Administer broad-spectrum antibiotics (account for penicillin allergy)
- Emergent surgical consultation – this is a surgical emergency
- Reassess after resuscitation; persistent peritoneal signs mandate immediate operative intervention

Abdominal Pain and a Rash in a Child

Opening Scenario

A 6-year-old male is brought in by his mother with vomiting since yesterday, abdominal pain, bloody diarrhea, and difficulty walking due to leg pain.

Initial Assessment

Vitals: BP 96/63, HR 136, RR 28, T 36.1°C. Weight: 23 kg

Uncomfortable, mildly distressed. Tachycardia with borderline hypotension for age indicates early compensated shock.

Immediate actions: Continuous monitoring, large-bore IV, 20 mL/kg (460 mL) NS bolus.

History

- HPI: Hematemesis, one episode bloody diarrhea, bilateral knee/ankle pain with difficulty walking, decreased oral intake. No fever, sick contacts, foreign travel, or raw meat consumption.
- PMHx: ADHD, prior strep throat 1 year ago

Physical Examination

- General: Uncomfortable, sunken eyes (moderate dehydration)
- HEENT: Palpebral purpura, tonsillar enlargement
- Cardiovascular: Tachycardic, no murmurs, weak peripheral pulses
- Abdomen: Epigastric tenderness, no rebound or guarding, decreased bowel sounds
- MSK: Antalgic gait, tender joints (knees, ankles)
- Skin: Palpable purpura on bilateral elbows, lower extremities, and buttocks (non-blanching, raised)
- Rectal: Hemoccult-positive stool

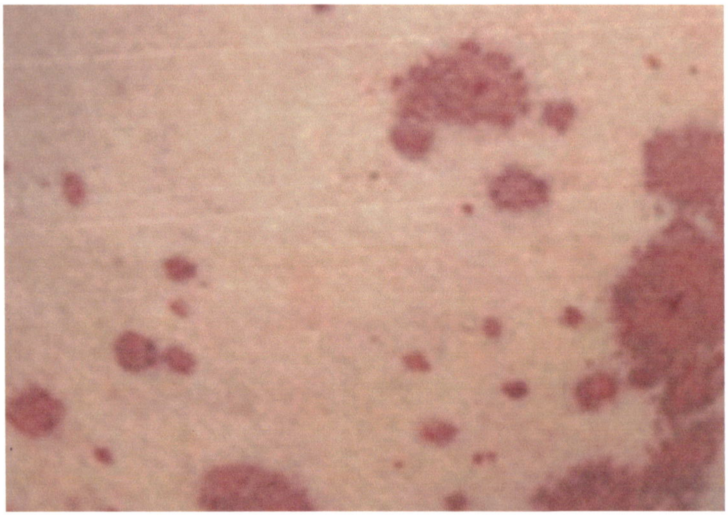

Diagnostic Studies

- CBC: WBC 15.3, Hct 35.1%, Plt 595 (elevated – rules out thrombocytopenic purpura)
- BMP: BUN 15, Cr 2.6, Na 138, K 3.8, HCO_3 21
- UA: SG 1.025, protein 3+ (renal involvement), ketones positive
- IgA level: 299 (elevated, supportive but not required for diagnosis)

- Abdominal US: No intussusception, no free fluid
- Abdominal XR: Non-specific bowel gas, no free air

Management

Diagnosis: Henoch-Schonlein Purpura (IgA Vasculitis) – classic tetrad of palpable purpura, arthritis, abdominal pain, and renal involvement. Differential includes intussusception (ruled out by US), appendicitis, IBD, TTP, and HUS.

- Repeat 20 mL/kg bolus if still tachycardic, then maintenance IV fluids
- Corticosteroids (methylprednisolone IV or prednisone) for severe GI involvement (hematemesis)
- Analgesia: Avoid NSAIDs (GI bleeding, renal involvement); use acetaminophen or opioids
- Abdominal Ultrasound: normal peristalsis without signs of intussusception
- Consult pediatric surgery if intussusception identified or peritoneal signs develop

Reassessment

After fluid bolus: HR improves to 110, BP 102/70. Proteinuria on UA indicates renal involvement (glomerulonephritis) requiring monitoring. No surgical abdomen on imaging – continue medical management.

Disposition

Admit to general pediatric floor for observation, hydration, steroids, pain management, and renal monitoring. Counsel family: HSP is self-limited IgA vasculitis, excellent prognosis but needs monitoring. Abdominal pain needs evaluation for intussusception risk – HSP can cause ileo-ileal intussusception (bloody stools, decreased urine output, edema). Arrange nephrology consult for proteinuria.

Critical Actions

- Recognize compensated shock and initiate fluid resuscitation
- Identify palpable purpura with abdominal pain, arthritis, and proteinuria as HSP (IgA Vasculitis)
- Order abdominal US to rule out intussusception
- Recognize thrombocytosis rules out thrombocytopenic purpura
- Identify proteinuria as renal involvement requiring monitoring
- Administer corticosteroids for severe GI symptoms
- Avoid NSAIDs given GI bleeding and renal involvement
- Admit for observation; do not discharge.

Altered Mental Status

Opening Scenario

An 85-year-old male is brought in by ambulance. His wife reports progressive disorientation over 2 days; this morning he did not know his address or phone number. He is awake but confused.

Initial Assessment

Vitals: BP 135/70, HR 88, RR 13, SpO_2 98% RA, T 36.0°C

Sleeping but arousable and cooperative. Speaking in full sentences. Pale and cool skin, regular rhythm, pulses 2+, normal cap refill. Fingerstick glucose: 107.

Immediate actions: Cardiac monitor, two large-bore IVs, O_2 via NC, fingerstick glucose.

History

- HPI: In usual state of health until 3 days ago when he fell in the bathroom and struck his head. Brief headache, no LOC, did not seek care. Over 2 days developed progressive confusion and forgetfulness. Constant midfrontal headache worse than baseline. Denies neck pain, photophobia, nausea, vomiting, vision changes, chest pain, SOB, or fever.
- PMHx: Hypertension, hypercholesterolemia
- PSHx: Umbilical hernia repair
- Meds: Metoprolol, simvastatin, aspirin
- Allergies: None
- Social: Lives with wife, drinks beer 1-2x/month, no tobacco/drugs, baseline independent in ADLs

Physical Examination

- General: Alert, oriented to person and place only, comfortable
- HEENT: No ecchymoses or lacerations; PERRL, EOMI, fundoscopic normal
- Neck: No rigidity
- Cardiovascular: Regular rate/rhythm, no murmurs
- Pulmonary: Clear
- Abdomen: Normal, non-tender
- Neuro: Oriented to self/place only; 5/5 strength bilaterally; sensation intact; CN II-XII intact; reflexes symmetric; no focal deficits; normal assisted gait

Diagnostic Studies

- CBC: WBC 9.2, Hct 41.5%, Plt 223
- BMP: Na 137, K 4.2, Cl 108, HCO_3 23, BUN 20, Cr 0.6, Glucose 110
- Coags: PT 13.0, PTT 29, INR 1.1
- LFTs: AST 24, ALT 33, Alk Phos 120, T Bili 0.9, Albumin 3.1
- UA: Normal
- ECG: NSR, no ischemic changes
- CXR: Normal
- Non-contrast Head CT: Crescent-shaped hyperdense extra-axial collection over right cerebral hemisphere with midline shift and compression of right lateral ventricle. Ventricular effacement on affected side. Consistent with subdural hematoma.

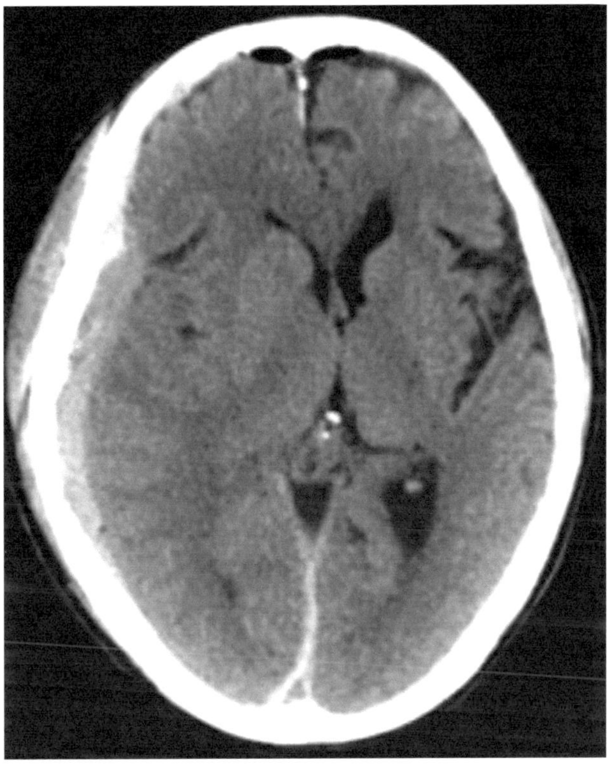

Reassessment

Subdural hematoma with midline shift is a neurosurgical emergency. Re-evaluate ABCs and neuro status. Contact neurosurgery immediately for operative drainage. Continuous monitoring for airway compromise.

Patient Communication

Meet with the patient's wife:

- Acknowledge distress and concern
- Explain in plain language: CT shows bleeding around the brain from the fall 3 days ago, causing pressure; aspirin may have contributed to continued bleeding
- Explain need for emergency surgery (burr holes/craniotomy) to drain blood and relieve pressure
- Honestly discuss surgical risks in an 85-year-old vs. risks of non-operative management (herniation, permanent brain damage, death)
- Involve wife in shared decision-making; offer to contact PMD

Disposition

Admission to neurosurgical ICU with continuous monitoring.

Critical Actions

- Immediate fingerstick glucose in any altered patient
- Elicit history of fall and aspirin use
- Obtain non-contrast head CT promptly
- Recognize subdural hematoma with midline shift as neurosurgical emergency
- Consult neurosurgery for operative drainage
- Counsel family regarding diagnosis and need for surgery
- Admit to ICU

Confusion

Opening Scenario

A 58-year-old male with type 2 DM and PVD is brought in by ambulance with altered mental status and abdominal pain. Spouse reports 12 hours of increasing confusion and 2 days of abdominal discomfort. One episode non-bilious emesis today; refusing oral intake.

Initial Assessment

Vitals: BP 94/58, HR 124, RR 26, SpO_2 93% RA, T 39.1°C

Cachectic, ill-appearing. Lying motionless with knees flexed. Diaphoretic, mottled lower extremities. Opens eyes only to painful stimuli. Airway patent. Tachypneic, lungs clear. Cap refill 4 seconds, thready pulses.

Physical Examination

- General: Lethargic, arousable to voice, oriented to person only
- HEENT: Dry mucous membranes, pupils equal/reactive
- Cardiovascular: Tachycardic, no murmurs, flat JVP
- Pulmonary: Clear bilaterally
- Abdomen: Soft, diffusely tender (worst epigastrium/RUQ), hypoactive bowel sounds, no rebound/guarding initially (limited by AMS), Murphy not obtainable initially
- Extremities: Cool, mottled, bilateral edema, delayed cap refill
- Neuro: Confused, moves all extremities equally, no focal deficits

Diagnostic Studies

- CBC: WBC 19.4 with 22% bands, Hgb 11.2, Plt 412
- BMP: Na 138, K 3.2, Cl 102, HCO_3 18, BUN 34, Cr 2.3, Glucose 412
- LFTs: AST 45, ALT 38, Alk Phos 480, T Bili 2.8, D Bili 1.9
- Lipase: 48 (normal); Lactate: 5.4
- UA: Ketones positive, glucose positive
- Blood cultures: Obtained
- CXR: No free air, no infiltrates
- Bedside RUQ US: GB wall 5.2 mm, pericholecystic fluid, no gallstones, sonographic Murphy positive

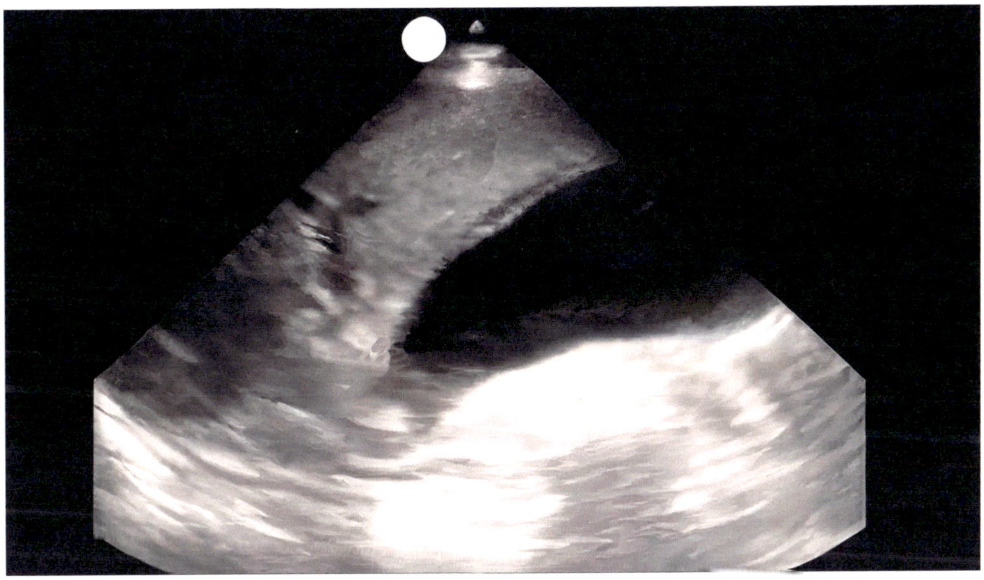

Management

- 30 mL/kg crystalloid resuscitation, broad-spectrum antibiotics (piperacillin-tazobactam) within 1 hour
- Blood cultures prior to antibiotics if possible without delay
- Recognize concurrent DKA (glucose 412, ketonuria, HCO_3 18, AG metabolic acidosis): start insulin infusion 0.1 units/kg/hr, replete K (3.2) before or with insulin, serial POC glucose q1-2h

Reassessment

Despite resuscitation and antibiotics: remains hypotensive (BP 78/52). Now reports severe RUQ pain with new guarding, rebound, and positive Murphy sign. Start vasopressors for septic shock refractory to fluids.

CT abdomen/pelvis with IV contrast: Emphysematous cholecystitis with intramural gas in GB wall, pericholecystic fluid. No perforation or abscess yet.

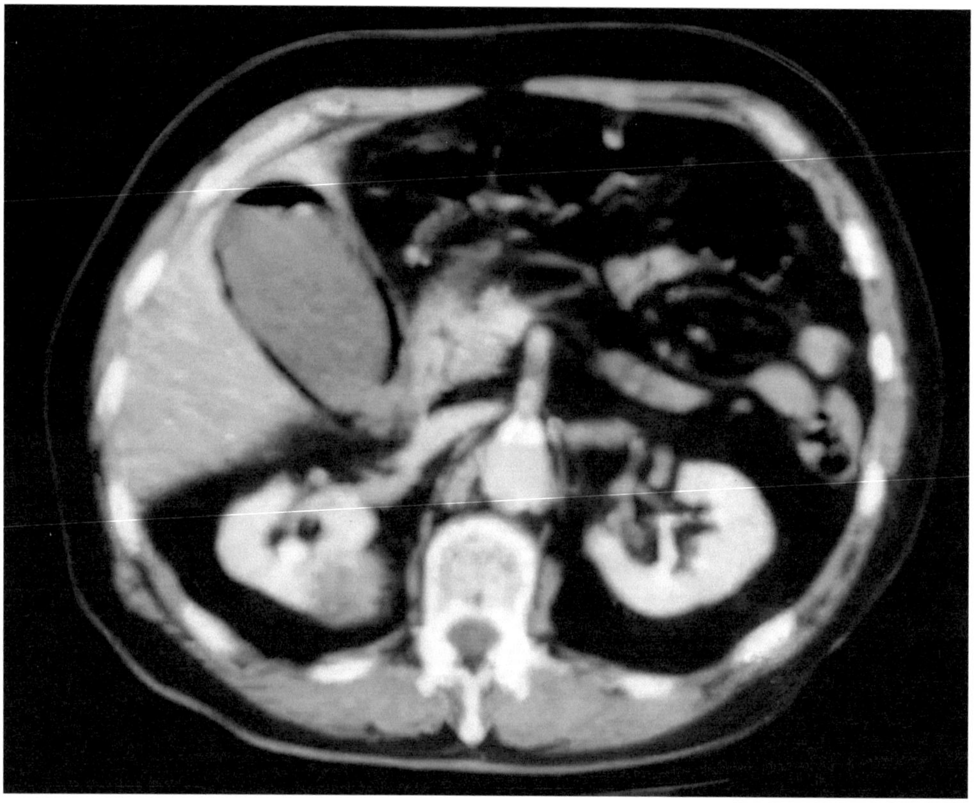

Patient Communication

Patient (now more alert but confused) refuses surgery citing "bad experience with anesthesia." Spouse distressed.

- Explain life-threatening nature of emphysematous cholecystitis in diabetics (high mortality without intervention)
- Discuss emergent cholecystectomy vs. percutaneous cholecystostomy tube as temporizing measure
- Explain risks of delay given sepsis and DM
- ICU admission required regardless of surgical decision

Critical Actions

- Early sepsis recognition and 30 mL/kg fluid resuscitation
- Blood cultures and broad-spectrum antibiotics within 1 hour
- Bedside RUQ US performed and interpreted
- Vasopressors for septic shock refractory to fluids
- Recognize and manage concurrent DKA (insulin infusion, K repletion)
- CT abdomen when clinical picture suggests complicated cholecystitis
- Emergent general surgery consultation for emphysematous cholecystitis
- ICU admission; discuss percutaneous cholecystostomy as alternative if patient refuses OR

Penetrating Chest Trauma with Decompensation

Opening Scenario

EMS arrives with a 31-year-old male who sustained a gunshot wound to the left chest 20 minutes ago during an altercation. Initially alert and speaking in full sentences on scene, his respiratory status deteriorated during transport. EMS placed a non-rebreather mask at 15 L/min. He is diaphoretic, sitting upright, speaking in two-word phrases, and appearing anxious.

Initial Assessment

Vitals: BP 82/48, HR 136, RR 36, SpO_2 87% on NRB, T 36.9°C, GCS 14 (E4 V4 M6)

- General: Muscular male, diaphoretic, using accessory muscles with intercostal retractions. Small-caliber presumed entry wound at left 4th ICS, mid-clavicular line, with minimal external bleeding. No second wound visible.
- Airway: Patent, speaking in short phrases, no stridor or gurgling
- Breathing: Severe respiratory distress with nasal flaring. Breath sounds markedly diminished on left, normal on right. Left hemithorax hyperresonant to percussion. Tracheal deviation to the right.
- Circulation: Rapid, thready pulses. Capillary refill 4 seconds. JVD present despite upright positioning. Skin cool and clammy.
- Disability: Pupils equal, round, reactive. Moving all extremities spontaneously.
- Exposure: No other injuries on log roll; no posterior wounds.

Immediate actions: Recognize tension pneumothorax (hypotension, JVD, tracheal deviation away from affected side, absent breath sounds, obstructive shock) and proceed with immediate decompression without awaiting radiographic confirmation.

Management

- Needle thoracostomy at left 5th ICS, mid-axillary line (or 2nd ICS, mid-clavicular line) – rush of air audible upon entry
- Two large-bore peripheral IVs (18-gauge or larger)
- 1 L crystalloid bolus (LR or NS)
- Continuous cardiac monitoring, pulse oximetry, automated BP cuff
- Prepare for emergent tube thoracostomy

History

- Allergies: NKDA
- Medications: None
- PMHx: No significant history
- Last Meal: Dinner 3 hours ago
- Events: Shot during altercation; no LOC; denies head or abdominal pain

Physical Examination

Post-decompression secondary survey:

- HEENT: Normocephalic, pupils reactive, no Battle sign or raccoon eyes
- Neck: Trachea midline, no subcutaneous emphysema, no step-offs
- Chest: Entry wound at left 4th ICS MCL; needle thoracostomy site in left mid-axillary line; breath sounds slightly diminished on left vs. right; no crepitus

- Heart: Regular rhythm, no murmurs/rubs/gallops; normal PMI
- Abdomen: Soft, non-distended, no tenderness or peritoneal signs
- Back: No posterior wounds, no step-offs or tenderness
- Extremities: Moving all four extremities; distal pulses palpable
- Neuro: Alert, oriented, appropriate; cranial nerves intact; strength 5/5 bilateral

Definitive management:

- Tube thoracostomy: 28-36 Fr chest tube at left 5th ICS, mid-axillary line, directed posteriorly and superiorly. Connect to Pleur-Evac at -20 cm H_2O suction. Returns air and 200 mL serosanguineous fluid.
- CXR: Left lung re-expanded, chest tube in good position, no foreign body, no mediastinal widening
- Labs: CBC, BMP, PT/PTT/INR, type and crossmatch 4 units PRBCs, lactate, blood alcohol
- Consult thoracic surgery
- Morphine 4 mg IV (titrate carefully given hemodynamics)
- Cefazolin 2 g IV; tetanus toxoid IM

Reassessment

5 minutes post-decompression: Vitals: BP 118/72, HR 96, RR 22, SpO_2 96% on NRB. Patient reports improved breathing. Trachea midline. Breath sounds diminished on left but air entry present.

45 minutes later: Patient awaiting CT chest/abdomen/pelvis on 2 L NC with SpO_2 94%.

Nurse reports: “Doctor, his pressure is dropping again.”

Vitals: BP 76/44 (falling from 118/72), HR 142, RR 28, SpO_2 89% on 2 L NC, T 37.1°C

Must systematically evaluate for: recurrent tension pneumothorax (tube malfunction), massive hemothorax, pericardial tamponade, hemorrhagic shock from intra-abdominal injury.

Findings on reassessment:

- Chest tube kinked at insertion site where patient rolled onto his side
- Left breath sounds again markedly diminished
- Trachea midline (tube partially functional)
- Neck veins flat (suggesting blood loss rather than obstruction)

Intervention: Straighten kinked chest tube – immediate return of 1,200 mL fresh blood followed by steady output of 200 mL/hour. Patient reports relief; SpO_2 improves to 96% on 2 L NC.

This represents massive hemothorax (initial output >1,500 mL or >200 mL/hour for 2-4 hours). The 1,200 mL initial output with ongoing 200 mL/hour meets criteria for emergent thoracotomy.

- Initiate Massive Transfusion Protocol (1:1:1 PRBCs:FFP:Platelets)
- Second 1 L crystalloid bolus
- Second large-bore IV or central venous access if needed

Disposition

Thoracic surgery evaluates at bedside and accepts for emergent operative intervention. Communicate handoff: mechanism, interventions, blood products administered, hemodynamic status. Patient transferred directly to OR.

Critical Actions

- Clinically diagnose tension pneumothorax (hypotension, JVD, tracheal deviation, absent breath sounds, obstructive shock) without awaiting CXR
- Perform immediate needle decompression at appropriate anatomical location on the affected side

- Place definitive chest tube (28-36 Fr) connected to suction
- Complete head-to-toe secondary survey including posterior wound inspection
- Consult thoracic surgery early for penetrating chest trauma
- Recognize deterioration at 45 minutes (dropping BP, hypoxia) and systematically troubleshoot
- Identify chest tube malfunction (kinked tube) and massive hemothorax on unkinking
- Initiate Massive Transfusion Protocol and arrange emergent operative intervention
- Communicate with patient during instability; coordinate team for monitoring, medications, and blood products
- Failure points: awaiting CXR before decompression, ignoring deteriorating vitals, failing to troubleshoot tube issues, not notifying trauma surgery or cardiothoracic surgery

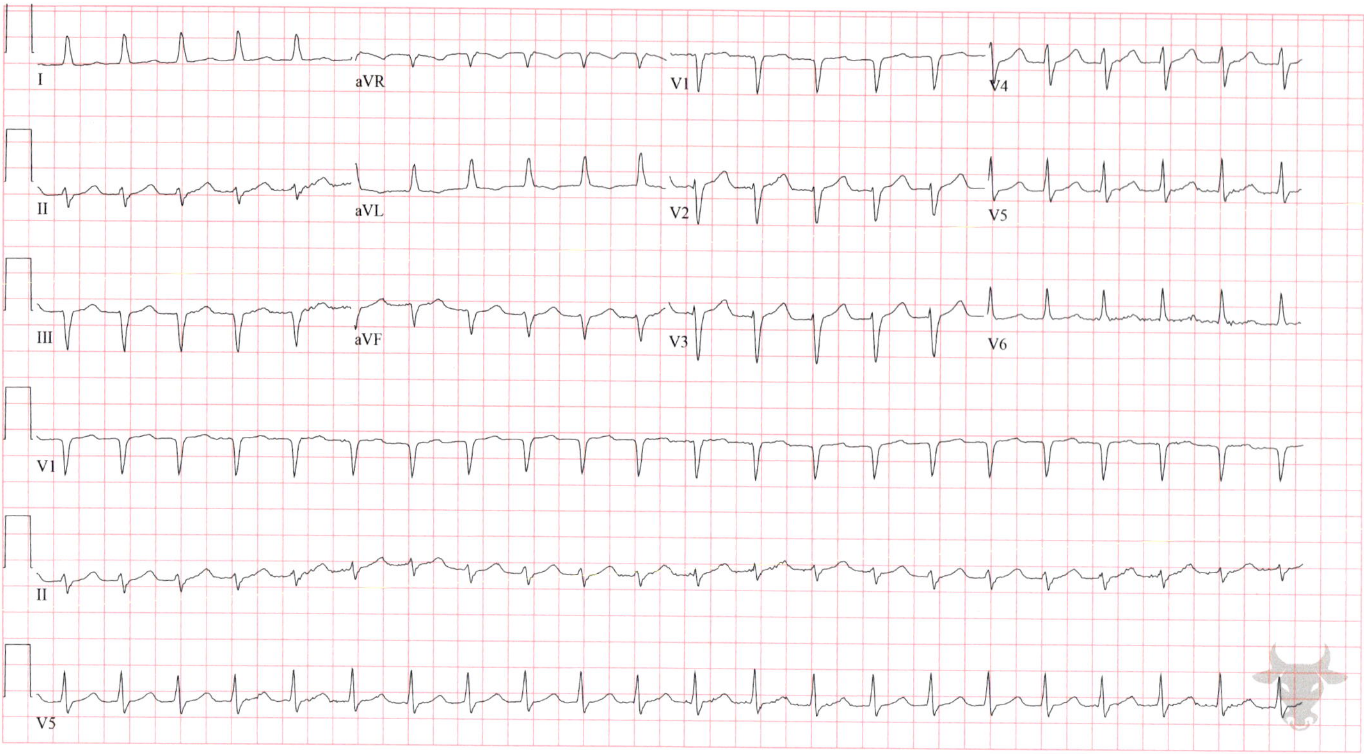

Chest and Back Pain

Opening Scenario

You are working as the attending physician in a high-volume academic emergency department. The charge nurse notifies you that an 82-year-old male has just arrived by private vehicle with his daughter. The patient was reportedly in his usual state of health this morning when he suddenly developed severe back pain while reading the newspaper. He became diaphoretic and lightheaded, prompting his daughter to drive him immediately to the hospital. The patient has been triaged to a monitored bed, and preliminary vitals have been obtained.

Chief Complaint

82-year-old male with acute, severe thoracolumbar back pain radiating to the groin

Vital Signs:

BP: 106/68 mmHg (left arm, supine)
HR: 108 beats/min (regular)
RR: 22 breaths/min
T: 36.7°C (oral)
SpO_2: 96% on room air

Initial Assessment

Patient appears older than stated age, diaphoretic and pale, clutching his lower back, lying in a position of comfort with knees drawn up. He is alert but in obvious distress, occasionally moaning with discomfort.

Primary Survey

Airway: Patent, speaking in full sentences with clear voice
Breathing: Non-labored, clear to auscultation bilaterally, no accessory muscle use
Circulation: Cool, clammy skin peripherally; capillary refill 3 seconds; radial pulses palpable but thready

Initial Actions

- Place patient on continuous pulse oximetry and cardiac monitoring
- Establish two large-bore peripheral IVs (14 gauge or 16 gauge)
- Draw stat labs: CBC, CMP, PT/PTT/INR, type and crossmatch (4-6 units PRBC), lactate, troponin
- Administer 1L normal saline bolus via rapid infuser
- Obtain 12-lead ECG
- Place Foley catheter for urine output monitoring (may defer if AAA strongly suspected)

History

HPI: Patient reports sudden onset of "tearing" pain in his lower back that began abruptly 90 minutes ago while at rest. Pain radiates to the left groin and lower abdomen. He describes it as the worst pain he has ever experienced (10/10). He denies chest pain, syncope, or shortness of breath. He reports mild nausea but no vomiting. He noticed his urine appeared "tea-colored" this morning. He denies recent trauma, heavy lifting, or straining.

PMHx: Hypertension, hyperlipidemia, coronary artery disease (prior MI 3 years ago), peripheral vascular disease
PSHx: Coronary artery stenting (3 years ago), appendectomy (childhood)
Allergies: NKDA
Meds: Aspirin 81mg daily, atorvastatin 40mg daily, metoprolol 50mg BID, amlodipine 5mg daily
Social: Lives with daughter; former smoker (quit 5 years ago, 40 pack-year history); denies alcohol or illicit drugs
FHx: Father died of sudden cardiac death in his 70s; mother had stroke

Reassessment After Initial Fluid Bolus

After 1L NS bolus:

- BP: 102/64 mmHg
- HR: 106
- RR: 20
- SpO_2: 97% on nasal cannula 2L
  Patient reports pain unchanged, still severe.

ECG shows: Sinus tachycardia at 135 bpm, normal axis, no ST changes, no Q waves, unchanged from baseline.

Physical Examination

General: Alert, oriented x3, moderate distress, diaphoretic
HEENT: Pale conjunctivae, anicteric sclera, mucous membranes moist
Neck: Supple, no JVD, no carotid bruits
Chest: Clear to auscultation bilaterally, symmetric expansion
Heart: Regular rate and rhythm, II/VI systolic murmur at right upper sternal border, no rubs or gallops
Abdomen: Soft, obese, mild epigastric tenderness without guarding or rebound; upon specific examination request, a pulsatile mass is appreciated in the epigastrium/umbilical region approximately 4-5 cm in diameter
Back: Thoracolumbar tenderness to palpation; subtle ecchymoses noted on the left flank upon closer inspection
Extremities: Cool bilaterally, DP pulses palpable but weak, no edema
Neuro: Cranial nerves intact, motor strength 5/5 bilateral lower extremities, sensation intact to light touch

Urgent Interventions

- Administer fentanyl 50mcg IV for pain control (reassessment with repeat dosing as needed)
- Perform bedside ultrasound of abdominal aorta
- Consult vascular surgery immediately (or general surgery if vascular unavailable)
- Activate massive transfusion protocol or ensure blood bank prepares 6-10 units PRBC and FFP
- Place arterial line for continuous monitoring
- Prepare for potential operative intervention

Reassessment

After morphine and during ultrasound preparation:

- BP: 94/58 mmHg (trending down from 102/64)
- HR: 112
- RR: 24
- Patient reports severe pain persists ("like I'm being ripped apart from inside")

Diagnostic Studies

Bedside Ultrasound: Shows abdominal aorta with diameter >5cm without visible dissection flap; free fluid in Morrison's pouch suggesting rupture/hemorrhage.

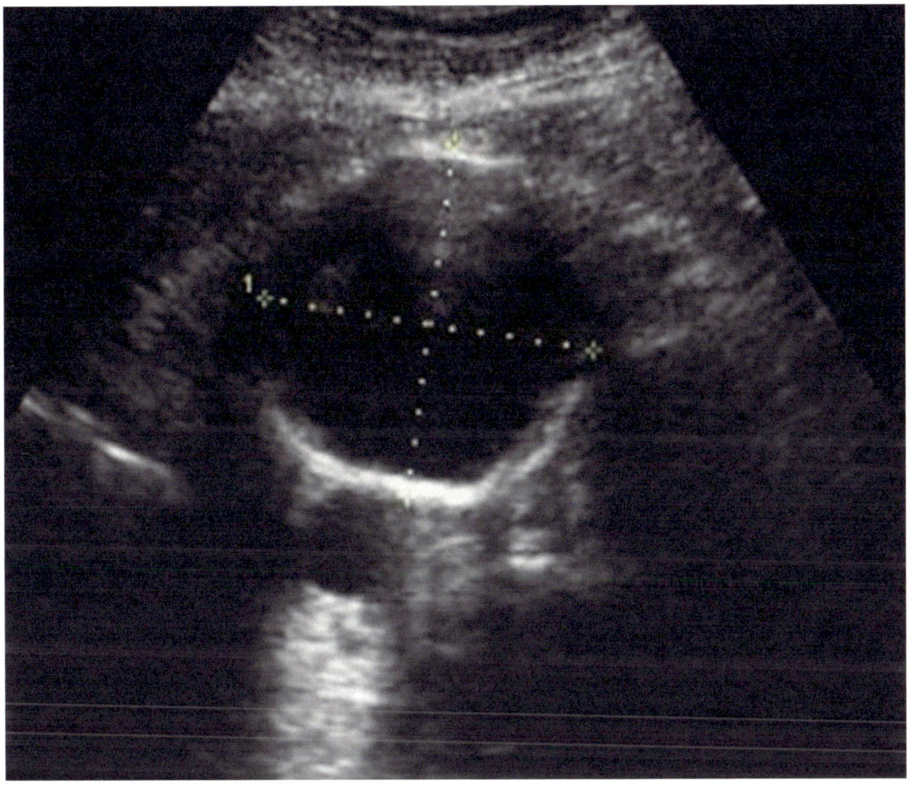

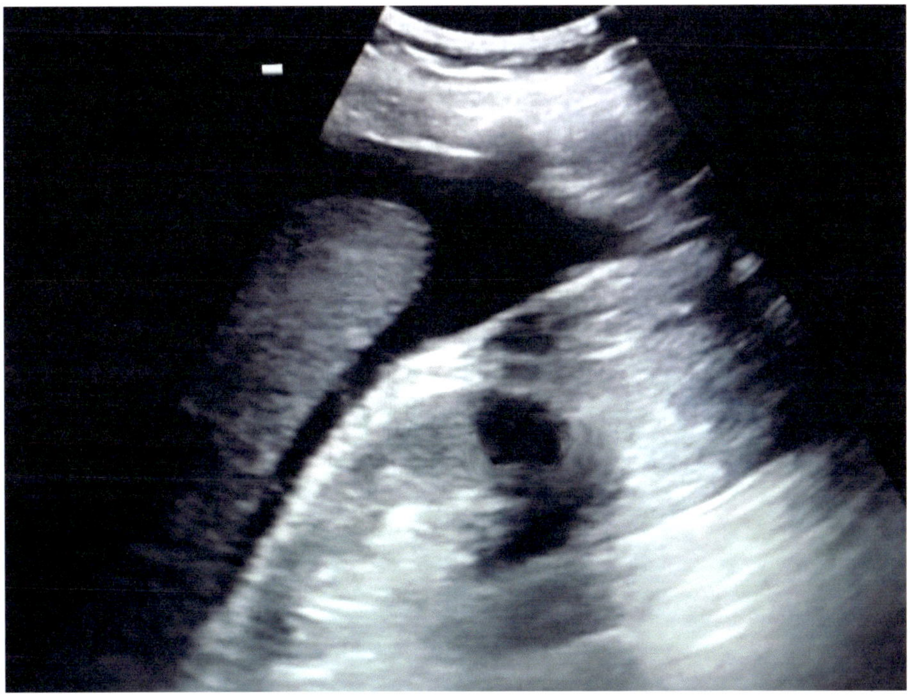

Labs:

- CBC: WBC 11.2, Hgb 9.8 (Hct 29.4%), Plt 198
- BMP: Na 138, K 4.3, Cl 102, HCO_3 18, BUN 38, Cr 1.6, Glucose 156
- Coags: PT 13.5 sec, PTT 28 sec, INR 1.1
- Lactate: 3.4 (elevated)

- Troponin: 0.04 (baseline)
- UA: 2+ blood, 1+ protein; RBCs seen on microscopic exam

Definitive Management

- Immediate vascular surgery consultation for emergent repair
- Transfuse 2 units O-negative or type-specific uncrossmatched blood immediately if crossmatch delayed
- Continue fluid resuscitation with blood products (1:1:1 ratio if massive transfusion initiated)
- Notify operating room for emergent case
- Update patient and family regarding critical nature of condition and need for immediate surgery
- Prepare vasopressor support for impending hemodynamic collapse

Diagnosis

Ruptured abdominal aortic aneurysm with retroperitoneal hemorrhage

Critical Actions

- Early Recognition of hemorrhagic shock: Identified hypotension, tachycardia, and cool extremities as signs of hemodynamic compromise requiring immediate large-bore IV access and fluid resuscitation.
- Bedside Ultrasound Utilization: Performed point-of-care ultrasound to rapidly diagnose AAA rather than delaying care with CT imaging in an unstable patient.
- Surgical Consultation: Early involvement of vascular surgery without awaiting definitive imaging in the setting of clinical deterioration.
- Hemorrhage Management: Initiated blood product transfusion (uncrossmatched if necessary) and preparation for massive transfusion protocol.
- Physical Examination Precision: Specifically sought and identified pulsatile abdominal mass and Grey-Turner's sign (flank ecchymosis) indicating retroperitoneal hemorrhage.
- Reassessment: Recognized worsening hemodynamics despite initial fluid resuscitation (drop in BP from 106→94) and adjusted management to include blood products and expedited surgical care rather than continuing with crystalloid alone.
- Differential Diagnosis: Appropriately differentiated AAA from renal colic/nephrolithiasis despite presence of hematuria (which can occur in AAA due to ureteral irritation or contamination).

Chest Pain and Vomiting

Opening Scenario

A 26-year-old male is triaged to the acute care area with severe chest pain. The charge nurse reports: "He says he started vomiting after a big meal last night and now has crushing chest pain. He's diaphoretic."

Initial Assessment

Vitals: BP 118/72 (orthostatic symptoms), HR 112, RR 22, T 38.2°C, SpO_2 97% RA

- General: Alert and oriented, severe distress, clutching chest, diaphoretic, leaning forward, reluctant to lie flat
- Airway: Patent, speaking in full sentences, no stridor
- Breathing: Tachypneic, no increased WOB, breath sounds equal bilaterally
- Circulation: Rapid but full pulses, capillary refill 2 seconds, skin warm and moist
- Disability: No focal neurologic deficits; anxious but appropriate

Immediate actions: Continuous monitoring, two large-bore IVs, 2 L LR bolus (tachycardic with borderline BP and vomiting history), supplemental O_2 via NC at 2 L/min, 12-lead ECG, stat labs (CBC, CMP, lipase, lactate, blood cultures x2, type and screen), analgesia (IV morphine or fentanyl), ondansetron, NPO status.

History

- HPI: Sudden onset severe, sharp retrosternal chest pain 6 hours ago after forceful retching and vomiting following a bachelor party dinner (heavy meal with alcohol). Pain 10/10, constant, radiates to back and shoulders, pleuritic. SOB when lying flat. Denies hematemesis, cocaine, tobacco, recent travel.
- PMHx/PSHx: None
- Allergies: NKDA
- Medications: Occasional OTC antacids
- Social: Occasional binge drinking, denies tobacco/illicit drugs
- FHx: Non-contributory

Physical Examination

- General: Diaphoretic and anxious, sitting upright
- HEENT: Mucous membranes dry; oropharynx clear without blood
- Neck: Full ROM; subcutaneous emphysema palpable bilaterally in supraclavicular fossae (crepitus); no JVD
- Chest: Mild sternal tenderness, no costochondral tenderness; symmetric expansion; clear bilaterally
- Cardiovascular: Tachycardic, regular rhythm, no murmurs/rubs/gallops
- Abdomen: Soft, non-distended, normal bowel sounds, no peritoneal signs; mild epigastric tenderness
- Skin: Warm, diaphoretic; no track marks

Diagnostic Studies

- ECG: Sinus tachycardia, no ST elevations or depressions

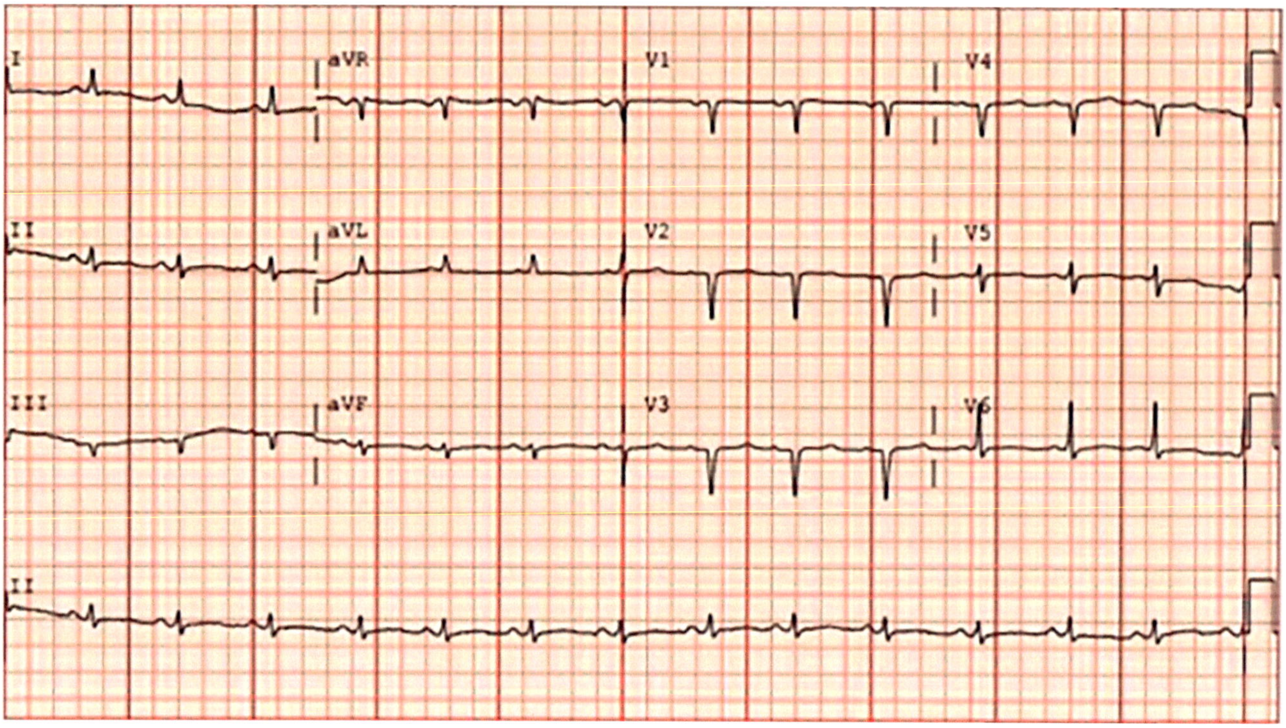
I
aVR
V1
V4
II
aVL
V2
V5
III
aVF
V3
V6
II

- CXR (portable, upright): Possible small left pleural effusion; no definite pneumothorax, mild widening of mediastinum

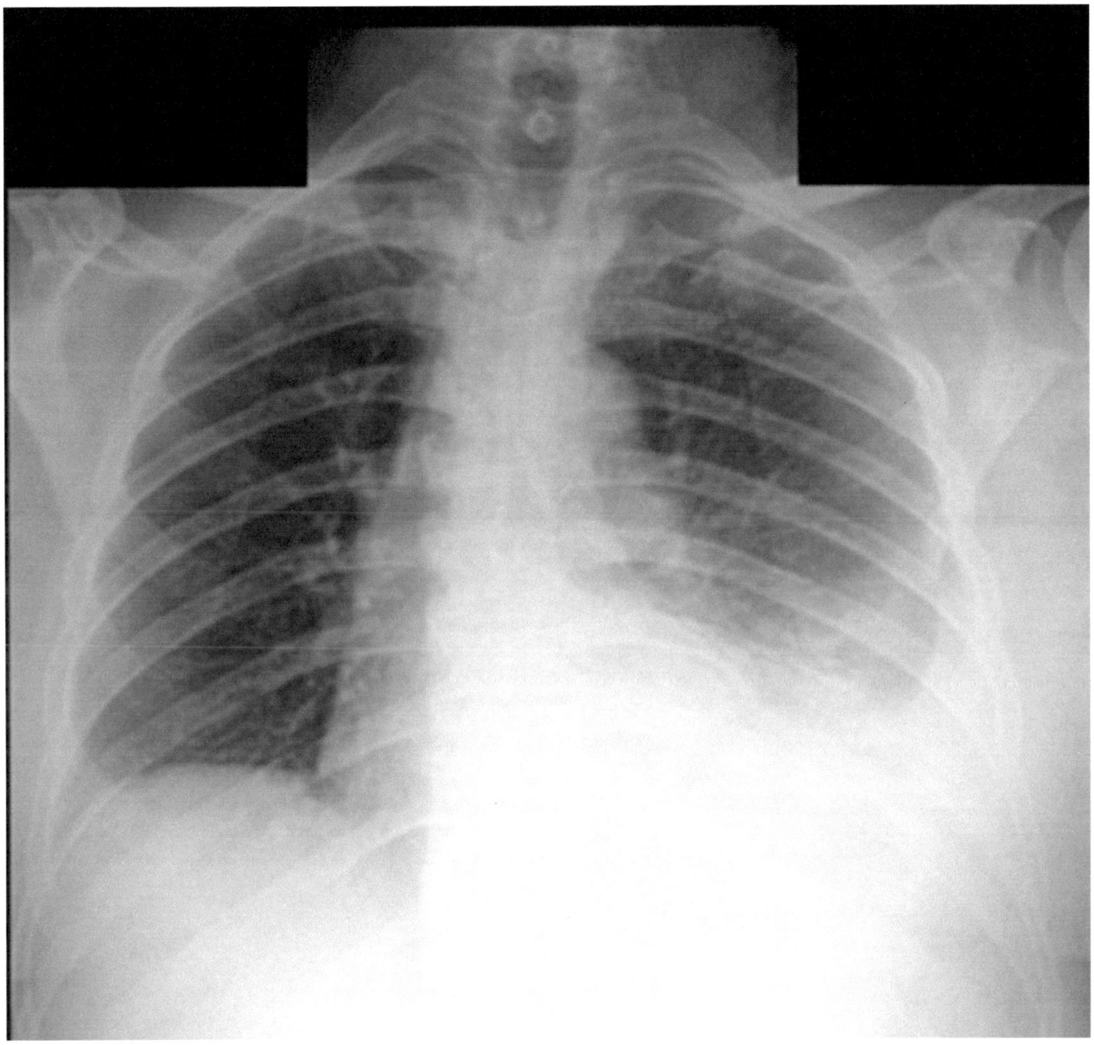

- CBC: WBC 16.2 (left shift), Hgb 14.8, Hct 44%, Plt 255
- BMP: Na 138, K 3.8, Cl 104, HCO_3 22, BUN 18, Cr 1.0, Glucose 102
- Lipase: 180 (mildly elevated)
- Lactate: 2.8 (elevated)
- Troponin I: <0.04 (negative); D-dimer: Negative
- Blood cultures: Pending
- CT Chest/Abdomen/Pelvis with IV contrast: Distal esophageal perforation (left posterolateral wall, just above GE junction), pneumomediastinum, subcutaneous emphysema in neck and chest wall, small left pleural effusion with possible early mediastinitis

Reassessment

If CT not ordered causing missed diagnosis of esophageal perforation:

- 2 hours: Worsening tachycardia (HR 130s) and hypotension (BP 90/60)
- 4 hours: Febrile to 39.5°C, confused, hypotensive (BP 75/40) requiring vasopressors
- 6 hours: Respiratory distress with hypoxia despite 15L NRB - intubation required

If managed appropriately (aggressive fluids, antibiotics, surgical consultation): Patient stabilizes with improved perfusion after 2L fluids, remains hemodynamically stable pending operative intervention. If intubation occurs prior to vasopressor administration and hemodynamic stabilization the patient has a cardiac arrest and the case ends.

Critical Actions

- Recognize sepsis/mediastinitis risk and initiate aggressive IV fluid resuscitation (minimum 2 L crystalloid) early
- Perform thorough neck and chest exam to identify subcutaneous emphysema (crepitus), pathognomonic for esophageal rupture
- Include Boerhaave syndrome in the differential for chest pain with vomiting/retching, especially with pneumomediastinum on imaging
- Order CXR followed by CT chest with contrast to confirm and locate perforation
- Initiate broad-spectrum IV antibiotics immediately covering oral flora (Gram-positives, Gram-negatives, anaerobes; e.g., piperacillin-tazobactam or ceftriaxone + metronidazole + vancomycin)
- Maintain NPO status and arrange emergent surgical consultation (thoracic surgery or GI for endoscopic vs. operative repair)
- Reassess hemodynamic status frequently for deterioration (hypotension, rising lactate, AMS) indicating septic shock progression
- Rule out other life-threatening causes of chest pain (MI, aortic dissection, PE, tension pneumothorax) while pursuing diagnosis

Painful Red Eye

Opening Scenario

A 67-year-old woman is brought by her daughter with sudden onset of severe right-sided headache and eye pain that began two hours ago while watching television. Triage nurse placed the patient in a darkened room due to photophobia.

Initial Assessment

Vitals: BP 174/102, HR 98, RR 16, T 36.8°C, SpO_2 99% RA, Pain 9/10 (right eye)

- General: Elderly Asian female, uncomfortable and anxious, sitting upright with head resting against right hand, guarding right eye
- Airway: Patent, speaking clearly without stridor
- Breathing: Non-labored, clear breath sounds
- Circulation: Radial pulses 2+, skin warm and dry, capillary refill <2 seconds

History

- CC: "My eye feels like it's going to explode"
- HPI: Sudden onset severe right periorbital pain and blurred vision 2 hours ago. Rainbow-colored halos around lights. Associated frontal headache, nausea, two episodes of non-bloody vomiting. No trauma. Worsened despite OTC acetaminophen.
- PMHx: Hypertension, type 2 DM
- PSHx: Cataract surgery (left eye only, 5 years ago)
- Medications: Metformin, amlodipine, lisinopril
- Allergies: NKDA
- FHx: Mother with primary open-angle glaucoma
- Social: Retired teacher, non-smoker, no alcohol

Physical Examination

- General: Moderate distress due to pain, no respiratory compromise
- Head: Normocephalic, atraumatic, temporal arteries non-tender
- Eyes:
  - Right: Marked conjunctival injection, hazy/steamy cornea preventing fundoscopy, pupil mid-dilated (~5mm) and fixed, globe rock-hard to palpation, shallow anterior chamber on penlight exam
  - Left: Normal appearance, clear cornea, reactive pupil, normal fundoscopy
  - EOMs: Intact bilaterally, painful on right
  - Visual acuity: Right – count fingers at 1 foot; Left – 20/30 with correction
- Cardiovascular: Regular rate and rhythm, no murmurs, no carotid bruits
- Neurological: CN II-XII intact except right CN II deficit as noted, no facial asymmetry, no focal deficits

Management

- Position supine with HOB elevated 30 degrees to reduce episcleral venous pressure
- Peripheral IV access; ondansetron 4mg IV for nausea/vomiting
- Emergent IOP reduction protocol (multi-modal):

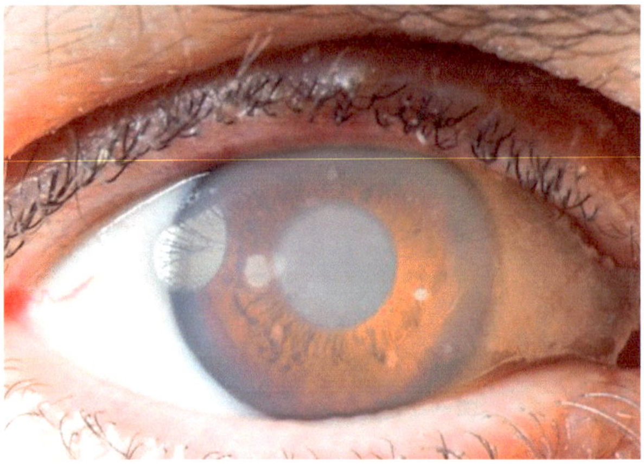

    - Topical timolol 0.5 – 1 drop right eye (reduce aqueous production)
    - Topical brimonidine 0.2 – 1 drop right eye (reduce aqueous production)
    - Acetazolamide 500mg IV (decrease aqueous secretion)
    - Mannitol 1-2g/kg IV over 45 minutes (osmotic gradient)
    - Prednisolone acetate 1 – 1 drop right eye (reduce inflammation, prevent synechiae)
- Protective shield over right eye (no pressure patch)
- Emergent ophthalmology consultation
- Baseline BMP given DM and planned diuretic therapy

Diagnostic Studies

- BMP: Na 138, K 3.8, Cl 102, HCO_3 24, BUN 22, Cr 1.1, Glucose 142
- CBC: WBC 7.2, Hgb 13.8, Plt 245
- Coags: PT 12.8, PTT 28.5, INR 1.0
- Intraocular pressure (Tonopen): Right eye 62 mmHg (normal <21); Left eye 14 mmHg

Reassessment

30 minutes post-treatment:

- Repeat IOP: Right eye 38 mmHg (improved but still critically elevated)
- Pain improved to 6/10; vision slightly improved to hand motion at 2 feet
- Nausea resolved; hemodynamically stable

Additional interventions now that IOP <40 mmHg:

- Pilocarpine 2 – 1 drop right eye every 15 minutes x2 doses (promotes aqueous outflow via trabecular meshwork; withheld at higher IOP to avoid paradoxical worsening)
- Continue topical beta-blocker and alpha-agonist
- Consider repeat acetazolamide 500mg IV in 6 hours if surgery delayed

Disposition

- NPO pending emergency laser peripheral iridotomy
- Continuous cardiac monitoring during osmotic therapy
- Ophthalmology bedside evaluation for immediate surgery vs. continued medical management with admission

Diagnosis: Acute primary angle-closure glaucoma

Critical Actions

- Identify acute angle-closure glaucoma based on painful red eye, fixed mid-dilated pupil, steamy cornea, and markedly elevated IOP in a patient with risk factors (Asian descent, older age, hyperopic eyes)
- Initiate simultaneous multi-modal IOP reduction (beta-blockers, alpha-agonists, carbonic anhydrase inhibitors, mannitol) without awaiting labs
- Withhold pilocarpine until IOP drops below 40 mmHg to avoid paradoxical shallowing of anterior chamber and worsening angle closure
- Recognize critical contraindications: acetazolamide absolutely contraindicated in sickle cell disease; avoid mannitol in CHF or renal failure; caution with non-selective beta-blockers in reactive airway disease
- Obtain emergent ophthalmology consultation for laser peripheral iridotomy within 1-2 hours to prevent permanent optic nerve damage
- Monitor IOP every 30-60 minutes to assess treatment efficacy and guide dosing
- Maintain upright or semi-upright positioning to maximize venous drainage
- Ensure NPO status, adequate analgesia/antiemetics, and patient understanding of the sight-threatening nature of the condition

Limping Teenager

Opening Scenario

A 16-year-old male presents with his father, complaining of progressive right leg pain and a limp that began yesterday during football practice. He describes a dull ache in the anterior thigh and medial knee that started insidiously six weeks ago but acutely worsened during athletics. He has difficulty bearing weight and ambulates with his right foot externally rotated. Denies trauma, fever, night sweats, or recent infections. No PMHx, no medications, NKDA.

Initial Assessment

Vitals: BP 124/78, HR 86, RR 16, T 36.9°C, SpO_2 99% RA. Weight 96 kg, Height 176 cm, BMI 31.

Physical Examination

- General: Obese adolescent male, no acute distress, alert and oriented, significant antalgic gait requiring father's assistance; right lower extremity held in external rotation and slight hip flexion
- Right knee: No effusion, erythema, or warmth; full active and passive ROM without pain; no crepitus; negative Lachman, anterior/posterior drawer, varus/valgus stress at 0 and 30 degrees; negative McMurray, no patellofemoral apprehension, no tibial tubercle tenderness
- Left knee: Normal
- Right hip: Pain with passive internal rotation and flexion beyond 90 degrees; internal rotation ~10 degrees vs. 40 degrees contralateral; no pain with external rotation; prefers flexed and externally rotated position
- Left hip: Full ROM, no pain
- Neurovascular: 5/5 strength all lower extremity groups; sensation intact L2-S1; 2+ DP and PT pulses bilaterally; capillary refill <2 seconds

Reassessment

Initial considerations (meniscal tear, patellofemoral syndrome, Osgood-Schlatter) are inconsistent with the completely normal knee exam despite significant functional limitation. The hip findings – pain with internal rotation, external rotation gait, absent knee pathology – redirect focus to hip pathology with referred pain to the knee.

Diagnostic Studies

- Right knee radiographs (AP and lateral): Normal alignment, no fractures, no effusion, no osteochondritis dissecans
- Bilateral hip radiographs (AP pelvis and frog-leg lateral): Widening of right capital femoral physis with posterior-medial displacement of femoral head relative to neck consistent with SCFE; Klein's line fails to intersect lateral quadrant of right femoral head; subtle contralateral physeal irregularity indicating bilateral disease

Patient Communication

Explain that despite the knee pain, the actual source is the hip growth plate. Discuss SCFE: not a fracture but growth plate displacement requiring urgent stabilization. Address the rationale for hip examination when the knee hurts, the association with obesity and mechanical stress, the need for immediate non-weight-bearing status, and urgent orthopedic surgery. Counsel regarding AVN risk with delayed treatment and need for endocrinologic evaluation.

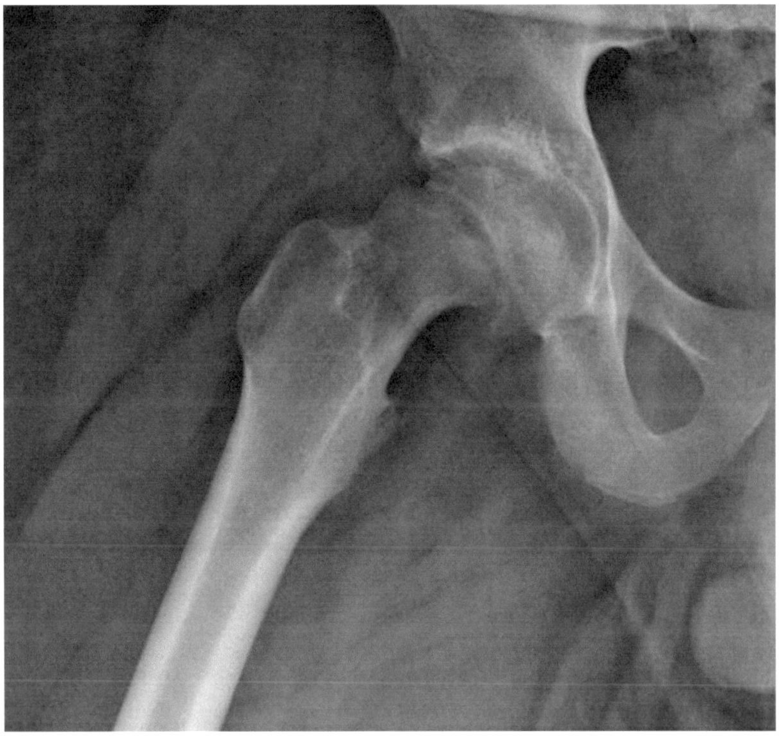

Critical Actions

- Recognize that knee pain in an adolescent male may represent referred pain from ipsilateral hip pathology rather than primary knee disease
- Perform comprehensive hip examination including assessment of internal rotation and observation of gait pattern
- Reassess initial diagnostic hypothesis when objective physical findings contradict the presumed diagnosis (normal knee exam despite significant symptoms)
- Obtain bilateral hip radiographs including lateral views (frog-leg or cross-table lateral) to evaluate for SCFE rather than isolating imaging to the knee
- Identify radiographic findings consistent with slipped capital femoral epiphysis including physeal widening and violation of Klein's line
- Institute immediate strict non-weight-bearing status on the affected extremity to prevent further slippage and reduce risk of avascular necrosis
- Obtain emergent orthopedic consultation for definitive surgical management (percutaneous in-situ pinning)
- Communicate effectively with patient and family regarding the counterintuitive nature of referred pain, the urgency of surgical treatment, and the association with obesity requiring lifestyle modifications and metabolic screening
- Recognize the potential for bilateral disease and ensure contralateral hip evaluation

Snake Bite

Opening Scenario

A frantic father carries his 14-year-old son into the resuscitation bay, reporting a rattlesnake bite 45 minutes ago while hiking. A tightly wrapped bootlace tourniquet is around the boy's right calf. The father demands to "cut out the poison" and produces a pocketknife.

Initial Assessment

Vitals: BP 94/58, HR 124, RR 24, T 37.1°C, SpO_2 97% RA, Pain 8/10 (right leg)

- General: Anxious adolescent male holding right leg immobile in slight flexion. Father pacing with heightened anxiety.
- Airway: Patent, speaking in full sentences, no stridor or hoarseness
- Breathing: Mild tachypnea, clear bilateral breath sounds, no cyanosis
- Circulation: Radial pulses 2+ bilaterally; right DP pulse weak/thready vs. left; capillary refill 4 seconds right great toe, 2 seconds left
- Skin pale and cool distal to tourniquet on right lower extremity

History

- CC: "Something bit my leg and it burns"
- HPI: 14-year-old male hiking on a desert trail felt sudden sharp pain to right calf. Father witnessed a 2-foot snake with triangular head and rattle strike once before retreating. Patient walked 50 yards to parking area with progressive tightness, burning pain, and nausea. Father applied bootlace tourniquet immediately. No prior snake exposure or antivenom allergies.
- PMHx: None significant. PSHx: Appendectomy age 10
- Medications: None
- Allergies: NKDA, no asthma or atopy
- FHx: No bleeding disorders
- Social: High school freshman, no substance use, avid hikers

Physical Examination

- General: Alert, anxious, moderate distress due to pain, no respiratory compromise
- Head: Normocephalic, atraumatic, pupils equal and reactive to light and accommodation
- Neck: Supple, no jugular venous distension, no lymphadenopathy
- Chest: Clear to auscultation bilaterally, symmetric chest expansion, no crepitus
- Cardiovascular: Tachycardic, regular rhythm, no murmurs or gallops, peripheral pulses present but diminished distal to tourniquet on right lower extremity
- Abdomen: Soft, non-tender, non-distended, normal bowel sounds, no hepatosplenomegaly
- Extremities: Right calf with two distinct puncture wounds 1.5 cm apart surrounded by early ecchymosis, moderate swelling extending from ankle to mid-knee, skin tense but compartments compressible. Tourniquet (tight ace wrapping and pant leg) tightly applied in the field above the knee causing distal pallor and coolness. Left leg normal with intact compartments.
- Skin: Cool and dry, no urticaria, no angioedema
- Neurological: Cranial nerves II-XII intact, grossly normal sensation to light touch bilaterally, strength limited to 3/5 in right foot dorsiflexion and plantarflexion due to pain and swelling, 5/5 strength in all

other extremities

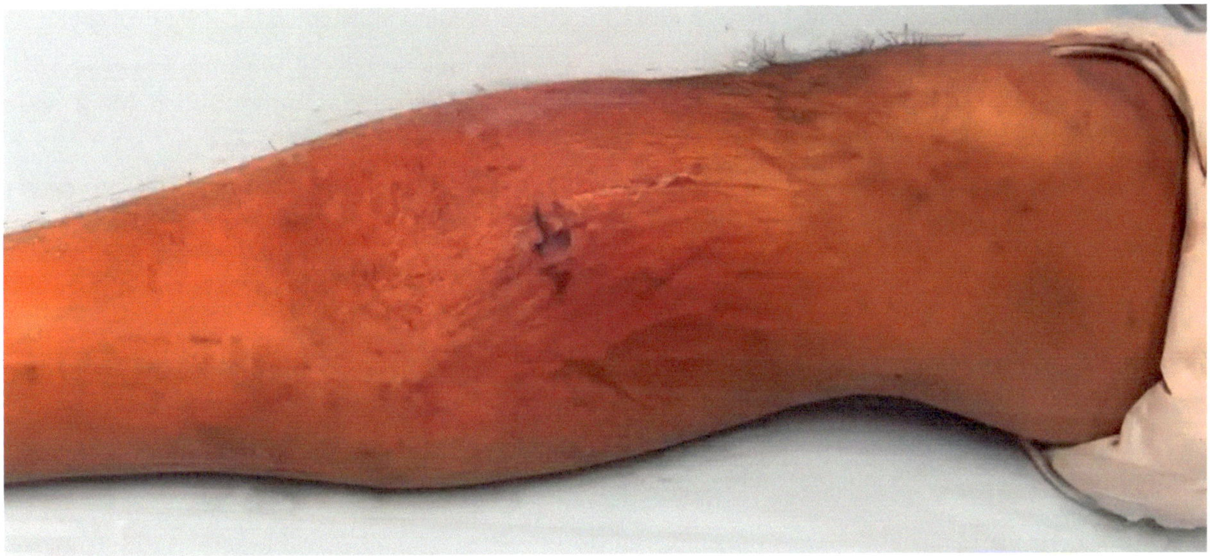

Management

- Immediately remove tourniquet to restore distal perfusion and prevent ischemic compartment syndrome
- Two large-bore IVs with NS at maintenance rate
- Emergent labs: CBC with platelets, CMP, PT/PTT/INR, fibrinogen, D-dimer, type and screen, UA for myoglobin
- Contact regional Poison Control Center for envenomation consultation
- Immobilize right lower extremity in neutral position at heart level (reduce lymphatic spread)
- Morphine 0.1 mg/kg IV for pain (avoid NSAIDs due to potential coagulopathy)
- Tetanus update if not current within 5 years
- Mark leading edge of edema/ecchymosis with skin marker and time for serial monitoring
- Foley catheter for UOP monitoring (rhabdomyolysis/hemolysis)
- Prepare for risk-benefit discussion regarding CroFab antivenom

Diagnostic Studies

- CBC: WBC 16.8, Hgb 14.2, Hct 42%, Plt 78 (severe thrombocytopenia)
- Coags: PT 19.2, PTT 48, INR 1.5, Fibrinogen 95 (hypofibrinogenemia), FSPs elevated
- BMP: Na 136, K 4.1, Cl 104, HCO_3 20, BUN 22, Cr 1.0, Glucose 156
- UA: 3+ blood on dipstick with 0-2 RBCs/HPF (hemoglobinuria from hemolysis), SG 1.025
- Type and Screen: O-positive, antibody negative

Reassessment

15 minutes post-tourniquet removal: Distal pulses return to 2+, capillary refill normalizes. Swelling progresses to knee and ankle within 20 minutes. New nausea with one episode clear emesis. Vitals: HR 118, BP 102/64.

45 minutes post-arrival: Classify as moderate envenomation: progressive swelling crossing two joints, severe thrombocytopenia, coagulopathy, systemic symptoms (nausea, hemolysis). Discuss with family that antivenom is indicated to halt tissue destruction, reverse coagulopathy, and prevent permanent disability. Address concerns about hypersensitivity and serum sickness; obtain informed consent for CroFab.

Antivenom administration: No routine premedication (low anaphylaxis risk with Fab fragments); epinephrine at bedside. CroFab 4-6 vials in NS over 60 minutes with continuous monitoring. Mark new edema border every 30 minutes.

2 hours post-arrival: Pain decreased to 5/10, swelling stabilized below proximal thigh. Plt improved to 145, fibrinogen 180. UOP 1.5 cc/kg/hour, hemoglobinuria clearing. No compartment syndrome (soft compartments, intact neurovascular status).

Disposition

ICU admission for continued antivenom (additional 6 vials at 6, 12, 18 hours) and monitoring for recurrent coagulopathy. NPO, limb elevation, surgical consultation if hemorrhagic vesicles progress to necrosis.

Diagnosis: Moderate Crotalinae (pit viper) envenomation with hematologic toxicity (thrombocytopenia, hypofibrinogenemia, coagulopathy) and systemic effects (hemolysis, nausea)

Critical Actions

- Immediately remove tourniquets/constricting bands to prevent iatrogenic ischemia and compartment syndrome
- Obtain complete envenomation panel (platelets, fibrinogen, coags) before antivenom to establish baseline severity
- Serial edema marking, compartment assessment, and repeat labs every 4-6 hours to guide antivenom redosing
- Risk-stratify: moderate-severe indications (edema crossing joints, Plt <150K, fibrinogen <100, systemic symptoms, hemodynamic instability) mandate antivenom
- Shared decision-making: communicate antivenom risks (hypersensitivity, serum sickness) vs. benefits (halt necrosis, correct coagulopathy) to obtain informed consent
- Avoid contraindicated therapies: no prophylactic antibiotics, no incision/suction, no fasciotomy without documented compartment hypertension, no aggressive fluids without shock
- Contact Poison Control for dosing guidance; maintain in monitored setting capable of managing anaphylaxis

Right Lower Quadrant Pain in a Young Woman

Opening Scenario

A 26-year-old female is triaged to a monitored bed with progressive right lower quadrant pain, nausea, and anorexia.

Initial Assessment

Vitals: BP 118/76, HR 102, RR 16, T 37.9°C, SpO_2 99% RA, Pain 8/10

- General: Lying supine with knees flexed and hips externally rotated, speaking in full sentences
- Skin warm and dry, mildly pale, no diaphoresis
- Radial pulses 2+, capillary refill <2 seconds

History

- HPI: Vague periumbilical discomfort began 18 hours ago, migrated to RLQ 6 hours ago. Worsens with movement, coughing, deep inspiration. Anorexia, nausea, two episodes non-bloody/non-bilious emesis. Denies diarrhea, constipation, dysuria, hematuria, vaginal discharge/bleeding.
- GYN: LMP 10 days ago, regular 28-day cycles. G0P0. Sexually active with husband, consistent OCP use.
- PMHx/PSHx: None. No prior surgeries or hospitalizations
- Medications: OCPs only
- Allergies: NKDA
- Social: No recent travel, sick contacts, or unusual food intake

Physical Examination

- General: Alert and oriented, moderate distress due to pain, reluctant to move
- Head, Eyes, Ears, Nose, Throat: Normocephalic, atraumatic, mucous membranes moist
- Cardiovascular: Tachycardic, regular rhythm, no murmurs, rubs, or gallops
- Respiratory: Clear to auscultation bilaterally, no accessory muscle use
- Abdomen: Soft, flat, tender to palpation maximal at McBurney's point with positive McBurney's tenderness; voluntary guarding and rebound tenderness present; positive Rovsing sign; negative psoas and obturator signs; bowel sounds diminished in right lower quadrant; no hepatosplenomegaly; negative Murphy sign
- Pelvic: External genitalia normal; speculum examination reveals no cervical discharge or blood; bimanual examination shows no cervical motion tenderness; uterus normal size, midline, non-tender; no adnexal masses or tenderness appreciated
- Rectal: Normal sphincter tone; no masses palpated; stool brown, hemoccult negative
- Extremities and Skin: No clubbing, cyanosis, or edema; no rashes or bruising
- Neurologic: Grossly intact, alert and oriented

Management

- Two large-bore IVs (18-gauge), 1 L LR bolus over 30 minutes, NPO
- Morphine 4 mg IV, ondansetron 4 mg IV
- Continuous cardiac monitoring and pulse oximetry

Diagnostic Studies

- CBC: WBC 14.2 (82% neutrophils), Hgb 13.2, Hct 38.5%, Plt 245

- BMP: Na 138, K 4.1, Cl 102, HCO_3 24, BUN 12, Cr 0.9, Glucose 95
- LFTs: Within normal limits
- UA: Yellow, clear, SG 1.020, pH 6.0, negative for protein/glucose/ketones/bilirubin/blood/LE/nitrites, no bacteria/crystals
- Urine pregnancy test: Pending (stat but delayed)

Reassessment

After 30 minutes: Vitals: BP 122/78, HR 88, T 37.8°C, Pain 4/10. RLQ tenderness persists with guarding but improved comfort. Urine pregnancy test negative.

CT abdomen/pelvis with IV contrast: Dilated, non-opacified appendix measuring 11 mm with wall enhancement and periappendiceal fat stranding; no perforation, abscess, or free fluid; no alternative pathology.

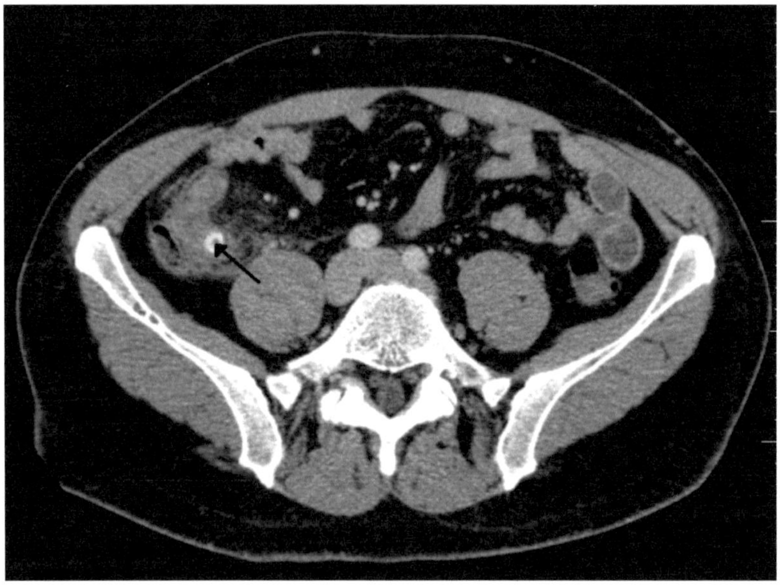

Patient Communication

- Discuss findings of acute appendicitis requiring surgical intervention
- Address patient anxiety regarding laparoscopic versus open surgical approach
- Explain risks of non-operative management including progression to perforation, abscess formation, and peritonitis
- Discuss fertility considerations and the low risk of tubal damage with laparoscopic approach
- Obtain informed consent for surgical consultation and operative management

- Provide opportunity for questions and ensure understanding of post-operative expectations

Disposition

- Consult general surgery for emergent laparoscopic appendectomy
- Administer preoperative antibiotics: Ceftriaxone 1 g IV and metronidazole 500 mg IV
- Continue intravenous fluids and maintain NPO status
- Update primary care physician (Dr. Martinez) on admission status
- Transfer to operating suite when team available

Critical Actions

- Prioritize urine pregnancy testing in all women of childbearing age prior to radiation exposure
- Generate appropriate differential: appendicitis, ectopic pregnancy, ovarian torsion, ruptured cyst, PID, nephrolithiasis, mesenteric adenitis
- Recognize visceral-to-somatic pain migration (periumbilical to RLQ) as classic for appendicitis
- Select imaging based on clinical scenario and pregnancy status (avoid CT if pregnancy test positive; use US instead)
- Interpret leukocytosis with left shift as supportive of surgical pathology
- Reassess after analgesia/fluids to verify persistence of peritoneal signs; persistent pain indicates need for definitive intervention
- Provide adequate analgesia (not masked by surgical findings concern); maintain NPO; administer preoperative antibiotics
- Communicate empathetically about surgery, fertility concerns, and surgical options using jargon-free language; obtain informed consent with teach-back
- Consult surgery based on clinical and radiographic findings without awaiting symptom resolution

Thigh Swelling

Opening Scenario

EMS brings a 62-year-old woman from a skilled nursing facility with severe right thigh pain and swelling that began 18 hours ago and rapidly worsened. Paramedic reports the patient appears toxic, moaning, with HR in the 140s. She is confused and unable to provide history.

Initial Assessment

Vitals: BP 88/56, HR 142, RR 28, T 38.9°C, SpO_2 94% RA

- General: Diaphoretic, confused to time and place, clutching right thigh
- Airway: Patent, speaking in short phrases
- Breathing: Tachypneic, clear bilaterally, no increased WOB
- Circulation: Weak, thready radial pulses; capillary refill 4 seconds; skin mottled on lower extremities
- Disability: Confused, moves all extremities spontaneously
- Exposure: Right thigh markedly swollen with bronze discoloration and several 3-4 cm hemorrhagic bullae

Immediate actions: NRB mask, two large-bore IVs, labs (CBC, BMP, lactate, coags, blood cultures), 2 L crystalloid bolus, POC glucose 48 – D50 25 grams IV.

History

- HPI: Nursing home resident. Staff noticed mild right thigh redness yesterday evening. Over 12 hours: severe pain, rapid swelling, skin blistering. Confused and refusing meals since this morning. Denies trauma or falls.
- PMHx: Type 2 DM (HbA1c 9.2), PAD, CKD (baseline Cr 1.8), HTN. No prior surgeries.
- Medications: Metformin (held due to poor PO intake), amlodipine, atorvastatin, gabapentin
- Allergies: NKDA

Physical Examination

- General: Lethargic but arousable, severe distress due to pain
- Cardiovascular: Tachycardic, regular rhythm, no murmurs
- Respiratory: Clear to auscultation bilaterally, no crackles or wheezes
- Abdomen: Soft, non-tender, normal bowel sounds
- Skin: Right thigh – extensive erythema from inguinal ligament to knee, marked edema, crepitus palpable in medial thigh, multiple hemorrhagic bullae with serosanguinous drainage, 5 cm dusky necrotic area near medial knee. Left leg – chronic venous stasis changes only.
- Neuro: Confused to date and situation, moves all extremities, diminished sensation in lower extremities bilaterally (chronic diabetic neuropathy)

Diagnostic Studies

- CBC: WBC 18.2 (22% bands), Hgb 11.2, Plt 89 (thrombocytopenia)
- BMP: Na 132, K 5.6, BUN 68, Cr 3.4 (AKI from baseline 1.8), Glucose 72 (post-dextrose)
- Lactate: 6.8
- ABG: pH 7.28, PCO_2 28, HCO_3 14, PaO_2 88 on 2L NC
- INR: 1.4; Fibrinogen: 450
- XR right thigh: Soft tissue gas in medial compartment tracking along fascial planes

- 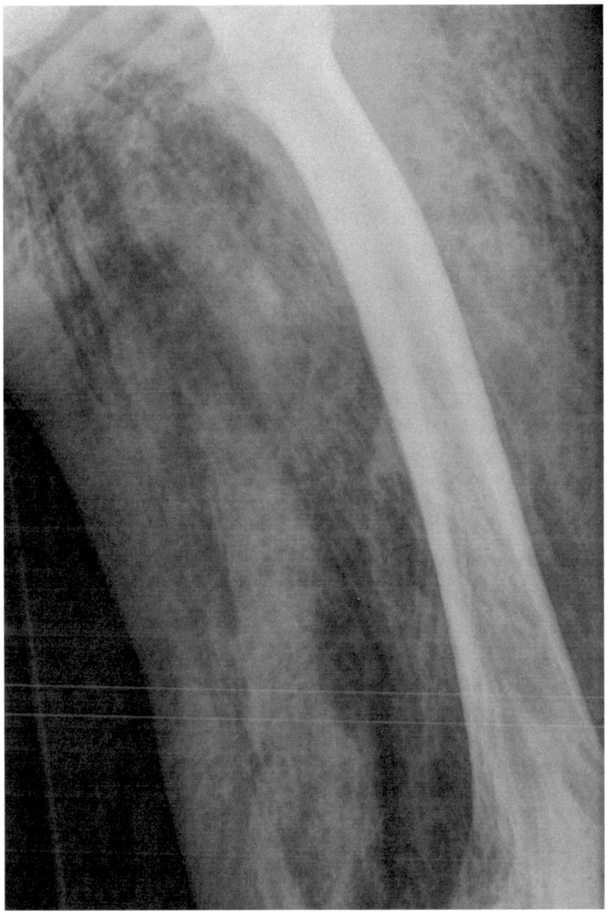
- Bedside US: Subcutaneous edema with cobblestoning

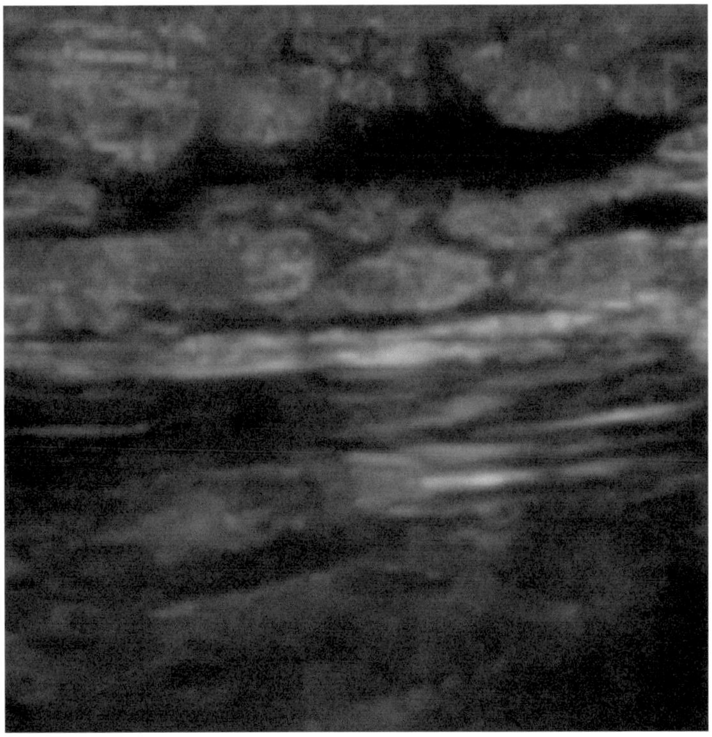

Management

Differential: Necrotizing fasciitis (most likely), severe cellulitis with sepsis, gas gangrene (clostridial myonecrosis), pyomyositis, septic arthritis with extension. Necrotizing fasciitis is the leading diagnosis based on: rapid progression (<24 hours), pain out of proportion, hemorrhagic bullae/necrosis (vascular thrombosis), crepitus and radiographic gas (polymicrobial gas-forming organisms), systemic toxicity with sepsis/acidosis/AKI.

- Broad-spectrum antibiotics covering Gram-positives (including MRSA), Gram-negatives, and anaerobes: vancomycin plus piperacillin-tazobactam or carbapenem; alternative: vancomycin plus ceftriaxone plus metronidazole
- Aggressive fluid resuscitation (balance septic shock needs against CKD fluid overload risk)
- Lactate elevation and metabolic acidosis indicate tissue hypoperfusion requiring continued resuscitation

Reassessment

After initial fluid resuscitation (2 liters) and antibiotic administration, the nurse notifies you that the patient's mental status has worsened. She is now minimally responsive to painful stimuli.

Repeat vitals: BP 72/48, HR 156, RR 32, SpO_2 91% on NRB. Patient now minimally responsive to pain.

- Recognize progression to septic shock despite initial resuscitation
- Vasopressor support (norepinephrine) while balancing limb perfusion risk
- Definitive therapy is surgical source control, not additional medical management
- Consider airway protection if mental status continues declining
- Plan ICU admission

Managing Conflict

The surgery resident requests CT to "confirm and define extent" before OR, stating the patient is "stable enough for imaging."

- The clinical presentation is pathognomonic for necrotizing fasciitis; imaging is unnecessary for diagnosis
- Mortality increases significantly with each hour of delay to surgical debridement
- Negotiate for immediate bedside evaluation or direct OR transfer without imaging
- CT delay risks cardiac arrest during transport in profound shock
- If imaging is deemed essential, perform in the OR as a scout only if it will not delay incision

Critical Actions

- Recognize septic shock and initiate aggressive fluid resuscitation (minimum 30 mL/kg crystalloid)
- Correct hypoglycemia promptly with IV dextrose
- Initiate broad-spectrum antibiotics (MRSA, Gram-negatives, anaerobes) within one hour; adjust dosing for AKI
- Recognize necrotizing fasciitis clinically (crepitus, bullae, rapid progression, pain out of proportion, systemic toxicity) without requiring imaging confirmation
- Radiographic gas in soft tissues confirms diagnosis and obviates CT
- Recognize deterioration despite initial intervention and escalate to vasopressors while balancing limb perfusion
- Maintain focus on emergent surgical debridement as only definitive therapy
- Effectively communicate urgency to surgery using specific clinical findings; resist inappropriate imaging delay; cite mortality data regarding time to debridement

The Weak Dialysis Patient

Opening Scenario

A 68-year-old female arrives by ambulance with severe generalized weakness and palpitations for six hours. History of ESRD on HD (T/Th/Sat), DM, HTN. Missed dialysis two days ago.

Initial Assessment

Vitals: BP 156/94, HR 52 (irregular), RR 24, T 37.1°C, SpO_2 94% RA

- General: Fatigued but alert, speaking in full sentences, slight confusion about current date
- Airway: Patent, handling secretions normally
- Breathing: No increased WOB, clear bilaterally
- Circulation: Warm and dry, peripheral pulses bradycardic and irregular, capillary refill 2 seconds

History

- HPI: Gradual weakness over 3 days since missing dialysis. Decreased urine output, mild ankle swelling. Nausea and "fluttering" chest sensation. Denies chest pain, SOB at rest, fever, vomiting, new medications/supplements.
- PMHx: ESRD on HD (3 years), type 2 DM, HTN, PVD
- Medications: Amlodipine, insulin glargine, sevelamer, aspirin
- Allergies: Not reported

Management

- Must obtain 12-lead ECG within 5 minutes. If delayed: HR drops to 38, BP 88/52, patient becomes lethargic.
- Immediate recognition of hyperkalemia presentation with empiric administration of 2g of calcium gluconate for cardiac stabilization
- Administration of calcium prior to remainder of physical exam
- ECG findings: Sinus bradycardia with peaked T waves (II, III, aVF, V2-V6), PR interval 240 ms, QRS 160 ms, absent P waves in some leads (developing sine wave pattern).

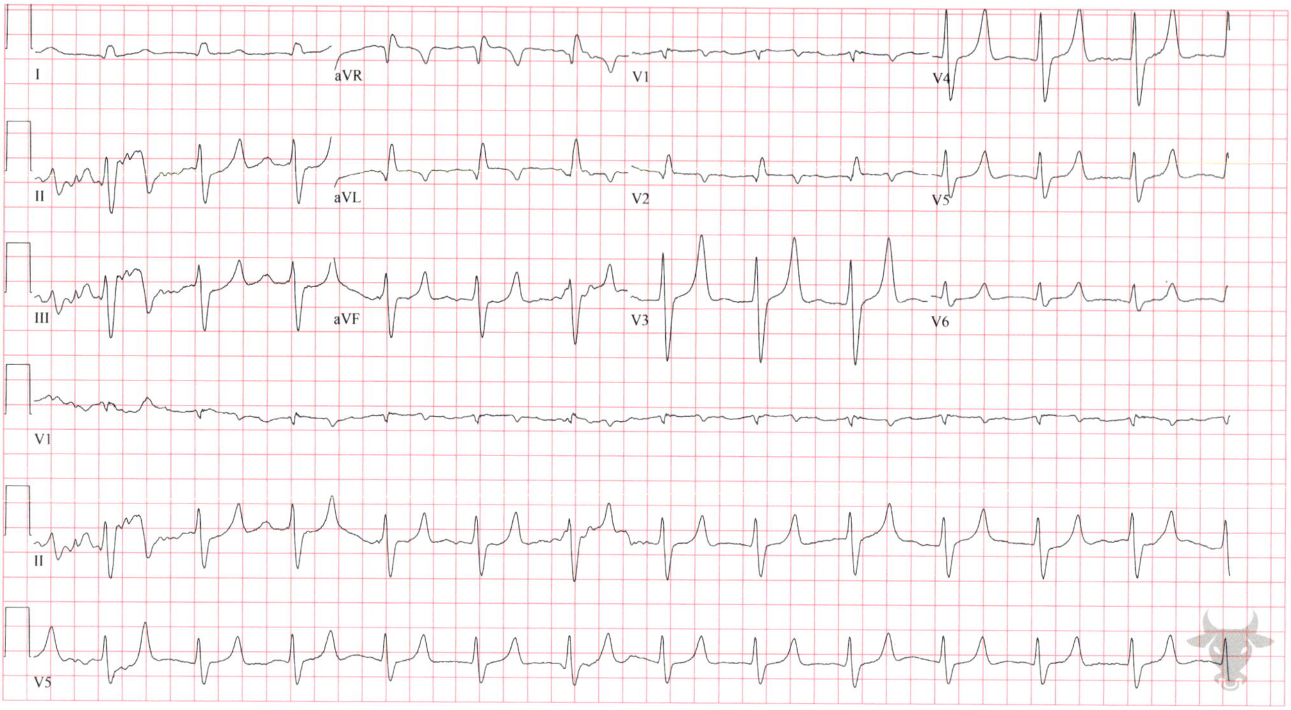

Physical Examination

- HEENT: Dry mucous membranes, pupils equal and reactive
- Cardiovascular: Bradycardic, irregular rhythm, no murmurs or rubs, no JVD
- Pulmonary: Clear to auscultation bilaterally, no wheezes or crackles
- Abdomen: Soft, non-tender, no guarding, normal bowel sounds
- Extremities: No edema, pulses diminished but palpable bilaterally
- Neurological: Alert and oriented to person and place, not time, cranial nerves intact, motor strength 4/5 bilaterally

Diagnostic Studies

- BMP: Na 140, K 8.1, Cl 108, HCO_3 16, BUN 92, Cr 6.8 (baseline 4.2), Glucose 178
- Repeat ECG if no calcium gluconate given (below)

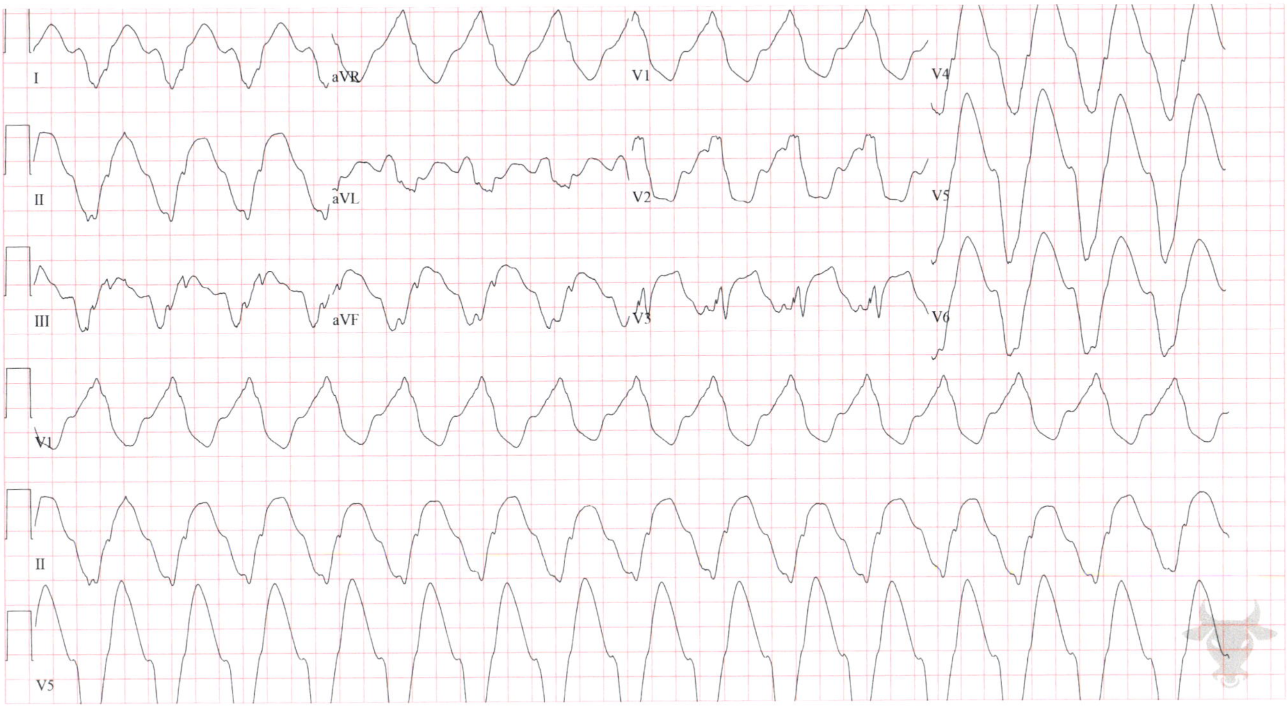

Critical Actions

- Obtain 12-lead ECG promptly (before lab confirmation); recognize hyperkalemia ECG progression (peaked T waves, PR prolongation, QRS widening, sine wave)
- Bradycardia in a dialysis patient is hyperkalemia until proven otherwise
- Administer calcium chloride or gluconate immediately to stabilize cardiac membranes (does not lower K+)
- Cardiac monitor and IV access
- Initiate potassium shifting: insulin with glucose, beta-agonist therapy, sodium bicarbonate if acidotic
- Do not rely on potassium binders such as sodium zirconium cyclosilicate (Lokelma) as sole/immediate therapy for life-threatening hyperkalemia with renal failure
- Contact nephrology for emergent dialysis (definitive therapy); diuretics ineffective in anuric/oliguric ESRD
- Prioritize treatment based on ECG over waiting for lab confirmation
- Plan immediate dialysis unit

Collapse While Working

Opening Scenario

EMS brings a 78-year-old male after his wife found him collapsed in their garden 30 minutes ago. He felt "faint" and fell to his knees. Denies LOC but cannot stand without assistance. History of AFib, HTN, type 2 DM.

Initial Assessment

Vitals: BP 108/58, HR 38 (regular), RR 20, T 36.4°C, SpO_2 95% RA

- General: Lethargic but arousable to voice, confused to time and place
- Airway: Patent, handling secretions, speaking in short phrases
- Breathing: Non-labored, bilateral breath sounds clear and equal
- Circulation: Pale, cool, mottled extremities; capillary refill >3 seconds; weak radial pulses

History

- HPI: Progressive weakness and dizziness over 4 hours since morning medications. Mild substernal chest pressure without radiation, nausea without vomiting. Denies SOB at rest, fever, recent illness. Wife notes confusion this morning and possible double-dose of medications. Denies falls, head trauma, visual changes.
- PMHx: AFib, HTN, type 2 DM, hyperlipidemia
- Medications: Metoprolol succinate 100mg daily, apixaban 5mg BID, lisinopril, metformin, atorvastatin

Physical Examination

- General: Alert to person only, moderate distress, unable to follow complex commands
- Head: Normocephalic, no trauma
- Eyes: Pupils equal and reactive, extraocular movements intact
- Neck: Supple, no jugular venous distension, no carotid bruits
- Cardiovascular: Regular rhythm, rate 38, no murmurs, rubs, or gallops appreciated
- Pulmonary: Clear to auscultation bilaterally, no wheezes or crackles
- Abdomen: Soft, non-tender, normal bowel sounds
- Extremities: Cool distal extremities, weak dorsalis pedis and posterior tibial pulses bilaterally, no edema
- Neurological: Confused, follows simple commands, moves all extremities equally, no focal deficits
- Skin: Cool, diaphoretic, no rashes or lesions

Management

Must obtain continuous monitoring and 12-lead ECG within 3 minutes. If delayed: patient becomes lethargic, BP 82/46, HR 32.

ECG: Sinus bradycardia rate 38, no acute ST changes, normal PR, narrow QRS. Remains hypotensive despite supine positioning.

Atropine 0.5mg IV: No response after 5 minutes. If transcutaneous pacing not prepared after atropine failure: HR drops to 28, unresponsive, BP unobtainable and patient arrests..

Diagnostic Studies

- Fingerstick glucose: 142
- BMP: Na 138, K 4.8, Cl 102, HCO_3 22, BUN 28, Cr 1.4 (baseline 1.1), Glucose 156
- CBC: Within normal limits

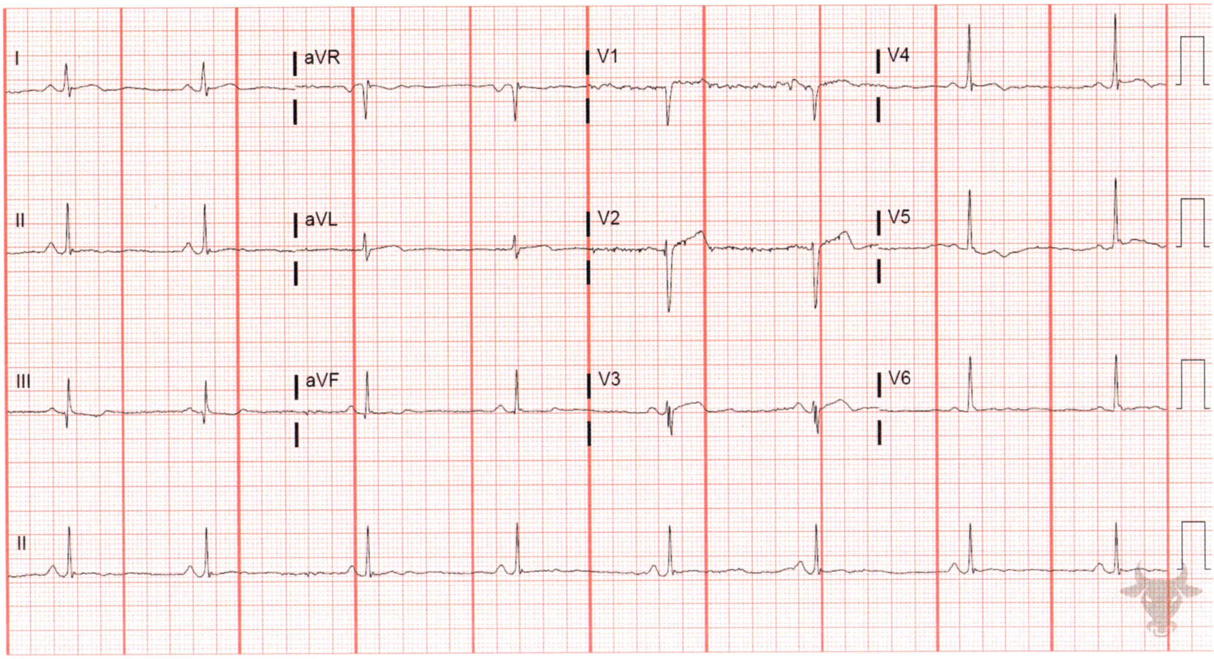

- Troponin: Pending
- CXR: Clear lung fields, normal cardiac silhouette, no pulmonary edema

Reassessment

After interventions: HR 36, BP 94/52 despite crystalloid bolus, increasingly somnolent. Recognize possible medication-induced bradycardia (possible beta-blocker toxicity from possible double-dose).

Next steps:

- Transcutaneous pacing pads, initiate pacing at 60-80 bpm
- Glucagon 5-10mg IV bolus
- Calcium gluconate 3gm IV
- Prepare for transvenous pacing if transcutaneous pacing fails
- Early cardiology consultation for emergent transvenous pacemaker
- Be able to describe transcutaneous pacing setup to obtain electrical and mechanical capture

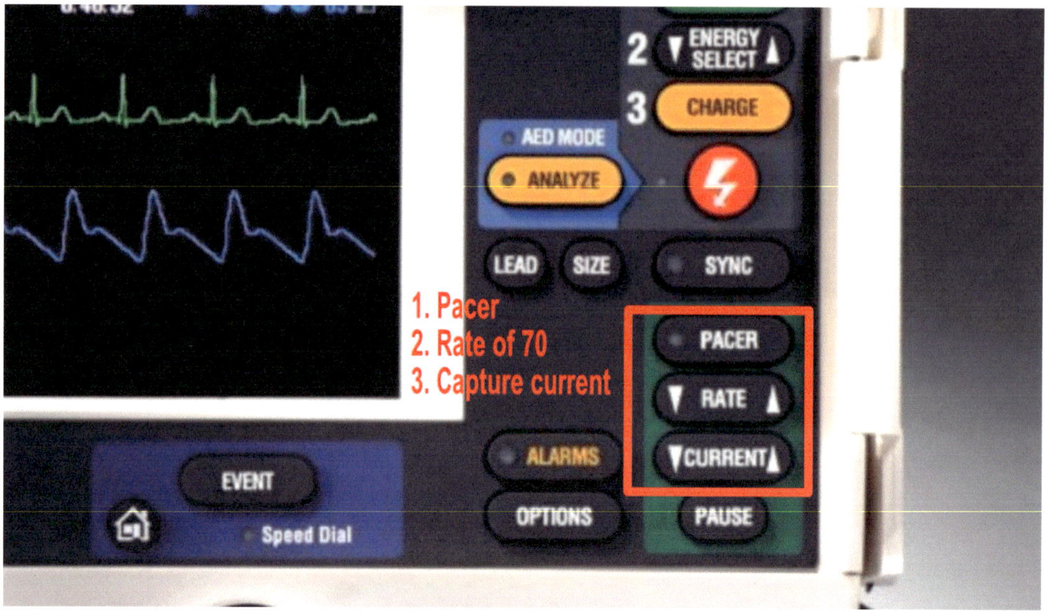

.

Critical Actions

- Recognize symptomatic bradycardia with poor perfusion (hypotension, AMS, cool extremities)
- Obtain 12-lead ECG immediately to differentiate rhythm (sinus bradycardia vs. heart block)
- Identify medication error/double-dose as likely etiology; obtain fingerstick glucose to exclude hypoglycemia
- Cardiac monitoring and large-bore IV access immediately
- Atropine 0.5mg IV (may repeat q3-5min, max 3mg) while recognizing limited efficacy in beta-blocker toxicity
- Prepare transcutaneous pacing early (pads placed before decompensation)
- Recognize atropine failure and escalate: glucagon for beta-blocker overdose, transcutaneous pacing, prepare for transvenous pacing
- Prioritize pacing over waiting for lab confirmation; beta-blocker toxicity causes atropine-refractory bradycardia
- Call cardiology early for transvenous pacing capability

The Irritable Infant

Opening Scenario

A 5-week-old male is registered for "fussiness and not eating." Triage places in resuscitation bay for abnormal breathing. Decreased feeding, irritability, tactile fever over 36 hours.

Initial Assessment

Vitals: BP 54/26, HR 192, RR 68, T 38.6°C (rectal), SpO_2 91% RA, Weight 4.5 kg

- General: Lethargic with weak cry; "floppy" this morning per parents
- Airway: Patent but handling secretions poorly, weak cough reflex
- Breathing: Tachypneic, shallow, no flaring or retractions, clear lungs bilaterally
- Circulation: Capillary refill 4 seconds, weak brachial pulses, warm/flushed despite hypotension
- Neuro: Difficult to arouse, does not track, weak suck reflex

Patient Communication

The mother is crying and states, "He was fine yesterday, just a little warm. Now he won't wake up. Is he going to be okay?" The father asks, "Can't we just give him Tylenol and see if he gets better? We don't want him poked with needles if it's just a virus."

Management

- Peripheral IV (bilateral upper extremities); IO in proximal tibia if unsuccessful after 2 attempts
- NRB at 15 L/min
- POC glucose: 25 (critical hypoglycemia) – D10 0.5 g/kg IV (5 mL/kg)
- NS 20 mL/kg bolus (90 mL) wide open
- Recognize warm shock physiology (distributive/septic shock, not hypovolemic)
- Defer LP until hemodynamically stable; prioritize resuscitation over workup
- Empiric antibiotics covering GBS, E. coli, Listeria (infants <60 days)
- Consider airway protection given poor secretion handling and lethargy

Diagnostic Studies

- Post-dextrose glucose: 68
- CBC: WBC 19.8 (15% bands), Hgb 11.2, Plt 285
- BMP: Na 141, K 3.6, Cl 109, HCO_3 15, BUN 5, Cr 0.6, Glucose 58
- Lactate: 3.8
- VBG: pH 7.14, pCO_2 36, HCO_3 12

Reassessment

Post-resuscitation: BP 64/42 (improved, still hypotensive), HR 168 (from 192), RR 58 (from 68), SpO_2 97% on NRB, capillary refill 3 seconds. Opens eyes to voice, stronger cry.

- Second NS bolus 20 mL/kg for persistent hypotension
- Empiric antibiotics: Ampicillin 50 mg/kg IV and cefotaxime 50 mg/kg IV (avoid ceftriaxone – bilirubin displacement risk in young infants)
- NPO; consult PICU for admission
- Update parents: vital sign improvement but continued aggressive management needed

Critical Actions

- Recognize septic shock with hypoglycemia, AMS, and warm shock physiology in a young infant
- Correct hypoglycemia and initiate fluid resuscitation before diagnostic workup or LP
- Communicate with parents about life-threatening illness while addressing concerns about invasive interventions; obtain informed consent
- Defer LP in hemodynamically unstable patients until after stabilization
- Select appropriate empiric antibiotics covering GBS, Gram-negative enterics, and Listeria for infants <2 months
- Reassess hemodynamics after each intervention to guide resuscitation
- Recognize need for ICU-level monitoring; do not admit to general pediatric floor
- Persistent hypotension despite 40 mL/kg fluids indicates need for vasoactive support

Unresponsive Elderly Patient

Opening Scenario

EMS brings a 76-year-old female found unresponsive in her kitchen by a home health aide. Last seen normal 90 minutes ago. Agonal breathing on EMS arrival, GCS 3. Supraglottic airway placed, BVM ventilation in progress. Daughter waiting in family room.

Initial Assessment

Vitals: BP 165/58, HR 52, RR 8 (EMS-assisted), T 36.8°C, SpO_2 82% RA -> 94% with assisted ventilations

- General: Cachectic, pale, unresponsive to verbal/painful stimuli. Dried blood at left nare. No obvious head/neck trauma.
- Airway: King LT in place, adequate chest rise, occasional gurgling
- Breathing: Agonal initially, now mechanically assisted; clear bilaterally
- Circulation: Mottled, cool extremities; capillary refill 4 seconds; weak radial pulses
- Disability: GCS 3 (E1V1M1); pupils 4mm bilaterally, sluggish
- Exposure: Medical alert bracelet: "Atrial Fibrillation – On Blood Thinners"

Immediate actions: Prepare RSI with neuroprotective premedication, two large-bore IVs, labs (CBC, BMP, coags, type and screen), POC glucose, 1L NS, prepare for emergent non-contrast head CT.

History

- HPI: Found unresponsive. Last seen alert at lunch (90 min prior). Aide found her slumped against kitchen cabinet. Brief right arm "shaking" noted by aide, ceased before EMS. No prior headache or chest pain complaints. Independent at baseline.
- PMHx: AFib (on apixaban), HTN, type 2 DM, osteoarthritis
- Medications: Apixaban 5mg BID, metformin, amlodipine
- Allergies: NKDA
- Social: Lives alone with daily aide visits. Non-smoker, rare alcohol.

Physical Examination

- General: Intubated, sedated, no spontaneous movement
- HEENT: Normocephalic, no lacerations. Bilateral periorbital ecchymosis (raccoon eyes) noted upon closer inspection. Left mastoid ecchymosis (Battle's sign). Clear otorrhea from left ear with positive halo sign on gauze testing. No tongue lacerations.
- Neck: C-collar in place, no step-offs or midline tenderness
- Chest: Clear to auscultation bilaterally, no retractions, symmetric expansion
- Cardiovascular: Bradycardic, regular rhythm, no murmurs appreciated; weak distal pulses
- Abdomen: Soft, non-distended, no guarding or rebound
- Neurological: Flaccid paralysis all extremities. No withdrawal to pain. Absent corneal and gag reflexes.
- Skin: Multiple ecchymoses on forearms (chronic), fresh abrasion on left palm

Reassessment

20 minutes post-intubation: Vitals: BP 195/110, HR 48, RR 14 (vent-assisted), T 37.0°C, SpO_2 100% on 100% FiO_2.

Daughter reports mother had a "minor bump" to the head 2 days ago while cleaning cabinets but seemed fine and refused medical attention. Asks: "Is she going to be okay?"

- Head CT: Large left-sided subdural hematoma with 8mm midline shift and uncal herniation
- Labs: Hgb 11.2, Plt 245K, INR 1.1 (apixaban effect not reflected in INR), Cr 1.1

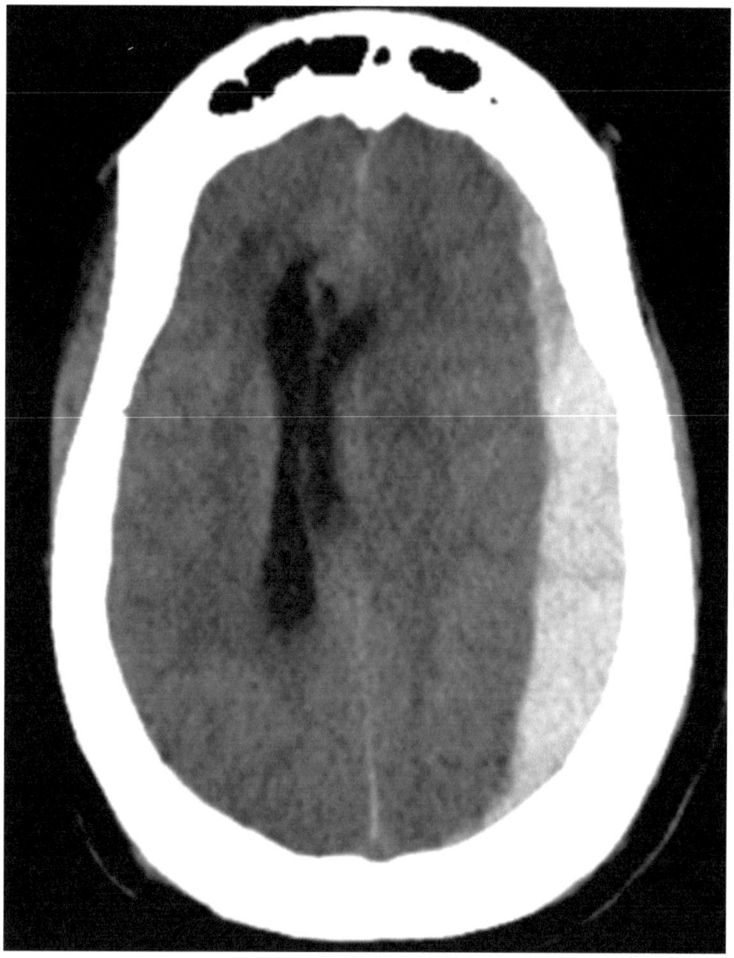

Patient Communication

- Explain critical nature of intracranial hemorrhage using clear, empathetic language
- Address daughter's guilt: subdural hematomas in anticoagulated patients can expand insidiously over days, even after minor trauma
- Discuss goals of care, prognosis, and code status given poor neuro exam and herniation on imaging
- Communicate neurosurgical urgency while remaining realistic about outcomes
- Obtain consent for interventions or facilitate understanding if transitioning to comfort care

Critical Actions

- Anticoagulation + AMS + trauma history mandates immediate non-contrast head CT before other diagnostics
- Identify basilar skull fracture signs (raccoon eyes, Battle's sign, CSF otorrhea) increasing TBI suspicion
- Recognize Cushing's reflex (bradycardia + hypertension) as critically elevated ICP and impending herniation
- Distinguish DOAC reversal (4-factor PCC or andexanet alfa for Xa inhibitors) from warfarin reversal (Vitamin K, FFP, PCC)
- Emergent neurosurgical consultation for possible decompressive hemicraniectomy or ventriculostomy
- Monitor for changing vitals indicating rising ICP; reassess neuro exam for pupillary changes or posturing

- Adjust anticoagulation reversal based on specific agent once medication history clarified

Fever and Thoracic Back Pain in a Spinal Cord Injury Patient

Opening Scenario

You are working as the attending physician in a high-volume emergency department. EMS brings in a 32-year-old female with a history of spinal cord injury who reports three days of progressive mid-back pain and fever. The triage nurse places the patient in a monitored bed and informs you that she appears flushed and uncomfortable, with a heart rate in the 130s. You have no previous records for this patient in your system.

History

- Three days of constant, aching pain in the mid-thoracic spine (T8-T10 region), worsening with movement and palpation
- Feverish sensation and chills beginning 48 hours prior to arrival
- Two episodes of non-bloody, non-bilious vomiting today
- Denies headache, neck stiffness, cough, or shortness of breath
- Denies recent trauma, falls, or invasive procedures
- Reports cloudy, foul-smelling urine for the past week but denies dysuria (has absent sensation below waist)

Initial Assessment

- General: Alert, oriented, diaphoretic, moderate distress due to back pain
- Vital Signs: Blood pressure 118/72 mmHg, Heart rate 132 beats/min, Respiratory rate 24 breaths/min, Oral temperature 38.9°C (102.0°F), SpO_2 98% RA

Past Medical History

- T12 complete spinal cord injury secondary to motor vehicle collision five years prior
- Neurogenic bladder managed with clean intermittent self-catheterization four to six times daily
- Chronic sensory deficits below T12 dermatome
- History of recurrent urinary tract infections (three in past year)
- No known drug allergies
- Current medications: oxybutynin, docusate sodium, aspirin 81 mg daily
- Social history: Former smoker (quit after injury), no alcohol or illicit drug use
- Lives with partner who assists with catheterization schedule

Physical Examination

- HEENT: Normocephalic, atraumatic, mucous membranes dry, neck supple, no meningismus
- Cardiovascular: Tachycardic with regular rhythm, no murmurs, rubs, or gallops, capillary refill 2 seconds
- Pulmonary: Clear to auscultation bilaterally, no accessory muscle use
- Abdomen: Soft, non-distended, normoactive bowel sounds, suprapubic tenderness absent (patient has no sensation), no costovertebral angle tenderness
- Back: Point tenderness over T9-T10 spinous processes, no step-off or deformity, no overlying skin changes or fluctuance
- Neurological: Cranial nerves II-XII intact, upper extremity strength 5/5 throughout, decreased rectal tone noted on voluntary attempt, decreased sensation to light touch and pinprick below T12 bilaterally, no new deficits per patient baseline
- Skin: Warm, dry, no pressure injuries or decubitus ulcers noted on sacral inspection

Diagnostic Studies

- CBC: WBC 26.8 with left shift, Hct 34, Plt 285
- BMP: Na 136, K 4.1, Cl 102, HCO_3 24, BUN 18, Cr 0.9, Glucose 142
- ESR: 9 (elevated)
- CRP: 32 (elevated)
- Urinalysis: Positive leukocyte esterase, positive nitrites, 15-20 WBCs per high-power field, many bacteria, specific gravity 1.025
- Blood cultures: Obtained prior to antibiotic administration (pending)
- Lactate: 1.8
- CT abdominal pelvis with IV contrast - no evidence of acute pathology

Reassessment

Thirty minutes after your initial evaluation, the patient reports new symptoms:

- Increasing back pain unrelieved by initial analgesia
- Nausea with dry heaving

Repeat vital signs: Blood pressure 102/64 mmHg, Heart rate 144 beats/min, Respiratory rate 26 breaths/min, Rectal temperature 39.4°C (102.9°F), Oxygen saturation 95 on room air.

Repeat focused examination reveals:

- New upper motor neuron findings: Increased tone in bilateral lower extremities (previously flaccid)
- New sensory level ascending to T6 dermatome (previously T12)
- Hyperreflexia at patellar and Achilles tendons (previously absent)
- Urinary retention with 800 mL output via catheter insertion (patient had not self-catheterized for 12 hours due to malaise)
- MRI Spine with and without contrast - new order due to changing neuro exam and fever. Indication on order is infectious spinous process such as spinal abscess
- Can reach out to neurosurgeon before MRI ordered but they will ask for order and agree to see the patient.

Patient Communication

After MRI confirms a T9-T10 epidural abscess with spinal cord compression, you contact neurosurgery who recommends emergent surgical decompression and drainage. Upon discussing the need for immediate surgery with the patient and her partner, the patient expresses refusal, stating: "I've had three surgeries since my accident and each one made my pain worse. I want to try antibiotics alone I don't want to lose what little function I have left.

You must navigate this conversation to ensure informed consent while respecting autonomy, addressing fears, and explaining the risk of permanent paralysis without surgical intervention. Also ask the surgeon to speak directly to the patient.

Critical Actions

- Recognizes spinal epidural abscess as a diagnostic consideration in a febrile patient with back pain and risk factors (neurogenic bladder, recurrent UTIs, spinal hardware history)
- Obtains rectal temperature to accurately assess for fever in a patient with autonomic dysfunction and unreliable oral temperatures
- Orders emergent MRI of the thoracic and lumbar spine with and without contrast as the definitive imaging study

- Initiates empiric broad-spectrum IV antibiotics (vancomycin plus ceftriaxone or cefepime, consider metronidazole) after obtaining blood cultures
- Consults neurosurgery emergently for operative intervention once diagnosis confirmed or highly suspected
- Demonstrates reassessment skills by identifying acute neurologic deterioration (ascending sensory level, autonomic dysreflexia signs, new spasticity) and understanding this represents a surgical emergency and requiring advanced imaging
- Employs patient-centered communication techniques including:
- Acknowledging the patient's previous traumatic surgical experiences

Exercise-Induced Syncope in an Adolescent Athlete

Opening Scenario

EMS brings a 14-year-old male who collapsed during track practice 45 minutes ago. Currently awake and alert. Coach reports 90 seconds of LOC immediately after crossing the finish line of a 400-meter sprint.

Initial Assessment

Vitals: BP 106/72, HR 88, RR 16, T 37.0°C, SpO_2 99% RA, Fingerstick glucose 102

- Airway: Patent, speaking in full sentences
- Breathing: Non-labored, symmetric chest rise, no cyanosis
- Circulation: Warm and dry, capillary refill <2 seconds, pulses 2+ bilaterally

History

- HPI: Previously healthy, no medications. Witnessed sudden collapse during 400m sprint without preceding chest pain or palpitations. No seizure activity, tongue biting, or incontinence. Regained consciousness spontaneously in 1-2 minutes. Now reports mild fatigue and vague chest "heaviness." Last meal 4 hours ago.
- PMHx: No prior syncope, seizures, cardiac murmur, or exercise intolerance
- FHx: Paternal uncle died suddenly at age 26 during recreational swimming. Mother has history of "fainting when startled" (no formal diagnosis).

Physical Examination

- General: Alert and oriented, mildly fatigued appearance, no acute distress
- HEENT: Normocephalic, atraumatic, pupils equal and reactive to light, mucous membranes moist
- Cardiovascular: Regular rate and rhythm, no murmurs, rubs, or gallops appreciated, radial and femoral pulses present and equal
- Respiratory: Clear to auscultation bilaterally, no wheezes, rales, or rhonchi, no accessory muscle use
- Neurological: Cranial nerves II-XII intact, motor strength 5/5 all extremities, sensation intact, gait not tested due to monitoring status
- Skin: No rashes, no signs of trauma, no diaphoresis

Diagnostic Studies

- 12-lead ECG shows sinus rhythm with heart rate 82, corrected QT interval approximately 510-520 ms (borderline first-degree AV block noted)
- Chest X-ray: Normal cardiac silhouette, no pulmonary edema, clear lung fields
- BMP: Na 141, K 4.0, Cl 105, HCO_3 24, BUN 12, Cr 0.7, Glucose 108
- Complete blood count and troponin pending

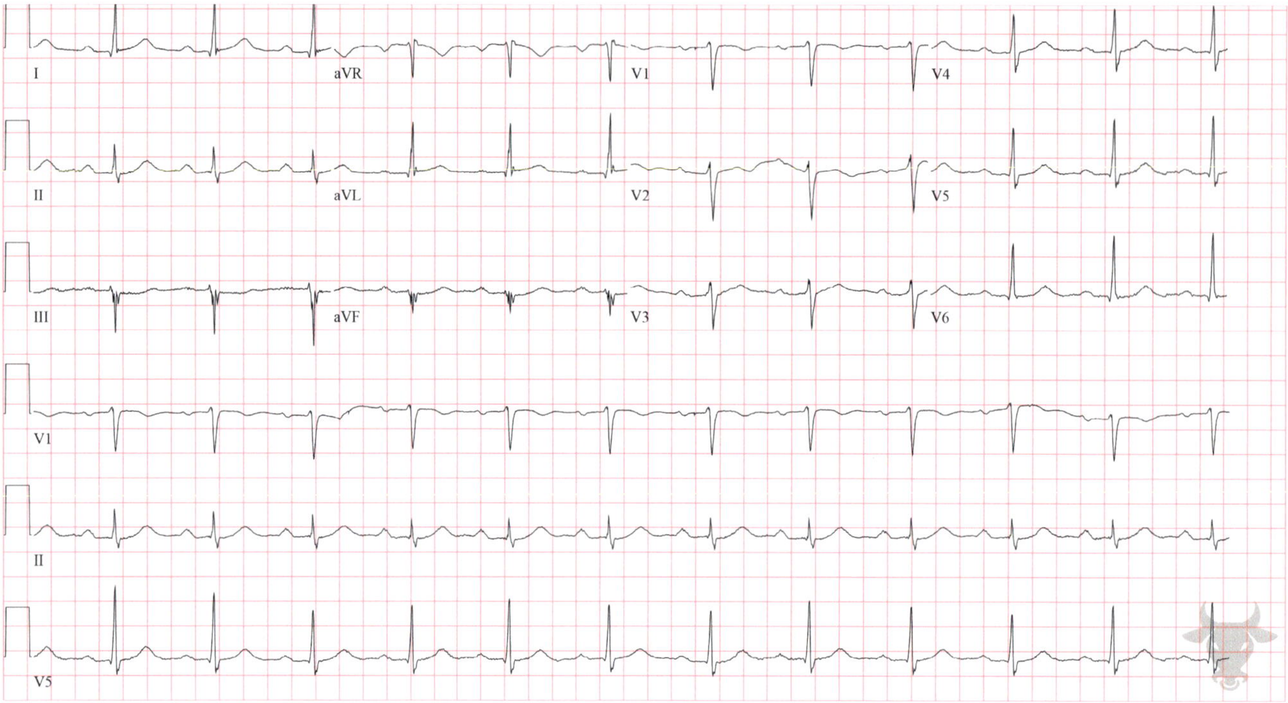

Management

- Exertional syncope in adolescents is high-risk requiring immediate cardiac workup
- ECG shows prolonged QTc (510-520 ms) consistent with congenital long QT syndrome
- Differentiate from vasovagal syncope based on exertional trigger and family history of sudden death
- Continuous cardiac monitoring, cardiology consultation
- Consider electrolyte replacement
- Plan admission to monitored setting

Reassessment

~15 minutes into evaluation: Patient suddenly loses consciousness. Apneic, pulseless. Monitor shows polymorphic VT with QRS twisting around baseline (torsades de pointes).

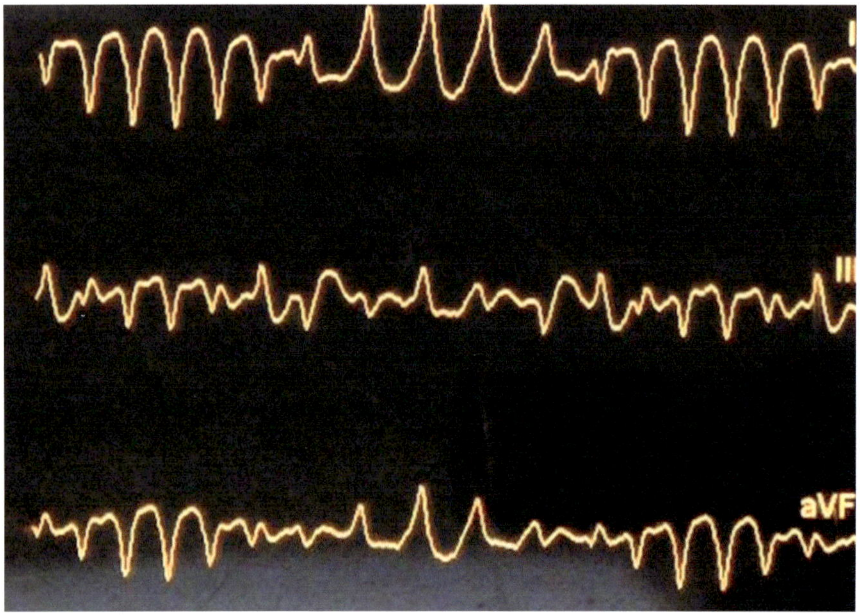

Resuscitation:

- Activate code, high-quality CPR at 100-120/min, BVM with 100% O_2
- Defibrillation at 2 J/kg (~100J for 50 kg adolescent), escalate to 4 J/kg (200J)
- Magnesium sulfate 2g IV push over 2 minutes (first-line for torsades)
- Second defibrillation required; ROSC achieved after second shock + magnesium
- Post-arrest: ETT, lidocaine infusion, ICU consultation

Patient Communication

- Discussion with parents regarding diagnosis of congenital long QT syndrome as cause of collapse
- Explanation of risk of sudden cardiac death and necessity of implantable cardioverter-defibrillator (ICD) evaluation
- Counseling regarding activity restrictions and disqualification from competitive athletics pending cardiology clearance
- Discussion of genetic testing implications for patient and first-degree relatives (cascade screening)
- Empathetic acknowledgment of family shock and provision of resources regarding sudden cardiac arrest in youth
- Clear communication regarding transition to ICU and ongoing need for antiarrhythmic therapy

Critical Actions

- Identify exertional syncope in adolescent as cardiac etiology until proven otherwise; obtain immediate 12-lead ECG
- Correctly measure and identify QTc prolongation (>500 ms) with associated torsades risk
- Recognize that channelopathy patients may deteriorate suddenly despite stable appearance; maintain continuous monitoring
- Identify polymorphic VT (torsades de pointes) on monitor and differentiate from monomorphic VT or VF
- Administer magnesium sulfate as first-line for torsades prior to or concurrent with defibrillation
- Deliver appropriate pediatric defibrillation dose (2-4 J/kg) for pulseless polymorphic VT; repeat if initial shock unsuccessful
- Communicate life-threatening diagnosis, hereditary implications, and ICD evaluation to family using empathetic language
- Discuss genetic testing for patient and first-degree relatives (cascade screening), activity restrictions pending cardiology clearance
- Arrange ICU admission with urgent cardiology consultation; understand post-resuscitation care requirements

Toddler with Fever

Opening Scenario

A 2-year-old female is brought by her father with fever and refusal to walk. Irritable for two days, began refusing to move neck this morning. Parents divorced; mother en route, calling to demand no "invasive procedures" without her consent.

Initial Assessment

Vitals: BP 98/62, HR 156, RR 32, T 39.8°C (rectal), SpO_2 97% RA, Weight 12 kg

- General: Toxic-appearing toddler sitting upright on father's lap, head in fixed neutral position, refusing to rotate or extend neck
- Airway: Patent, speaking in short phrases, slight pooling of secretions, no stridor at rest
- Breathing: Non-labored, clear bilaterally, no retractions
- Circulation: Capillary refill 2 seconds, warm and flushed, distal pulses intact
- Disability: Alert but irritable, moves all extremities, resists passive neck movement

Management

Differential: retropharyngeal abscess (leading), bacterial meningitis, cervical osteomyelitis, epidural abscess. Upright posture with neck extension suggests potential airway compromise.

- Continuous cardiorespiratory monitoring, two large-bore IVs, 20 mL/kg isotonic fluid bolus
- Prepare difficult airway equipment (video laryngoscopy, bougie)
- Lateral soft tissue neck radiograph (before CT with contrast)
- Empiric antibiotics covering oral flora, S. aureus, Streptococcus (ampicillin-sulbactam or clindamycin)
- Determine LP vs. advanced imaging based on presentation
- Bedside lateral neck xray show distortion of laryngeal space consistent with large retropharyngeal abscess
- Consult ENT after imaging results. They call back and request CT soft tissue neck with IV contrast since patient has stable vitals.
- Order broad spectrum antibiotics

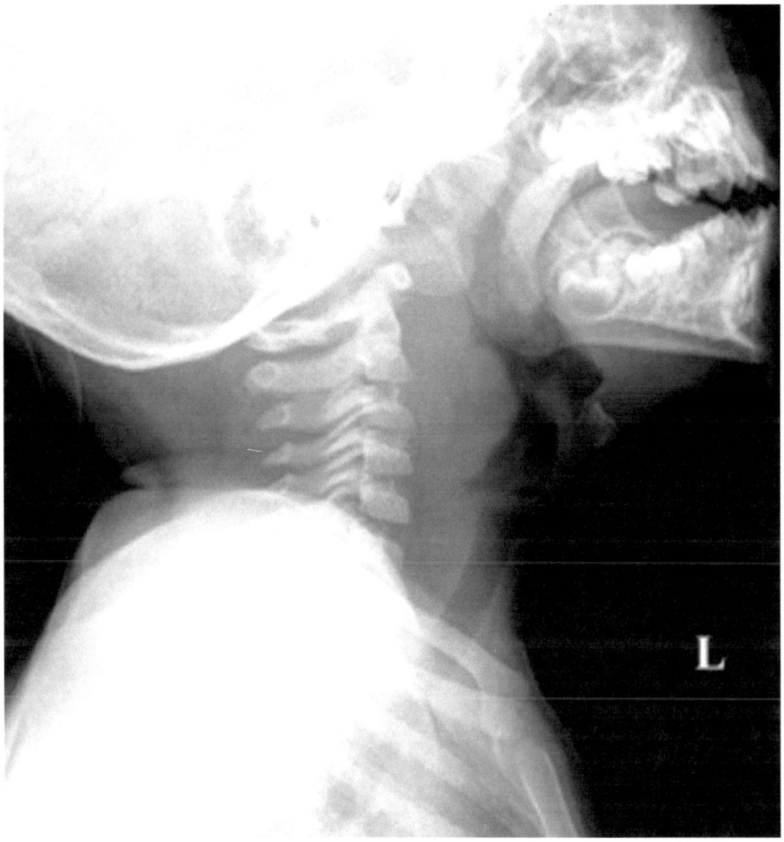

Patient Communication

- Father is present but mother technically has custody so he doesn't want to make any decisions without her permission.
- Navigate complex family dynamics while maintaining focus on the child's emergent needs.
- Engage both parents (father present, mother via phone) for unified understanding of the emergency
- Explain airway obstruction risk from deep space neck infection using clear, non-jargon language
- Maintain professional authority regarding standard of care while eliciting parental values

Reassessment

30 minutes: Vitals: BP 88/50, HR 178, RR 38, SpO_2 94% RA. Now drooling profusely, refusing supine position, assuming tripod position.

- Immediately reassess airway patency and WOB
- Recognize impending upper airway obstruction
- Abort CT if not yet performed and inform ENT on need for emergent surgery.
- Consider urgent awake fiberoptic intubation or surgical airway with ENT
- Re-evaluate antibiotics; consider vancomycin if toxic shock suspected
- Update both parents on critical change and need for immediate intervention

Critical Actions

- Recognize retropharyngeal abscess as leading diagnosis in toxic child with neck stiffness; do not misinterpret solely as meningismus
- Order lateral soft tissue neck X-ray as initial imaging before CT
- Initiate broad-spectrum antibiotics promptly; do not delay pending definitive imaging

- Consult ENT early for potential surgical drainage
- Identify deteriorating airway (new drooling, tachypnea, tripod positioning) and prioritize airway stabilization over imaging
- Change management plan when patient cannot tolerate supine position; abort CT due to airway concerns
- Communicate clearly with both parents about life-threatening condition; address radiation/procedure concerns empathetically and provide reassurance that ENT can coordinate definitive management
- Identify legal decision-maker quickly; mediate between parents without taking sides

Sudden Abdominal Pain

Opening Scenario

An 82-year-old male is brought by his daughter to a tertiary care ED with severe abdominal pain that began three hours ago. Placed in a resuscitation bay.

Initial Assessment

Vitals: BP 94/58, HR 108, RR 24, T 37.4°C, SpO_2 95% RA, Pain 9/10

- Elderly male appearing older than stated age, diaphoretic and pale
- Guarding abdomen with knees flexed, speaking in short phrases
- Airway: Patent, speaking, no stridor
- Breathing: Tachypneic, equal breath sounds, no wheezes or crackles
- Circulation: Delayed capillary refill (>3 seconds), cool extremities, weak radial pulses
- Disability: GCS 14 (confused to date, oriented to person and place)
- Exposure: No obvious trauma, rash, or bleeding

History

- HPI: Sudden onset of severe, diffuse abdominal pain while straining at stool. Began in the left lower quadrant, rapidly became generalized. Describes pain as "knifelike" and constant. Reports nausea, denies vomiting. Every bump in the car worsened pain significantly.
- PMHx: Hypertension, type 2 DM, CKD (baseline Cr 1.8), diverticulosis on prior colonoscopy. Prior inguinal hernia repair and appendectomy.
- Meds: Metformin, lisinopril, aspirin 81 mg daily, atorvastatin
- Allergies: NKDA
- Social: Lives independently, widowed, no tobacco or alcohol use. Last meal: breakfast four hours ago.

Physical Examination

- General: Alert, moderate distress, diaphoretic
- Cardiovascular: Tachycardic, regular rhythm, no murmurs, pulses 2+ but thready
- Respiratory: Clear bilaterally, tachypneic, using accessory muscles
- Abdomen: Distended, rigid with diffuse tenderness, absent bowel sounds, marked rebound tenderness and guarding throughout, no palpable masses or hernias
- Rectal: Normal tone, brown stool, hemoccult negative
- GU: No CVA tenderness, suprapubic non-tender
- Skin: Cool, clammy, poor turgor
- Neurological: Oriented x2, cranial nerves intact, strength symmetric

Diagnostic Studies

- CBC: WBC 14.2, Hgb 11.8, Plt 198
- BMP: Na 138, K 4.1, Cl 106, HCO_3 10, BUN 48, Cr 2.1, Glucose 142
- Lactate: 3.4
- VGG: pH 7.28, pCO_2 30 mmHg, HCO_3^- 16 mmol/L, BE −8 mmol/L
- Upright CXR: Free air under both hemidiaphragms (larger on left)

- CT Abdomen/Pelvis (if obtained): Large intraperitoneal free air, thickened sigmoid colon with pericolonic fat stranding, small pelvic free fluid

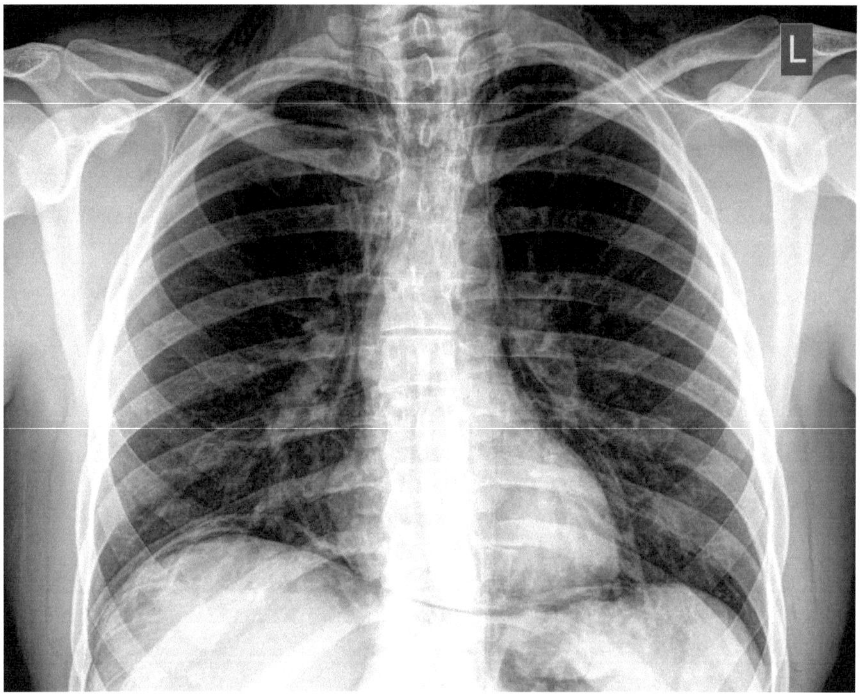

Management

- Two large-bore peripheral IVs established
- Broad-spectrum antibiotics (piperacillin-tazobactam)
- Emergent surgical consultation
- NPO status
- Analgesia with morphine titrated for pain control

Disposition

Emergent operative management following resuscitation. Discussion with family regarding severity and need for emergent surgery.

Critical Actions

- Recognize shock state (tachycardia, hypotension, delayed capillary refill) and initiate aggressive crystalloid resuscitation with two large-bore IVs
- Identify peritonitis (rigid abdomen, rebound, guarding, absent bowel sounds)
- Obtain upright CXR to evaluate for free air
- Interpret metabolic acidosis and elevated lactate as signs of sepsis
- Administer early broad-spectrum antibiotics covering gram-negative and anaerobic organisms
- Perform nasogastric decompression and declare NPO status
- Obtain immediate surgical consultation — free air + peritonitis = operative emergency regardless of etiology
- Avoid delaying surgical management for prolonged diagnostic workup in an unstable patient

Paroxysmal Cough in 9-Month-Old

Opening Scenario

A 9-month-old female is brought in by her mother for severe coughing spells. The mother states, "She turns blue and stops breathing during these coughing fits." The infant is currently calm with visible dried vomitus on her clothing.

Initial Assessment

Vitals: BP 88/52, HR 182, RR 34, T 37.1°C rectal, SpO_2 96% RA, Weight 8.2 kg

- Alert and interactive between coughing episodes; slightly pale with mild perioral cyanosis resolving with stimulation
- Bilateral subconjunctival hemorrhages
- Airway: Patent, occasional gagging with secretions
- Breathing: Irregular pattern with intermittent apneic pauses (3-5 seconds) following coughing paroxysms; no retractions at rest
- Circulation: Tachycardic, capillary refill 2 seconds, peripheral pulses palpable
- Fontanelle flat and soft; no rashes or edema

History

- HPI: Rhinorrhea and conjunctival injection 10 days ago attributed to a cold. Five days later developed harsh, staccato paroxysmal cough in bursts of 10-15 coughs, occurring 20-30 times daily, worse at night, followed by post-tussive vomiting and brief cyanotic episodes (5-10 seconds). Decreased oral intake over 48 hours with only two wet diapers today. No documented fevers. Family emigrated from Guatemala three months ago; immunization records unavailable. Mother states she "doesn't trust the vaccine schedule here yet."
- PMHx: None. Immunizations not up to date.
- Allergies: None

Physical Examination

- HEENT: Bilateral subconjunctival hemorrhages, clear rhinorrhea, oropharynx clear
- Neck: Supple, no lymphadenopathy
- Chest: Clear bilaterally with good air entry at rest; occasional scattered wheeze immediately following coughing paroxysm
- Cardiovascular: Regular rhythm, no murmurs
- Abdomen: Soft, non-distended, normoactive bowel sounds, no hepatosplenomegaly
- Neurological: Age-appropriate, symmetric tone and strength
- Skin: Pale, cool extremities, no mottling

Diagnostic Studies

- POC glucose: 98
- CBC: WBC 38.2 (82% lymphocytes, 12% neutrophils, 6% monocytes), Hgb 10.8, Hct 32%, Plt 312
- BMP: Na 138, K 3.6, Cl 102, HCO_3 18, BUN 28, Cr 0.4, Glucose 102
- CXR: Perihilar infiltrates with "shaggy" right heart border; no lobar consolidation, effusion, or pneumothorax
- Nasopharyngeal PCR: Pending for Bordetella pertussis

Management

- Continuous cardiorespiratory and pulse oximetry monitoring
- Peripheral IV access (24-gauge); supplemental O_2 via NC at 2 L/min (titrate to $SpO_2 > 94\%$)
- Respiratory isolation (droplet precautions)
- Initiate azithromycin to reduce transmission; all household contacts need prophylactic antibiotics

Reassessment

Twenty minutes in, the infant begins a severe paroxysmal coughing spell lasting 45 seconds. She becomes cyanotic, stops breathing for 15 seconds, and becomes limp. SpO_2 drops to 78%.

- Position head-up at 30 degrees, suction oropharynx
- BVM ventilation with 100% O_2 at 15 L/min
- Consider NPA if obstruction persists; prepare for RSI

Following 30 seconds of BVM, the infant resumes spontaneous respirations. SpO_2 returns to 97% on 4 L NC. Patient is lethargic for 5 minutes then returns to baseline.

Patient Communication

- Explain pertussis diagnosis: severe bacterial respiratory infection causing violent coughing spells; "whoop" and vomiting follow coughing fits
- Address vaccine hesitancy non-judgmentally; explain DTaP significantly reduces risk of severe disease, hospitalization, and death; provide information about local vaccine education resources
- Emphasize all household contacts need prophylactic antibiotics regardless of vaccination status
- Return precautions: apnea >30 seconds, persistent cyanosis, decreased responsiveness, or refusal to feed

Disposition

Admission to pediatric ward for continuous cardiorespiratory monitoring given witnessed apnea and cyanosis.

Critical Actions

- Recognize pertussis based on paroxysmal cough, post-tussive vomiting, marked leukocytosis with lymphocyte predominance, and unvaccinated status
- Implement droplet isolation precautions immediately
- Order CBC, CXR, and nasopharyngeal PCR for Bordetella pertussis
- Initiate macrolide antibiotic therapy (azithromycin); acknowledge that antibiotics in paroxysmal phase reduce transmission but do not alter clinical course
- Recognize acute deterioration (apnea/cyanosis) and execute BVM ventilation promptly; prepare for intubation if indicated
- Address vaccine hesitancy non-judgmentally with accurate risk-benefit information
- Recommend macrolide prophylaxis for all household contacts
- Admit for continuous monitoring given witnessed apnea in an infant

Left Sided Weakness

Opening Scenario

EMS arrives with a 68-year-old male found by his wife at 09:15 with acute confusion and left-sided weakness. He was at baseline at 06:30 when he took his morning medications. He skipped breakfast because he was fasting for a scheduled outpatient procedure.

Initial Assessment

Vitals: BP 158/92, HR 108, RR 16, T 36.6°C, SpO_2 99% RA, Fingerstick glucose: pending (obtain only if requested)

- Cachectic, diaphoretic male; awake but confused with slurred speech and pronounced left facial droop; left arm drift
- Airway: Patent, garbled speech
- Breathing: Unlabored, clear bilateral breath sounds
- Circulation: Tachycardic, cool and clammy skin, capillary refill 2 seconds

History

- HPI: Wife confirms he took glipizide at 06:30 but consumed no food afterward. No recent illness, fever, or trauma.
- PMHx: Type 2 DM, hypertension, hyperlipidemia, mild CKD
- Meds: Glipizide, metformin, amlodipine, simvastatin, low-dose aspirin
- Allergies: None known
- Social: Retired accountant, lives with wife, non-smoker, occasional alcohol use

Physical Examination

- General: Confused, diaphoretic, moderate distress
- Eyes: PERRL, no nystagmus, EOM intact
- Cardiovascular: Tachycardic, regular rhythm, no murmurs
- Respiratory: Clear bilaterally
- Abdomen: Soft, non-tender, non-distended
- Neurological: Confused to time and place; follows simple commands inconsistently. Left lower facial droop, dysarthria, visual fields full. Left arm drift with weak hand grip, left leg weakness; right side 5/5. Sensation intact bilaterally. Reflexes 2+ symmetric.

Diagnostic Studies

- Fingerstick glucose (if requested): 26
- BMP: Na 140, K 4.2, Cl 106, HCO_3 24, BUN 22, Cr 1.2, Glucose 32
- CBC: Hgb 12.8, Hct 38%, Plt 198, INR 1.0
- ECG: Sinus tachycardia, no acute ischemic changes
- CT Head (if ordered): Negative for acute hemorrhage or large vessel occlusion; age-appropriate atrophy

Management

- Two large-bore IVs established
- Administer D50 50 mL IV push immediately followed by by dextrose infusion and scheduled glucose checks.
- Obtain 12-lead ECG - NSR, mild LVH.

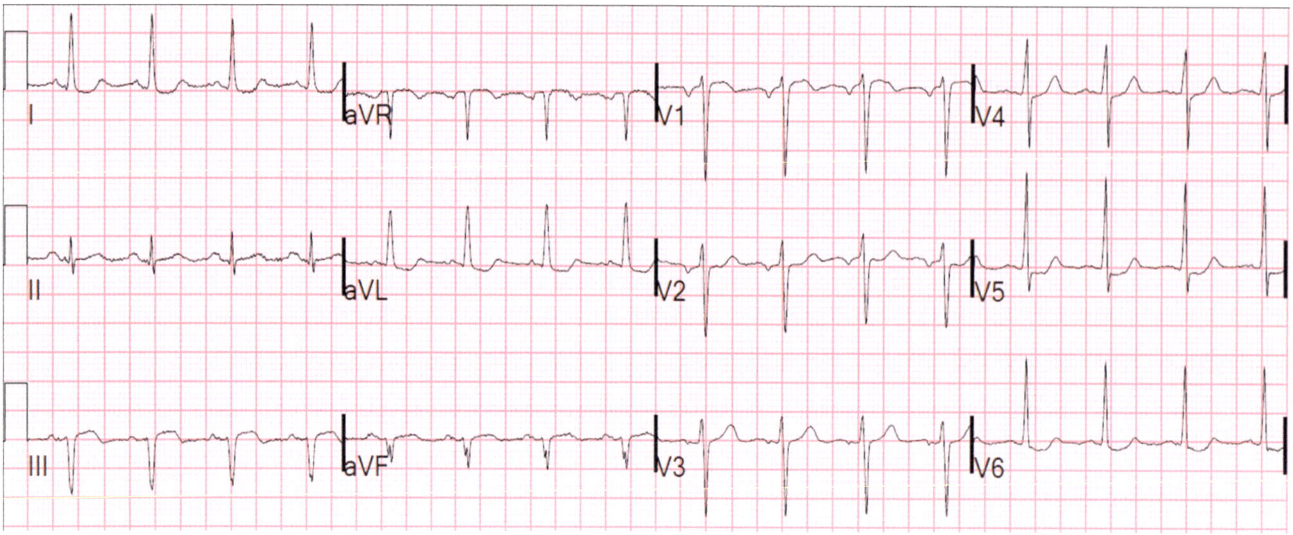

Reassessment

- Repeat fingerstick glucose: 94
- Patient becomes fully alert and oriented; left facial droop resolves, speech clears, motor strength 5/5 bilaterally
- Patient recalls taking medications but not eating
- Administer oral carbohydrate meal; continue D5W at maintenance rate
- Consider octreotide 50 mcg SQ for sulfonylurea toxicity
- Admit for serial glucose monitoring (rebound hypoglycemia risk with sulfonylureas lasts 12-24 hours)

Patient Communication

- Explain symptoms were caused by critically low blood sugar, not a stroke
- Glipizide stimulated insulin release without food intake, causing the episode
- Risk of recurrent hypoglycemia over 12-24 hours requiring admission
- Importance of eating when taking sulfonylureas and carrying glucose tablets
- Return precautions: recurrence of symptoms, confusion, sweating

Critical Actions

- Obtain point-of-care blood glucose immediately in any patient with altered mental status or acute focal neurologic deficits
- Recognize hypoglycemia as a stroke mimic before initiating stroke protocol
- Administer IV dextrose promptly for severe hypoglycemia (glucose <50)
- Reassess clinically and repeat glucose after treatment to confirm resolution
- Identify sulfonylurea-induced hypoglycemia as requiring admission due to prolonged hypoglycemia risk (12-24 hours)
- Implement prevention strategies (carbohydrate intake, D5W infusion, consider octreotide)

Choking Toddler

Opening Scenario

A 3-year-old male is brought in by his father, who carries the child upright against his chest. The child began choking suddenly while playing with his older sibling approximately 25 minutes ago. The father notes his lips "turned blue" briefly.

Initial Assessment

Vitals: BP 88/58, HR 132, RR 44, T 37.0°C, SpO_2 89% RA

- Well-nourished, anxious toddler in tripod posture on father's lap with prominent intercostal and supraclavicular retractions
- Pale mucous membranes with perioral cyanosis; frightened but interactive
- Airway: Patent but compromised; high-pitched inspiratory stridor at rest; pooling of oral secretions
- Breathing: Labored with nasal flaring and accessory muscle use; air entry diminished bilaterally
- Circulation: Pulses 2+ bilaterally, capillary refill <2 seconds, warm skin

History

- HPI: Father was in the kitchen while the child and 6-year-old sister played in the living room. Heard sudden coughing followed by crying. Found child grasping throat, unable to speak, face turning red then blue. Refuses to lie down; more distressed when separated from father. No witnessed ingestion, but small toy parts were present.
- PMHx: Full-term, no neonatal complications, immunizations current through 2-year visit
- Meds/Allergies: None / NKDA
- Social: Lives with both parents and older sister

Physical Examination

- General: Alert, anxious, prefers upright position, crying intermittently
- Oropharynx: Pooling secretions; no visible foreign body; lips cyanotic
- Neck: Mild subcutaneous emphysema in bilateral supraclavicular fossae; trachea midline
- Lungs: Inspiratory stridor audible without stethoscope; breath sounds markedly diminished on right compared to left; significant intercostal, subcostal, and supraclavicular retractions; grunting intermittently
- Heart: Tachycardic, regular rhythm, no murmurs
- Abdomen: Soft, non-tender, non-distended
- Neurological: Awake, alert, age-appropriate; no focal deficits
- Skin: Warm and dry; perioral cyanosis persistent

Diagnostic Studies

- CXR (AP): Radio-opaque circular foreign body at right mainstem bronchus.
- Lateral Neck X-ray: Foreign body at thoracic inlet (C7-T1); unclear if button battery or a coin and must assume a battery

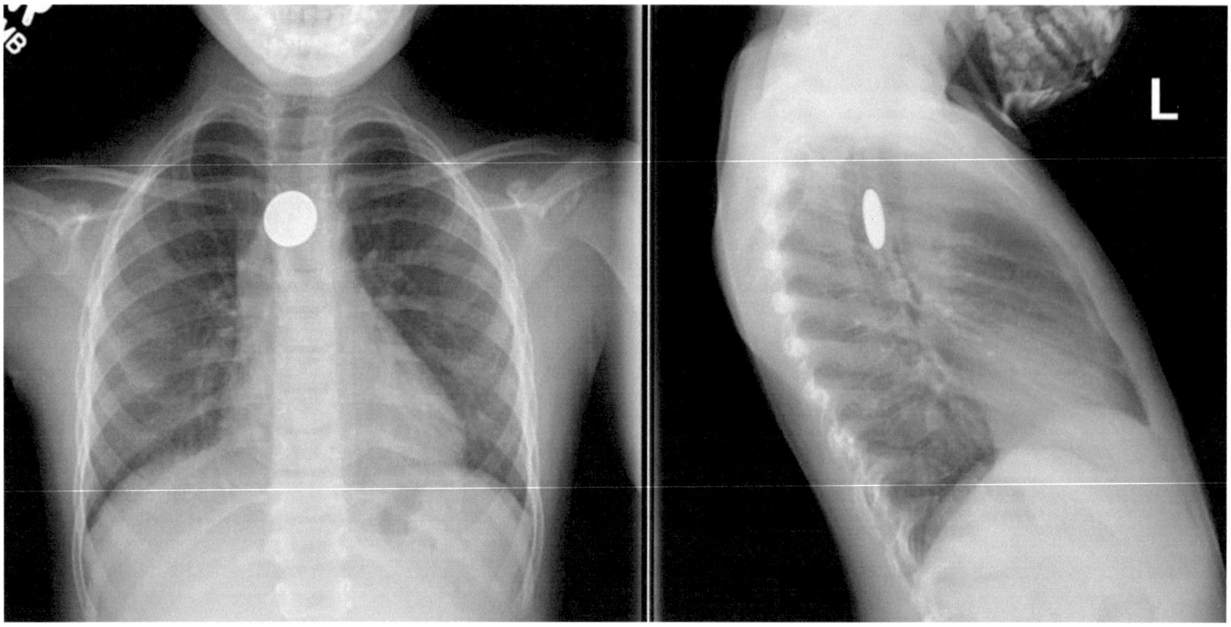

Management

- Supplemental O_2 via blow-by; allow child to remain in position of comfort on parent's lap
- Prepare for emergent airway management: assemble BVM, laryngoscope blades, ETT (cuffed 4.0/4.5), surgical airway equipment, and code medications at bedside
- Peripheral IV with minimal disturbance; continuous monitoring
- NPO status
- Emergent ENT consultation for rigid bronchoscopy
- Communicate with father: explain concern for foreign body aspiration with partial airway obstruction, imminent risk of complete obstruction, need for rigid bronchoscopy, and obtain informed consent

Reassessment

ENT performs bronchoscopy to assist in removal of foreign body (it was a coin). Stridor resolves; breath sounds equal and clear. Vitals: BP 92/60, HR 115, RR 28, SpO_2 98% on blow-by O_2.

30 minutes post-procedure: child develops new barking cough, mild inspiratory stridor, increasing retractions, SpO_2 declining to 92% on RA.

- Administer racemic epinephrine (2.25, 0.5 mL in 3 mL NS) via nebulizer
- Dexamethasone 0.6 mg/kg IV (max 10 mg)
- After 15 minutes: stridor improves, SpO_2 97% RA, patient comfortable

Disposition

Observe in ED for 3 hours post-treatment for rebound symptoms (post-procedural subglottic edema/croup).

Critical Actions

- Recognize partial upper airway obstruction and avoid actions that might convert to complete obstruction (agitation, forced supine positioning, blind finger sweeps)
- Provide supplemental oxygen while maintaining position of comfort with parent presence
- Treat post procedural laryngosoasm
- Prepare for definitive airway management including surgical airway backup without premature intubation attempts

- Obtain imaging to localize and characterize the foreign body while minimizing patient movement
- Communicate with parent regarding life-threatening nature, need for procedural intervention, and potential complications
- Reassess after foreign body removal to identify post-procedural complications (subglottic edema)
- Manage post-procedural airway edema with racemic epinephrine and systemic steroids

Paroxysmal Crying

Opening Scenario

A 10-month-old female infant is brought in by her father who reports the baby has been "screaming on and off" for the past 8 hours. She initially appeared well between episodes but has become increasingly difficult to arouse over the past hour.

Initial Assessment

Vitals: BP 82/56, HR 158, RR 28, T 37.9°C, SpO_2 97% RA, Weight 9.5 kg

- Pale, diaphoretic infant lying listlessly in father's arms; opens eyes briefly to loud voice then returns to somnolent state
- Airway: Patent, gag reflex intact
- Breathing: Tachypneic, clear bilaterally, no retractions or nasal flaring
- Circulation: Capillary refill 3 seconds, distal pulses weak but palpable, no mottling

History

- HPI: Paroxysmal crying spells for 8 hours, lasting 10-15 minutes each, during which the infant draws knees to abdomen and screams inconsolably. Pain-free intervals progressively shortening over the past 3 hours. Four episodes of non-bilious, non-bloody emesis. One episode of "reddish-brown" mucous-filled stool 2 hours ago. No fever, sick contacts, travel, or trauma. Immunizations up to date. Father's mother-in-law insisted this was "just colic," delaying arrival.
- PMHx: None significant
- Allergies: None

Physical Examination

- General: Lethargic, minimally responsive to painful stimuli
- HEENT: Anterior fontanelle slightly sunken, dry/sticky mucous membranes
- Neck: Supple, no meningismus
- Cardiovascular: Tachycardic, regular rhythm, no murmurs
- Respiratory: Clear bilaterally, good air entry
- Abdomen: Soft but diffusely tender with voluntary guarding. Palpable sausage-shaped mass in right upper quadrant with empty right lower quadrant (Dance's sign). Hypoactive bowel sounds.
- Rectal: Guaiac-positive stool
- Neurologic: Withdraws to pain, symmetric movement, pupils equal and reactive

Diagnostic Studies

- CBC: WBC 14.2, Hgb 11.2, Plt 298
- BMP: Na 138, K 4.1, Cl 103, HCO_3 19, BUN 18, Cr 0.4, Glucose 78
- Abdominal Radiograph: Nonspecific bowel gas pattern with paucity of gas in right lower quadrant, no free air
- Bedside Ultrasound: Target sign in RUQ consistent with ileocolic intussusception (ordering formal US is acceptable but ask for study to be done in ED due to concerns regarding patient's acute abdomen

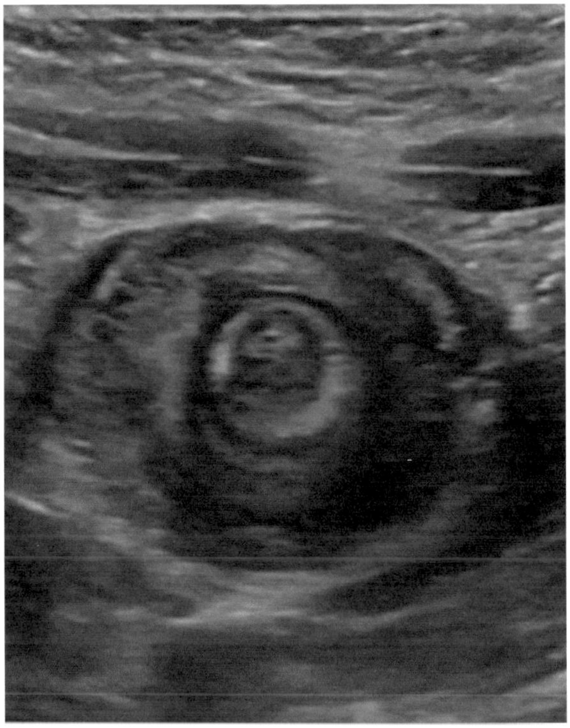

Management

- IV access and 20 mL/kg NS bolus
- Continuous monitoring
- Pediatric surgery consultation

Reassessment

Twenty minutes after NS bolus, the infant becomes increasingly lethargic and appears gray. Repeat vitals: BP 68/40, HR 182, capillary refill 4 seconds, T 38.4°C. Abdomen now rigid with rebound tenderness; patient groans with passive hip flexion. This represents hemodynamic deterioration with peritoneal signs indicating possible bowel ischemia, perforation, or sepsis – escalate to emergent operative intervention rather than therapeutic enema.

Patient Communication

The father expresses anxiety about surgery and voices his guilt for delayed arrival, and requests to speak with his wife via video call before consenting. The wife is described as "very against unnecessary medical interventions."

- Explain intussusception using accessible language (telescoping intestine)
- Validate father's concerns while emphasizing urgency of time-sensitive treatment
- Address guilt without casting blame
- Clearly communicate risks of perforation and shock to navigate request for delay
- Communicate with surgery and explain the need for surgical reduction since patient not stable to go for air enema.

Critical Actions

- Recognize classic intussusception presentation (paroxysmal abdominal pain, vomiting, lethargy, currant jelly stool) in appropriate age group (5-12 months)
- Initiate resuscitation with IV access and isotonic crystalloid bolus prior to imaging

- Interpret bedside ultrasound target sign as consistent with intussusception
- If formal ultrasound ordered ask for tech to perform US at bedside.
- Recognize hemodynamic deterioration and peritoneal signs – call pediatric surgery for emergent operative intervention rather than delayed enema
- Communicate effectively with father regarding diagnosis, urgency, and treatment plan
- Coordinate PICU admission with pediatric surgical consultation

Respiratory Failure

Opening Scenario

EMS arrives with a 67-year-old female with severe COPD (FEV1 35), CHF (EF 30), and pulmonary hypertension presenting with acute-on-chronic dyspnea worsening over 48 hours despite increased rescue inhaler use. Accompanied by her daughter, who holds healthcare proxy.

Initial Assessment

Vitals: BP 164/92, HR 108, RR 34, T 37.6°C, SpO_2 86% RA / 90% on 4L NC

- Alert, oriented, anxious, and fatigued; sitting upright, leaning forward, using accessory muscles; speaks in 2-3 word sentences; peripheral cyanosis and diaphoresis
- Airway: Patent, tachypneic with difficulty completing sentences
- Breathing: Diffuse wheezing bilaterally, decreased air movement at bases, coarse crackles in lower fields, paradoxical abdominal motion
- Circulation: Tachycardic, regular, capillary refill 2 seconds

History

- HPI: Symptoms began 3 days ago with increased cough productive of yellow-green sputum. Increased home O_2 from 2L to 4L without relief. Increased orthopnea over 24 hours. Denies fever, chest pain, or hemoptysis.
- PMHx: Severe COPD on home O_2, CHF with reduced EF, pulmonary hypertension, HTN
- Meds: Home O_2 2L NC, furosemide 40 mg daily, lisinopril, albuterol inhaler, tiotropium
- Allergies: Sulfonamides (rash)
- Social: Former smoker (quit 1 year ago, 50 pack-years), lives with daughter

Physical Examination

- General: Moderate respiratory distress, drowsy but arousable
- Cardiovascular: Tachycardic, regular rhythm, S3 gallop present
- Lungs: Decreased breath sounds at bases, prolonged expiratory phase, diffuse wheezing, scattered rhonchi
- Abdomen: Soft, non-tender, no hepatomegaly
- Extremities: 2+ pitting edema bilaterally
- Neurological: Alert to voice but drowsy, no focal deficits

Diagnostic Studies

- CBC: WBC 14.2, Hgb 13.8, Hct 41.2%, Plt 298
- BMP: Na 140, K 4.1, Cl 102, HCO_3 34, BUN 18, Cr 1.0, Glucose 112
- Troponin I: 0.04 (borderline), BNP: 850 pg/mL (elevated)
- VBG (on 4L NC): pH 7.28, $pCO_2$78, pO_2 62, HCO_3 32 (acute-on-chronic hypercapnic respiratory failure)
- CXR: Hyperinflation, bilateral infiltrates suggestive of pulmonary edema vs pneumonia, no pneumothorax
- Bedside ultrasound with multiple B-lines with intact lung sliding.

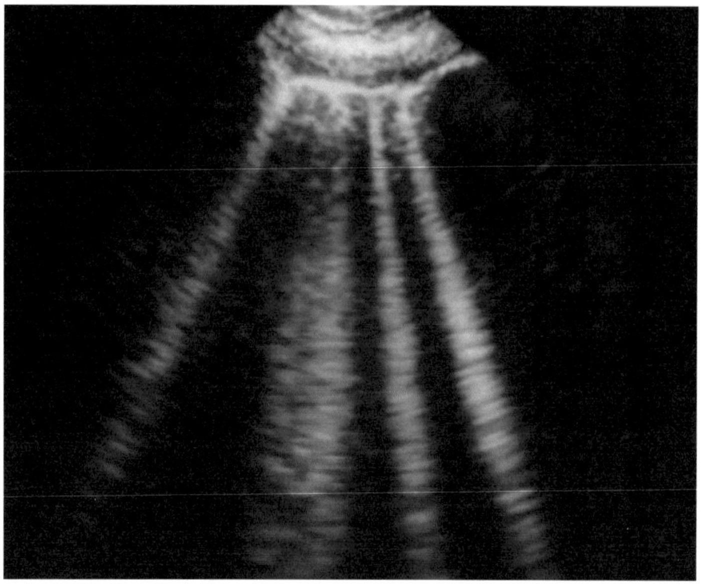

Management

- O_2 via NC titrated to SpO_2 88-92% (avoid 100% O_2)
- Two large-bore IVs, continuous monitoring
- Nebulized albuterol and ipratropium continuously
- IV methylprednisolone 125 mg
- IV furosemide 40 mg for fluid overload
- Antibiotics for suspected pneumonia triggering exacerbation
- ABG, ECG, portable CXR
- Initiate BiPAP (IPAP 12, EPAP 5, FiO_2 titrated to SpO_2 88-92%) given worsening somnolence and hypercapnia

Reassessment

After 20 minutes of therapy: mild subjective improvement but remains tachypneic. Vitals: BP 158/88, HR 102, RR 28, SpO_2 91% on 4L NC. Becoming increasingly somnolent.

After 30 minutes on BiPAP: patient pulls off mask, increasingly agitated and confused. Vitals: BP 148/76, HR 118, RR 36, SpO_2 82% RA. Asymmetrical chest rise and absent breath sounds on the right – suspect tension pneumothorax from BiPAP barotrauma.

- Bedside ultrsound of thorax on right shows no lung slide and barcode sign

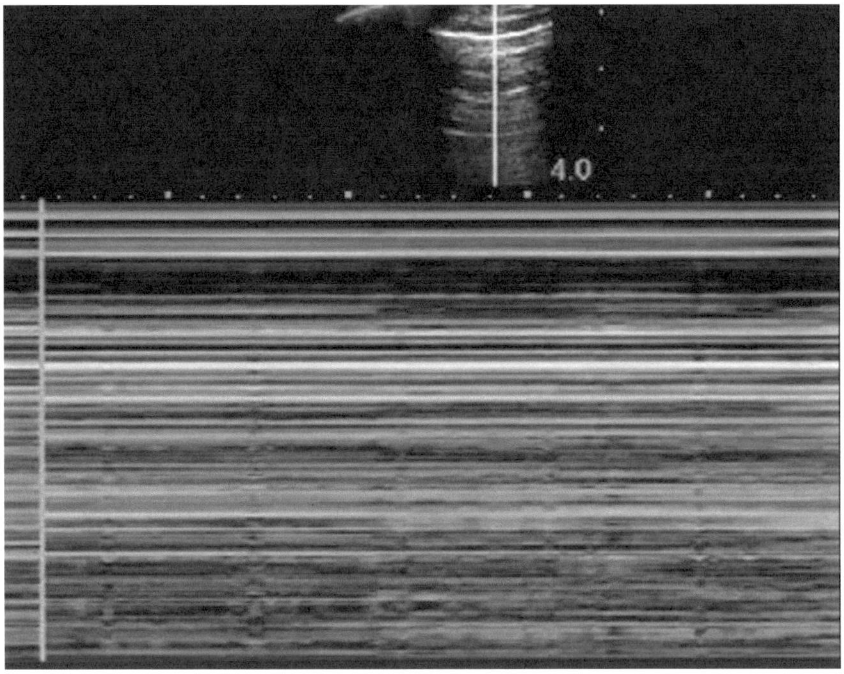

- Immediate needle decompression (14-gauge, right 2nd intercostal space, midclavicular line)
- Emergent bedside ultrasound shows no lung slide on the right with barcode sign (no sand on beach on m-mode)
- Prepare for chest tube thoracostomy
- Reapply BiPAP after decompression if stable; otherwise prepare for intubation

Patient Communication

- Explain severity of condition, lung infection triggering breathing problems and heart failure
- Discuss possibility of intubation if she tires further
- Discuss goals of care and code status; patient expresses fear of being "on a machine forever" but agrees to continue BiPAP
- Confirm daughter as surrogate decision-maker

Disposition

ICU admission for ongoing management.

Critical Actions

- Recognize acute-on-chronic hypercapnic respiratory failure requiring controlled O_2 therapy (target SpO_2 88-92%)
- Initiate bronchodilators and corticosteroids for COPD exacerbation
- Recognize need for BiPAP based on VBG results and clinical deterioration
- Recognize tension pneumothorax (asymmetric chest rise, absent breath sounds) and perform immediate needle decompression
- Recognize contraindications and complications of NIV (barotrauma)
- Disposition to ICU level care

Shallow Water Accident

Opening Scenario

EMS arrives with a 32-year-old male who dove headfirst into the shallow end of a lake 30 minutes ago. Bystanders pulled him from the water. He briefly lost consciousness but is now awake, alert, complaining of severe neck pain, and unable to move his arms or legs. C-collar and backboard in place.

Initial Assessment

Vitals: BP 88/42, HR 58, RR 22, T 36.1°C, SpO_2 96% RA

- Awake, alert, anxious, wet, supine on backboard
- Airway: Patent, speaking in full sentences
- Breathing: Shallow respirations, breath sounds equal bilaterally
- Circulation: Warm, dry skin; thready pulses; capillary refill <2 seconds
- Disability: Eyes open spontaneously, follows commands. Upper extremities: shoulder abduction and elbow flexion 3/5 bilaterally; no extension at elbows, wrists, or fingers. Lower extremities: 0/5. Sensory level at C5 bilaterally.
- Exposure: C-collar in place, priapism noted, no deformities or open wounds

History

- HPI: Dove into ~3 feet of water at a lakeside gathering, struck head on sandy bottom. Immediate neck pain and electric shock sensation radiating down arms and legs. Unable to move extremities since. Denies headache, chest pain, abdominal pain. Reports urinary retention.
- PMHx/Meds/Allergies: None / None / NKDA
- Social: Lives with partner, software engineer, occasional alcohol

Physical Examination

- General: Alert, oriented x3, anxious, on backboard
- Head: 5 cm occipital contusion, no lacerations or step-off
- Neck: C-collar in place, midline tenderness at C5-C6 spinous processes
- Chest: Clear bilaterally, no crepitus
- Cardiovascular: Regular rhythm, no murmurs, pulses 2+
- Abdomen: Soft, non-tender, non-distended
- Pelvis: Stable to compression
- Rectal: No anal sphincter tone, flaccid rectum, guaiac negative
- GU: Priapism present
- Neurologic: CN II-XII intact. UE: 3/5 shoulder abduction and elbow flexion (C5), 0/5 wrist extension/finger flexion/hand intrinsics. LE: 0/5 throughout. Sensory level C5. Upgoing Babinski bilaterally. DTRs absent in lower extremities.

Diagnostic Studies

- CBC: WBC 6.2, Hgb 13.8, Hct 41.2%, Plt 280
- BMP: Na 140, K 4.1, Cl 106, HCO_3 24, BUN 14, Cr 1.0, Glucose 118
- Coags: PT 12.4, PTT 28, INR 1.0
- UA: Unremarkable

- CT C-spine: C5 burst fracture with retropulsion into spinal canal causing severe central canal stenosis and cord compression
- CT Head: Negative for hemorrhage or skull fracture
- CT Chest/Abdomen/Pelvis: Negative for traumatic injury

Management

- Maintain spinal immobilization throughout
- Fluid resuscitation with 2L lactated Ringer's
- Emergent neurosurgery consultation
- Arterial line for continuous BP monitoring
- Foley catheter for urinary retention

Reassessment

20 minutes after arrival: increasing difficulty breathing. Vitals: BP 82/38, HR 52, RR 34, SpO_2 92% on 2L NC. Shallow, rapid breathing with intercostal retractions and paradoxical abdominal breathing. Unable to speak in full sentences.

- RSI with manual inline stabilization for respiratory failure from diaphragmatic fatigue (phrenic nerve C3-C5 involvement)
- Mechanical ventilation initiated
- Norepinephrine for neurogenic shock (warm shock with hypotension and bradycardia)

Disposition

Surgical ICU for neurosurgical evaluation and potential operative decompression and stabilization.

Critical Actions

- Maintain spinal immobilization throughout, including during intubation with inline stabilization
- Identify neurogenic shock (hypotension + bradycardia + warm/dry skin) and distinguish from hypovolemic shock
- Recognize cervical injuries at/above C5 can impair phrenic nerve function (C3-C5) causing diaphragmatic paralysis
- Intubate early based on respiratory muscle fatigue rather than waiting for arrest
- Manage neurogenic shock with fluids followed by vasopressors rather than excessive fluids alone
- Perform complete neurological exam including sensory level, motor grading, and rectal tone assessment
- Identify priapism and urinary retention as signs of spinal shock
- Obtain emergent neurosurgery consultation for burst fracture with cord compression
- Reassess frequently given risk of delayed respiratory compromise

Right Flank Pain with Clinical Deterioration

Opening Scenario

A 28-year-old female presents via private vehicle with severe right-sided flank pain. She is accompanied by her husband and is unable to sit still, constantly shifting positions on the stretcher.

Initial Assessment

Vitals: BP 148/92, HR 118, RR 18, T 37.6°C, SpO_2 98% RA, Pain 10/10

- Airway: Patent, speaking in full sentences, no stridor
- Breathing: Non-labored, clear breath sounds bilaterally, no cyanosis
- Circulation: Tachycardic, capillary refill <2 seconds, skin warm and dry
- Disability: Alert and oriented x4, no focal neurologic deficits
- Exposure: Diaphoretic, writhing on stretcher, unable to find comfortable position

Immediate actions: Two large-bore IVs, 1L LR bolus over 30 minutes, continuous cardiac and SpO_2 monitoring, ondansetron 4 mg IV, ketorolac 15 mg IV (after confirming no contraindications including pregnancy).

History

- HPI: Sudden onset severe right flank pain radiating to the right groin, began 8 hours ago at work. Constant, colicky, "worst pain ever." Three episodes of non-bloody, non-bilious emesis over 2 hours. Denies visible hematuria, fever/chills at home, dysuria, frequency, or urgency. No prior kidney stones. Denies chest pain, shortness of breath, or recent trauma.
- PMHx: No significant medical history, no prior surgeries
- Medications: Oral contraceptives, multivitamin
- Allergies: NKDA
- Social: Lives with husband, financial analyst. No tobacco, social alcohol (1-2 glasses wine weekly), no illicit drugs. Sexually active with husband only.

Physical Examination

- General: Improved comfort compared to arrival but still occasionally shifting position, diaphoresis resolved
- HEENT: Normocephalic, PERRL, EOMI, oropharynx clear
- Cardiovascular: Tachycardic, regular rhythm, no murmurs/rubs/gallops
- Pulmonary: Clear bilaterally, no wheezes or crackles
- Abdomen: Soft, non-distended, no rebound or guarding, normal bowel sounds, no hepatosplenomegaly
- Back: Moderate right CVA tenderness to percussion, no spinal step-offs or midline tenderness
- Genitourinary: Normal external genitalia, no discharge, no inguinal hernias
- Extremities: No edema, pulses 2+ bilaterally
- Neurologic: CN II-XII intact, normal sensation and strength, normal gait and reflexes

Diagnostic Studies

- CBC: WBC 11.2, Hgb 13.8, Hct 41.2%, Plt 280
- BMP: Na 138, K 4.0, Cl 102, HCO_3 22, BUN 18, Cr 0.9, Glucose 102
- Urinalysis: Amber, SG 1.025, pH 6.0, large blood, LE negative, nitrites negative, ketones negative, RBCs 100+, WBCs 6/hpf

Patient Communication

The patient asks about imaging options and expresses concern about radiation exposure from the CT scan. She read online that ultrasound can detect stones and questions whether she can avoid a CT scan.

- Bedside renal ultrasound: moderate right sided hydronephrosis without stone visualization

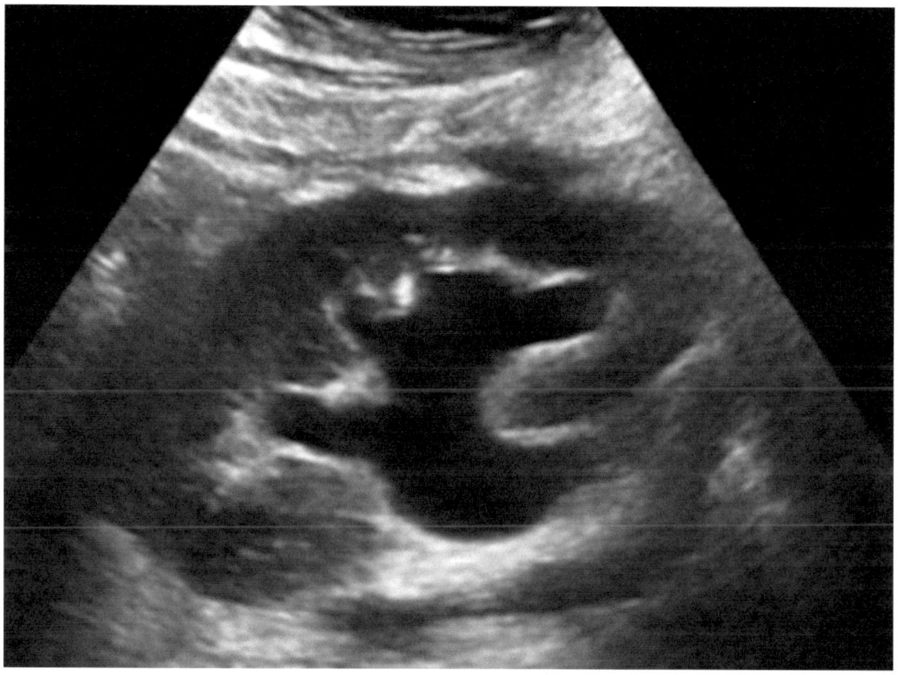

- Acknowledge and validate concerns regarding radiation exposure and desire for shared decision-making
- Explain that while ultrasound was diagnostic for hydronephrosis, a non-contrast CT remains the gold standard for first-time stone visualization due to superior sensitivity for stone size and location. Also discuss the concern for an infected stone and possible need for an intervention.
- CT Abdomen/Pelvis (non-contrast): 9 mm calculus at the right ureterovesicular junction with moderate right hydronephrosis and perinephric stranding
- Discuss need for antibiotics and urology consult since she has pyelonephritis with an obstructing stone.

Reassessment

Ninety minutes after initial analgesia, patient received morphine 4 mg IV in addition to ketorolac with good initial effect. She has received 2L of LR.

Vitals: BP 132/84, HR 98, T 38.5°C (new fever), SpO_2 97% RA, Pain 4/10 with increasing cramping

Physical exam now reveals new right lower quadrant tenderness with mild guarding and continued severe right CVA tenderness. Patient appears more flushed and anxious.

Managing Conflict

The patient becomes increasingly anxious upon learning of the fever. Urology is available at your hospital at night but she becomes increasingly anxious and wants to be transferred to an academic medical center, expresses frustration that "nothing is happening fast enough," and threatens to sign out AMA.

- Strongly counsel against leaving AMA given risk of rapid clinical deterioration and sepsis; document risks discussed and decision-making capacity
- Acknowledge her anxiety while providing clear explanation of the life-threatening nature of infected obstruction

Management

- Recognize fever with obstructing ureteral stone as infected obstruction (pyonephrosis/obstructive pyelonephritis) — a urologic emergency
- Obtain blood cultures prior to antibiotic administration if possible without delaying therapy
- Initiate broad-spectrum IV antibiotics (ceftriaxone 1 g IV or piperacillin-tazobactam 3.375 g IV)
- Contact urology immediately for emergent decompression (ureteral stent or percutaneous nephrostomy tube)
- Admit for continued IV antibiotics, monitoring, and definitive management

Critical Actions

- Provide immediate analgesia and antiemetics for suspected renal colic before extensive history gathering
- Obtain appropriate workup including urinalysis and non-contrast CT for first-time stone former with classic presentation
- Recognize new-onset fever with obstructing ureteral stone as infected obstruction requiring emergent intervention rather than outpatient management
- Reassess after initial stabilization, identify clinical deterioration, and change management plan accordingly
- Engage in shared decision-making regarding imaging while explaining medical necessity and radiation risks
- Manage conflict by acknowledging patient anxiety, explaining the life-threatening nature of infected obstruction, and establishing appropriate boundaries regarding AMA discharge
- Demonstrate knowledge of stone size passage rates (approximately 50 for 5 mm stones at UVJ)
- Initiate broad-spectrum antibiotics and urgent urology consultation once fever develops in obstructed system
- Do not discharge

Seizure

Opening Scenario

EMS arrives with a 38-year-old female actively seizing for 20 minutes despite 4 mg lorazepam IM en route. Her husband accompanies the ambulance and is visibly agitated, demanding answers about why his wife is not waking up.

Initial Assessment

Vitals: BP 168/95, HR 128, RR 22, T 37.2°C, SpO_2 94% RA, Fingerstick glucose 92

- Airway: Gurgling respirations with copious secretions, no cough or gag reflex during active convulsions
- Breathing: Tachypneic with accessory muscle use, bilateral air entry present but diminished at bases
- Circulation: Tachycardic, regular rhythm, strong radial pulses, capillary refill <2 seconds
- Disability: GCS 3 (E1, V1, M1) during seizure
- Exposure: Multiple old ecchymoses on extremities; fresh track marks on bilateral antecubital fossae; generalized tonic-clonic movements, frothy oral secretions with tongue laceration bleeding, cyanotic nail beds

Immediate actions: Left lateral decubitus positioning, high-flow O2 via NRB at 15 L/min, aggressive oropharyngeal suctioning, two large-bore IVs, continuous cardiac and SpO_2 monitoring, point-of-care glucose. Midazolam 10 mg IV push (and consider antiepileptic loading). Patient seizure ceases and she enters post-ictal state. Prepare for definitive airway management if seizure persists beyond 5 minutes despite adequate benzodiazepines and antiepileptic loading doses..

History

- HPI: Per husband, heavy daily alcohol consumption (6-8 beers daily). Attempted to quit "cold turkey" four days ago due to epigastric discomfort. First seizure began approximately 25 minutes ago at home. Husband denies witnessed head trauma, though patient fell during the event. No prior seizure history.
- PMHx: Hypertension, generalized anxiety disorder, alcohol use disorder
- PSHx: Laparoscopic appendectomy at age 16
- Medications: Lisinopril (not taken for past 3 days), occasional OTC ibuprofen
- Allergies: NKDA
- Social: Lives with husband and two school-age children. Currently unemployed. Tobacco 1 PPD. Husband denies illicit drug use, though track marks noted on exam.
- Family Hx: Father deceased from alcoholic cirrhosis; mother with hypertension

Physical Examination

- General: Post-ictal, confused and combative when stimulated, attempting to remove IV lines
- HEENT: 1 cm tongue laceration with active oozing, PERRL (3 to 2 mm), no Battle sign or raccoon eyes, TMs clear bilaterally
- Neck: Cervical collar in place, no step-offs, neck supple once seizure terminated
- Chest: Clear bilaterally, no wheezes or crackles
- Cardiovascular: Tachycardic, regular, no murmurs/rubs/gallops
- Abdomen: Soft, non-distended, mild epigastric tenderness, normoactive bowel sounds, no hepatosplenomegaly
- Musculoskeletal: No deformities; track marks on bilateral antecubital fossae with surrounding erythema

- Neurologic: GCS 10 (E3, V2, M5), localizes pain, no focal motor deficits post-ictally, facial symmetry intact
- Skin: Warm, diaphoretic, multiple old bruises in various stages of healing

Diagnostic Studies

- CBC: WBC 14.2, Hgb 13.8, Hct 41.2%, Plt 248
- BMP: Na 132, K 3.8, Cl 98, HCO_3 20, BUN 28, Cr 1.4, Glucose 110
- Coags: PT 12.8, PTT 28, INR 1.1
- LFTs: AST 45, ALT 32, ALP 110, T.Bili 0.8
- Lactate 8.4, EtOH <10, acetaminophen <5, salicylate <2
- Urine toxicology: Positive for benzodiazepines (expected), cocaine metabolites (unexpected)
- ECG: Sinus tachycardia at 125, no ST changes
- CT Head (non-contrast): No acute intracranial hemorrhage, no mass effect or midline shift, moderate cerebral edema
- Chest X-ray: Clear lung fields, no infiltrates or effusions

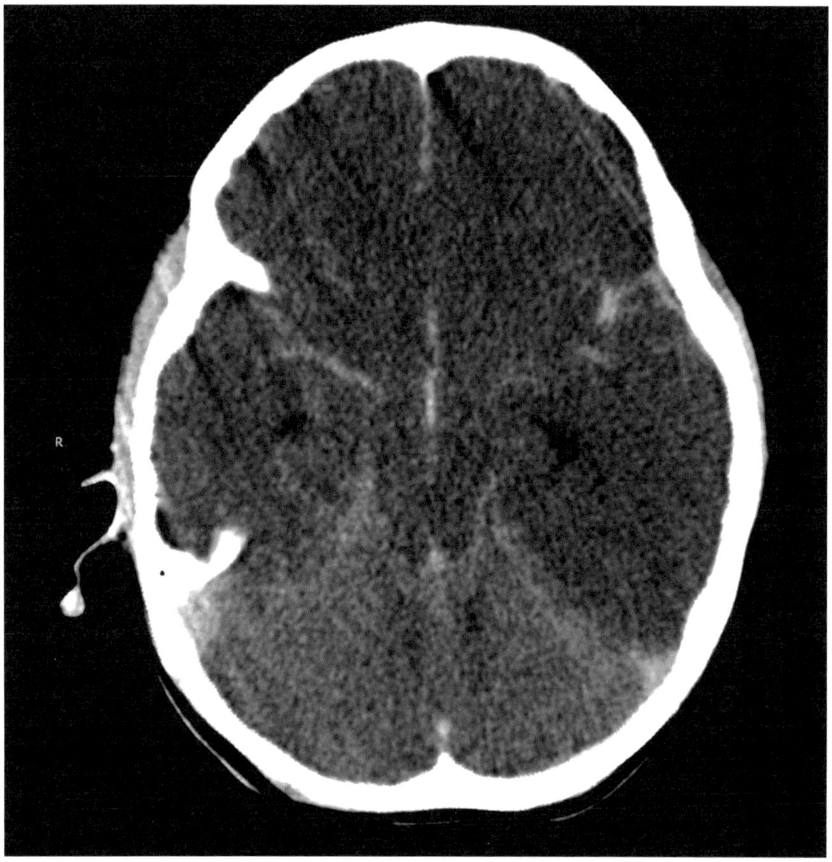

Reassessment

Ten minutes after seizure cessation:

- Increasingly somnolent, difficult to arouse
- RR drops to 10 with shallow respirations, SpO_2 88% on NRB
- GCS declines to 6 (E1, V1, M4), gag reflex diminished

Management: Prepare for RSI given declining mental status, respiratory depression, and inability to protect airway. Administer additional benzodiazepines or phenobarbital IV if seizure recurs. Consult neurology for continuous EEG monitoring if available. Notify ICU for admission.

Managing Conflict

The husband becomes confrontational when informed of the positive cocaine metabolites, stating: "She promised me she stopped that stuff years ago! I thought this was just from the alcohol!" He is angry and demands to know why she is not waking up normally.

- Acknowledge husband's distress and anger without becoming defensive
- Explain the pathophysiology of alcohol withdrawal seizures and risk of status epilepticus
- Address polysubstance use findings in a non-judgmental, factual manner
- Discuss potential for complicated withdrawal including delirium tremens
- Explain the necessity of intubation for airway protection given clinical deterioration
- Obtain informed consent for intubation and ICU admission

Critical Actions

- Recognize status epilepticus immediately and protect the airway during active seizure
- Dose benzodiazepines aggressively — alcohol withdrawal seizures often require >8 mg lorazepam for termination
- Administer thiamine due to the consideration of possible prevention of Wernicke encephalopathy
- Obtain comprehensive metabolic and toxicologic workup to exclude alternative etiologies while recognizing alcohol withdrawal as primary cause
- Correlate physical findings (track marks) with unexpected positive cocaine screen, recognizing polysubstance withdrawal
- Reassess mental status and respiratory drive; proceed to definitive airway management when indicated
- Manage conflict with family regarding unexpected substance use findings while maintaining therapeutic alliance
- Disposition to ICU for continuous monitoring, sedation, and alcohol withdrawal protocol
- Recognize seizure-related complications: tongue laceration, rhabdomyolysis risk, cerebral edema on imaging and need for MRI to categorize underlying cause

Lethargic Elderly Patient

Opening Scenario

EMS arrives with a 68-year-old male from an assisted living facility with fever and lethargy. He has a history of diabetes, peripheral vascular disease, and advanced dementia. He is accompanied by his daughter (medical power of attorney) and his estranged son, who arrived from out of state and is demanding immediate answers.

Initial Assessment

Vitals: BP 94/58, HR 124, RR 26, T 39.2°C (102.6°F), SpO_2 93% RA

- Airway: Patent, groaning, gurgling sounds noted
- Breathing: Tachypneic, clear breath sounds bilaterally
- Circulation: Weak radial pulses, capillary refill 4 seconds, mottling of lower extremities
- Disability: GCS 9 (eyes open to pain, withdraws, incomprehensible sounds)
- Exposure: Cachectic, toxic-appearing, diaphoretic, foul odor, discoloration in pelvic region

Immediate actions: Continuous cardiac monitoring and SpO_2, two large-bore IVs (14 or 16 gauge), aggressive fluid resuscitation with 30 mL/kg LR (~2L), supplemental O2 via NC at 4 L/min, 12-lead ECG.

Labs: CBC with differential, BMP, lactate, blood cultures x2, urine culture.

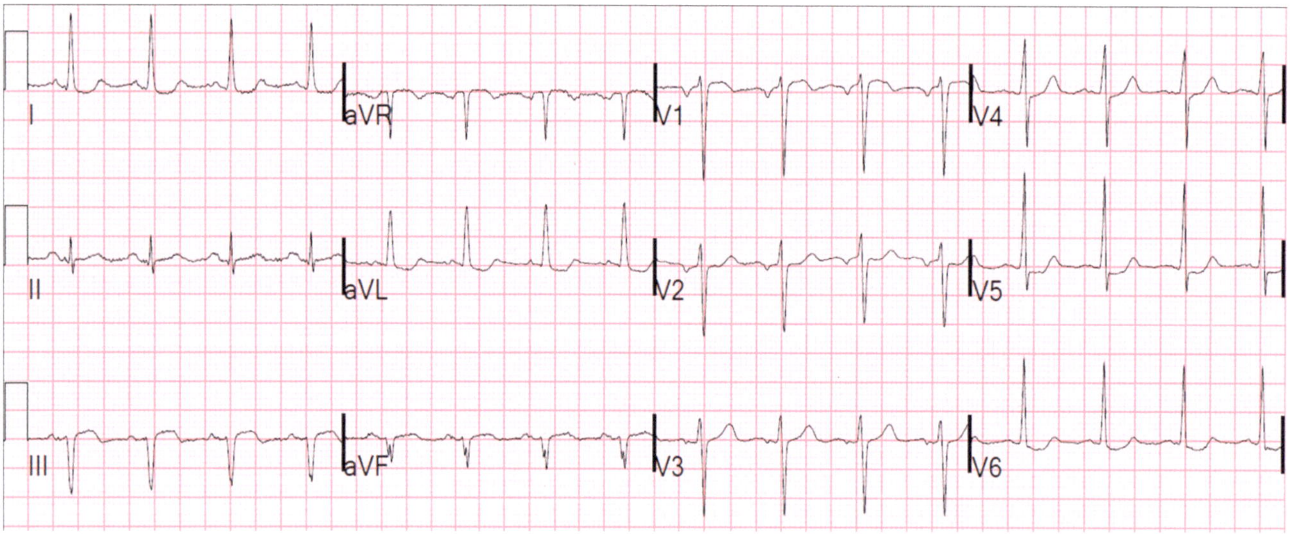

History

- HPI: 68-year-old male with progressive somnolence over 48 hours per assisted living staff. Developed fever and refused meals today. Daughter states he was at his baseline (nonverbal but responsive) three days ago. Son reports he "looks worse than I've ever seen him" and insists "everything possible must be done."
- PMHx: Type 2 diabetes mellitus (insulin-dependent), peripheral arterial disease, coronary artery disease (prior NSTEMI 2 years ago), vascular dementia, benign prostatic hyperplasia
- PSHx: Right femoral-popliteal bypass graft (18 months ago), cardiac catheterization with drug-eluting stent
- Medications: Aspirin 81 mg daily, Atorvastatin 40 mg daily, Insulin glargine 20 units nightly, Haloperidol 0.5 mg PRN agitation
- Allergies: No known drug allergies

- Social: Resides in assisted living, requires assistance with all activities of daily living. Daughter holds medical power of attorney per advanced directive. Son is estranged but present and emotional.

Diagnostic Studies

- CBC: WBC 19.4, Hgb 10.8, Plt 128 (low)
- BMP: Na 138, K 5.2 (high), BUN 42, Cr 2.1 (baseline 1.0), Glucose 398
- Lactate: 5.4
- ECG: Sinus tachycardia, no ST changes

Physical Examination

- General: Cachectic male, toxic appearance, guarding with movement
- HEENT: Normocephalic, dry mucous membranes, PERRL
- Neck: Supple, no JVD, no lymphadenopathy
- Cardiovascular: Tachycardic, regular, no murmurs/rubs/gallops
- Pulmonary: Clear bilaterally, no wheezes/rales/rhonchi
- Abdomen: Soft, non-distended, hypoactive bowel sounds, suprapubic tenderness without rebound or guarding
- Genitourinary/Rectal: Marked erythema and edema of scrotum extending to perineum; crepitus extending from scrotum to perineum and medial thighs bilaterally; black necrotic patches at perineal midline with purulent drainage; significant pain with gentle palpation
- Extremities: Diminished pedal pulses bilaterally, cool distal extremities, mottling on lower legs
- Skin: Warm trunk with diaphoresis, cool extremities
- Neurologic: Nonverbal, withdraws to pain, CN II-XII grossly intact

Management

- Broad-spectrum antibiotics immediately: piperacillin-tazobactam 4.5 g IV, vancomycin 25 mg/kg IV (renal dose adjustment required), clindamycin 900 mg IV (toxin suppression and anaerobic coverage)
- Vasopressor support with norepinephrine if hypotension persists after 30 mL/kg fluid resuscitation
- Emergent urology and general surgery consultation for operative debridement (if they ask for a CT ask if they can meet you at the patient's bedside since they are relatively hypotensive)
- Admit to ICU

Reassessment

Post-fluid vitals (if adequate resuscitation): BP 108/72, HR 112, RR 24, T 38.8°C, SpO_2 98% on 4L NC. Patient remains lethargic but less mottled.

If fluids inadequate: BP 78/48, HR 138, RR 30 — patient becomes increasingly obtunded, repeat lactate 6.8, progresses to require vasopressors and potential intubation.

Difficult Conversations

The son becomes verbally aggressive: "If you don't operate immediately, you're killing him!" The daughter cries: "I don't want him to suffer, but I don't know what he would want." They disagree about the level of intervention.

- Acknowledge son's distress while clarifying daughter's legal authority as power of attorney
- Redirect focus to patient's best interests and previously expressed wishes
- Explain diagnosis of Fournier gangrene with high mortality risk

- Describe necessary surgical intervention (extensive debridement, possible orchiectomy, potential colostomy) and that delay significantly increases mortality
- Establish code status based on prior advance directives and family consensus
- Involve social work or chaplaincy if available

Critical Actions

- Recognize septic shock and initiate immediate aggressive fluid resuscitation (30 mL/kg crystalloid)
- Perform complete physical examination including genital inspection to identify source of infection (crepitus indicates necrotizing fasciitis requiring emergent surgical intervention)
- Select appropriate broad-spectrum antibiotics covering anaerobes, Gram-negative enterics, and MRSA
- Obtain early surgical consultation for source control (debridement is time-critical; antibiotics alone are insufficient)
- Reassess after initial interventions to identify fluid-refractory shock requiring vasopressors
- Navigate difficult goals-of-care conversation with family regarding grave prognosis and surgical urgency
- Recognize that nonverbal patients with sepsis require thorough physical examination to locate source
- Recognize that Fournier gangrene in diabetic patients carries high morbidity and requires immediate operative consult prior to imaging.

HIV with Respiratory Failure

Opening Scenario

A 42-year-old male with known HIV/AIDS arrives via EMS with respiratory distress. He has been febrile and hypoxic during transport. He is anxious and refuses the surgical mask, stating "I can't breathe with that thing on."

Initial Assessment

Vitals: BP 98/52, HR 118, RR 28, T 39.1°C (102.4°F), SpO_2 85% RA, Weight 68 kg

- Airway: Patent, speaking in short phrases, no stridor
- Breathing: Tachypneic, bilateral crackles audible without stethoscope, paradoxical abdominal breathing
- Circulation: Tachycardic, weak radial pulses, capillary refill 3 seconds, warm and moist skin
- Disability: Alert and oriented x3, GCS 15
- Exposure: Cachectic, diaphoretic, tripod positioning with accessory muscle use, visible oral thrush, no rashes or Kaposi lesions

Immediate actions: 15L O2 via NRB, two large-bore IVs, continuous cardiac monitoring and SpO_2, point-of-care glucose. Labs: CBC with differential, CMP, lactate, blood cultures (aerobic/anaerobic), LDH, HIV viral load/CD4 count, UA and urine culture. Portable CXR. Prepare for potential advanced airway management.

History

- Chief Complaint: "I can't breathe and I'm burning up"
- History of Present Illness: Patient reports 5 days of progressive exertional dyspnea that has now become present at rest, associated with subjective fevers, night sweats, and a nonproductive cough. He notes white patches in his mouth for several weeks. Today he developed rigors and severe shortness of breath prompting EMS call. Denies hemoptysis, chest pain, headache, or neck stiffness. No recent travel, camping, or known sick contacts.
- Past Medical History: HIV diagnosed 8 years ago, last known CD4 count 6 months ago was 120 cells/µL. Not on antiretroviral therapy for past 4 months due to medication side effects and financial constraints.
- Surgical History: None
- Medications: None currently (noncompliant with prior ART regimen)
- Allergies: Sulfonamides (anaphylaxis—throat swelling and hives)
- Social History: Lives alone in apartment. Former smoker (1 pack/day for 15 years, quit 2 years ago). No alcohol or illicit drug use. Recently lost job and health insurance. Not currently sexually active.
- Family History: Non-contributory

Physical Examination

- General: Alert, oriented, moderate to severe respiratory distress, speaking in 2-3 word sentences
- HEENT: Poor dentition, thick white plaques on buccal mucosa and tongue consistent with thrush, no cervical lymphadenopathy, no JVD
- Eyes: Extraocular movements intact, pupils equal and reactive
- Neck: Trachea midline, no stridor, full range of motion
- Cardiovascular: Tachycardic, regular rhythm, no murmurs, rubs, or gallops
- Pulmonary: Decreased breath sounds bilaterally, diffuse fine inspiratory crackles throughout all lung fields, no wheezing, increased work of breathing with supraclavicular and intercostal retractions
- Abdomen: Soft, non-tender, non-distended, normoactive bowel sounds, no hepatosplenomegaly

- Extremities: No clubbing, cyanosis, or edema; pulses 2+ bilaterally
- Skin: Warm, diaphoretic, no Kaposi sarcoma lesions or rashes
- Neurological: Cranial nerves II-XII intact, no focal deficits, normal strength and sensation
- Psychiatric: Appropriate affect given situation, anxious but cooperative

Diagnostic Studies

- CBC: WBC 0.9 (critical — severely neutropenic), Neutrophils 82%, Lymphocytes 12%, Hgb 10.2, Hct 30.8%, Plt 198
- BMP: Na 138, K 3.8, Cl 102, HCO_3 20, BUN 48, Cr 1.4, Glucose 186
- ABG (on 15L NRB): pH 7.35, PaCO2 32, PaO2 58, HCO_3 18, A-a gradient 45 mmHg
- Lactate 3.2, LDH 485
- Urinalysis: Yellow, clear, negative for leukocytes/nitrites/blood
- Chest X-ray: Bilateral diffuse interstitial infiltrates with perihilar ground-glass opacities extending to periphery; no effusions, pneumothorax, or focal consolidation

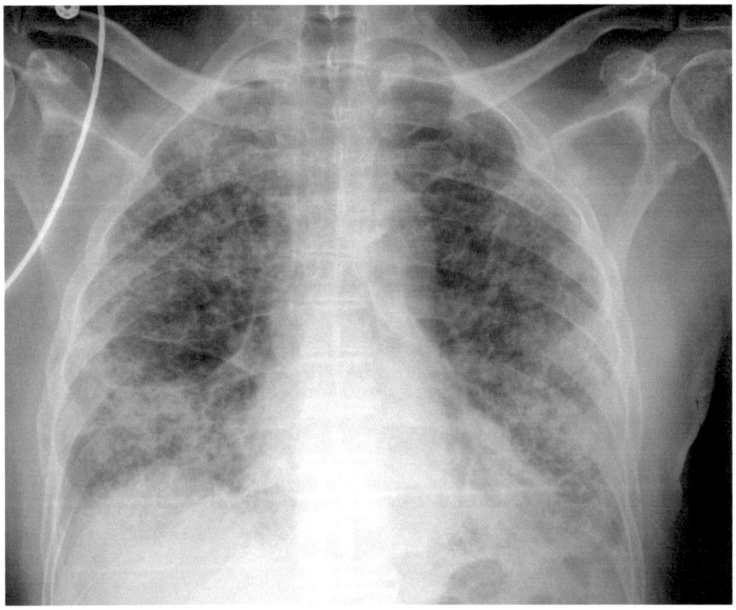

Managing Conflict

Upon learning of placement in a negative pressure isolation room, the patient becomes agitated: "I know what this means — you think I have tuberculosis and you're going to lock me away like a prisoner. I want to leave right now. I'd rather die at home than be treated like a leper."

- Acknowledge concerns without dismissing feelings
- Explain the room protects both the patient from hospital-acquired infections and staff from potential airborne pathogens while testing is pending
- Negotiate a compromise: door open when not performing procedures, frequent nursing check-ins, phone/computer access
- Address stigma directly: isolation is standard for this presentation, not a judgment of character
- Frame continued treatment as necessary for survival

Difficult Conversations

The patient asks: "Be honest with me — am I going to die?"

- Discuss the severity of PCP pneumonia with respiratory failure

- Address uncertainty of prognosis while awaiting treatment response
- Explain potential need for intubation and mechanical ventilation
- Establish code status and surrogate decision-maker given severity

Management

- Community acquired coverage + TMP/SMX for acute pneumonia (probably PJP)
- Corticosteroids due to elevated AA gradient
- Isolation due to airborne risk

Reassessment

Thirty minutes after initial interventions (oxygen, IV fluids, antibiotics, corticosteroids):

- Vitals: BP 102/58, HR 112, RR 26, SpO_2 90% on 15L NRB, T 38.8°C
- Patient remains tachypneic with increased work of breathing, paradoxical breathing pattern developing. States: "I still feel like I'm drowning. I can't keep this up." Persistent hypoxemia despite high-flow oxygen, rising PaCO2 on repeat ABG (48 mmHg, up from 32), MAP <65 mmHg.
- Management: Escalate to BiPAP to decrease work of breathing. If patient refuses BiPAP or SpO_2 remains <92%: prepare for RSI with etomidate and rocuronium.
- Initiate norepinephrine if MAP remains <65 after additional 500 mL crystalloid. Consult MICU for admission.

Critical Actions

- Recognize immunocompromised status (AIDS with CD4 <200) and prioritize differential: PCP pneumonia, bacterial pneumonia, tuberculosis, CMV pneumonitis, fungal infections
- Identify severe hypoxemic respiratory failure (PaO2 58 on 15L NRB) with widened A-a gradient consistent with PCP
- Initiate empiric therapy covering typical bacterial pathogens (ceftriaxone/azithromycin) and Pneumocystis jirovecii (atovaquone due to sulfa allergy)
- Recognize indication for adjunctive corticosteroids in severe PCP (PaO2 <70 on RA or A-a gradient >35)
- Place in appropriate isolation precautions (airborne/droplet) pending tuberculosis rule-out
- De-escalate patient's refusal of isolation through negotiation, education, and mutual respect while maintaining safety
- Initiate goals-of-care discussion and establish code status and surrogate decision-maker before potential loss of capacity
- Reassess systematically at 30 minutes; recognize inadequate response to supplemental oxygen (rising PaCO2, paradoxical breathing) and escalate to BiPAP or intubation
- Initiate vasopressor support for persistent hypoperfusion after adequate fluid resuscitation
- Consult ICU for admission

Tachycardia

Opening Scenario

EMS brings in a 42-year-old female who developed sudden palpitations and mild chest tightness at work 90 minutes ago. She appears anxious but speaks in full sentences. Prehospital ECG shows a regular narrow-complex tachycardia at approximately 170 bpm. She is frightened she is having a heart attack.

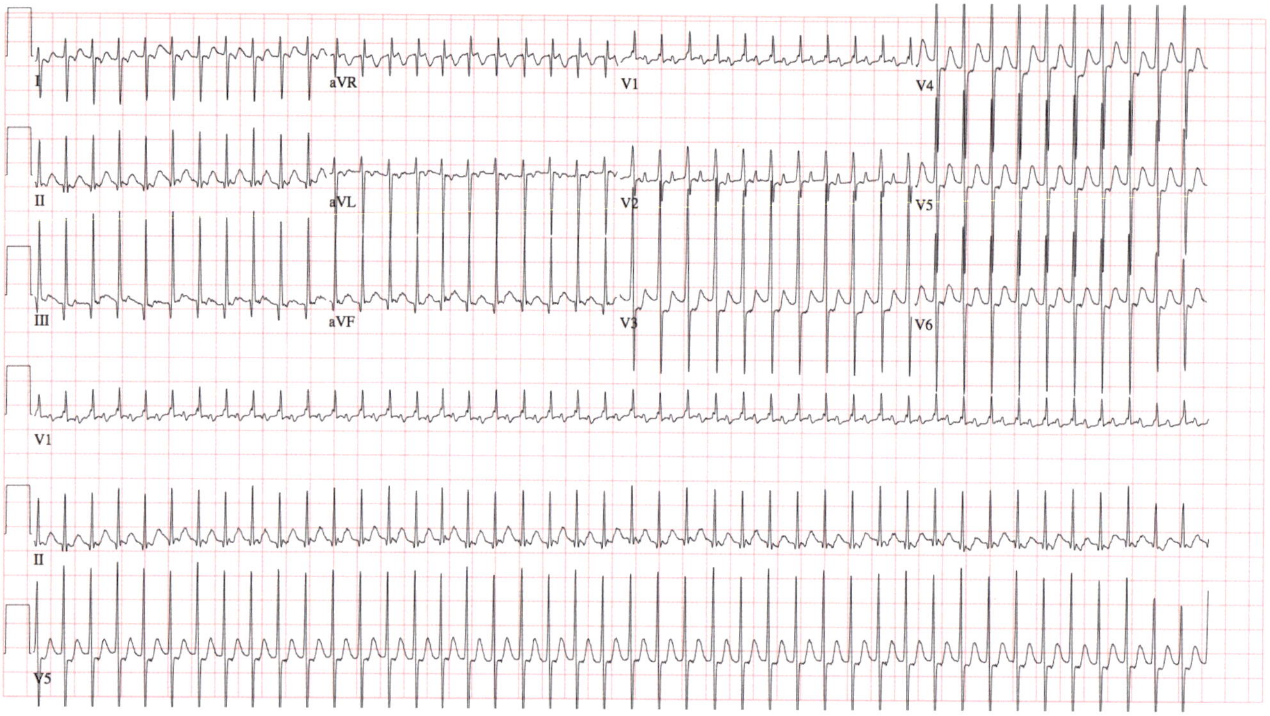

Initial Assessment

Vitals: BP 168/110, HR 172, RR 20, T 36.8°C, SpO_2 98% RA

- PMHx: Hypertension, generalized anxiety disorder
- Hemodynamically stable with mild dyspnea and chest tightness without radiation
- Denies syncope, presyncope, diaphoresis, nausea, caffeine excess, decongestant or stimulant use
- No family history of sudden cardiac death or arrhythmias

Immediate actions: Two large-bore IVs, continuous cardiac monitoring with SpO_2 and automated BP cuff, 12-lead ECG (narrow complex regular tachycardia at 172 bpm, absent P waves, normal QRS — consistent with SVT).

Physical Examination

- General: Alert, anxious, sitting upright, mildly uncomfortable
- Head/Neck: Normocephalic, no JVD, no thyromegaly, no carotid bruits
- Cardiovascular: Tachycardic, regular, no murmurs/rubs/gallops, pulses equal and strong, capillary refill <2 seconds
- Pulmonary: Clear bilaterally, no wheezes/crackles
- Abdomen: Soft, non-tender, non-distended
- Neurologic: CN intact, no focal deficits, alert and oriented x3
- Skin: Warm, dry, no rash

Diagnostic Studies

- CBC: WBC 7.2, Hgb 13.8, Plt 285
- BMP: Na 140, K 4.1, Cl 102, HCO_3 26, BUN 14, Cr 0.9, Glucose 108
- Troponin I: <0.04 (negative)
- TSH: 1.8 (normal)
- Urine HCG: Negative

Differential: SVT (AVNRT vs AVRT), sinus tachycardia, atrial flutter with 2:1, hyperthyroidism. Regular narrow-complex at 172 bpm at rest is most consistent with reentrant SVT. Hemodynamic stability allows vagal maneuvers before pharmacologic intervention.

Patient Communication

- Acknowledge fear of cardiac arrest; validate symptoms while reassuring stability
- Describe SVT as an electrical "short circuit"; differentiate from myocardial infarction
- Explain vagal maneuvers and adenosine as treatment options
- Obtain informed consent: warn about transient chest burning, flushing, nausea, and "impending doom" lasting 10-20 seconds

Management

Vagal maneuvers attempted sequentially (modified Valsalva with leg elevation, breath into a syringe) — maneuvers unsuccessful. Adenosine 6 mg rapid IV push via proximal large-bore IV with immediate 20 mL saline flush, rhythm strip running, defibrillator at bedside prior to adenosine administration .

Reassessment

Post-first dose: Brief asystole (6 seconds) then conversion to sinus rhythm at 86 bpm. Transient chest burning resolves within 20 seconds. Vitals: BP 148/92, HR 86, RR 16, SpO_2 99%.

Twenty minutes post-conversion: Return of palpitations. Vitals: BP 162/108, HR 158, RR 18. Repeat ECG confirms recurrent SVT, hemodynamically stable. Adenosine 12 mg rapid IV push — immediate conversion to sinus rhythm at 78 bpm.

Forty-five minutes observation without recurrence. Serial troponin negative at 3 hours. Final vitals: BP 138/88, HR 78, RR 14, SpO_2 99% RA.

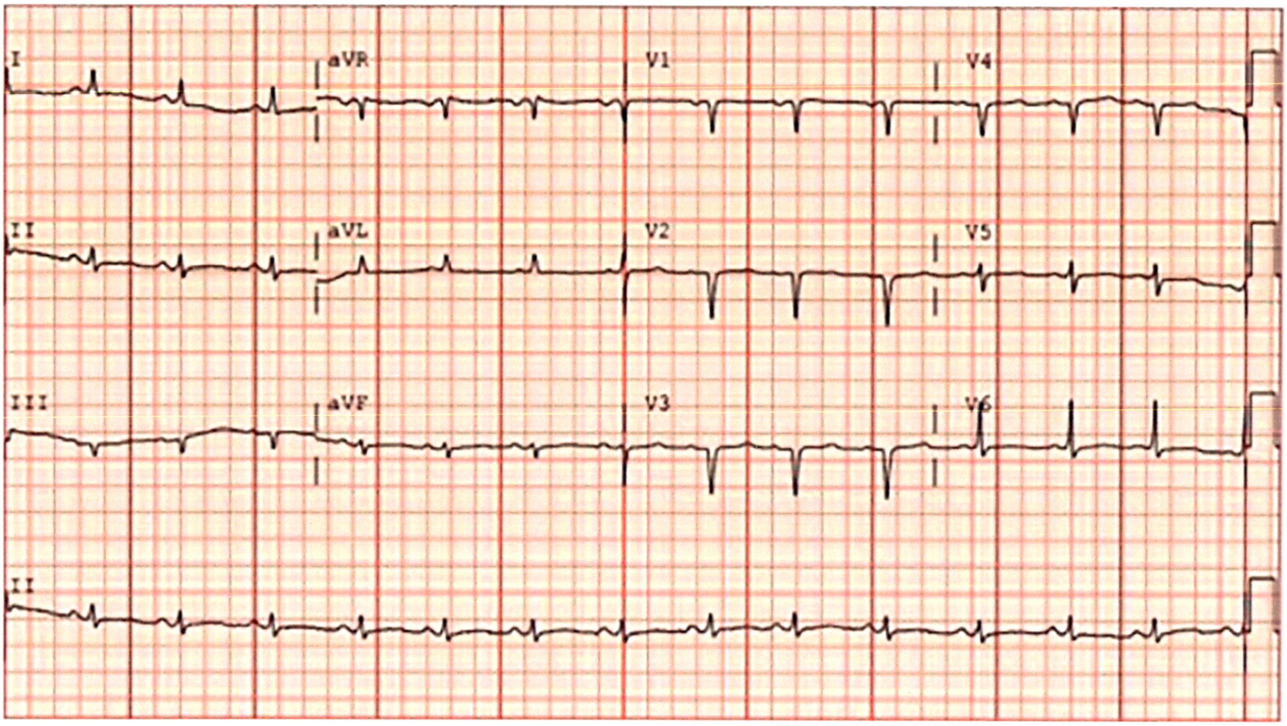

Disposition

- Discharge criteria met: hemodynamically stable, asymptomatic, negative biomarkers, normal repeat ECG
- Cardiology appointment within 48 hours for electrophysiology evaluation
- Teach vagal maneuvers for home use
- Return precautions: chest pain, syncope, sustained palpitations >30 minutes, severe dyspnea

Critical Actions

- Recognize hemodynamically stable narrow-complex regular tachycardia as SVT
- Attempt vagal maneuvers prior to pharmacologic therapy (carotid massage only after checking for bruits)
- Administer adenosine correctly: rapid IV push of 6 mg via proximal large-bore IV with immediate saline flush, rhythm strip running, defibrillator present
- Reassess rhythm and symptoms immediately after adenosine, recognizing successful conversion
- Recognize SVT recurrence and escalate to 12 mg adenosine
- Observe minimum 30-45 minutes to ensure sustained rhythm stability before discharge
- Address anxiety, explain diagnosis accessibly, obtain informed consent including side effect warnings
- Discharge with cardiology referral and clear return precautions

Severe Pneumonia with Septic Shock

Opening Scenario

EMS brings in a 52-year-old male with fever, productive cough, and worsening shortness of breath. During transport he became increasingly confused and hypotensive. A friend reports the patient has been ill for four days.

Initial Assessment

Vitals: BP 76/48, HR 128, RR 32, T 39.8°C (103.6°F), SpO_2 88% RA

- Airway: Patent, speaking in short phrases, no stridor
- Breathing: Tachypneic with bilateral crackles and decreased breath sounds at right base, accessory muscle use with intercostal retractions
- Circulation: Weak peripheral pulses, capillary refill 4 seconds, cool extremities with mottling on distal lower extremities
- Cachectic, diaphoretic, somnolent but opens eyes to verbal stimuli

Immediate actions: NRB targeting SpO_2 >92%, two large-bore IVs, blood cultures prior to antibiotics if possible without delay, 30 mL/kg isotonic crystalloid, continuous cardiac monitoring and SpO_2, prepare for potential emergent airway management.

History

The patient reports progressive symptoms over four days, beginning with fatigue and dry cough, evolving to high fevers with rigors and rust-colored sputum production. He developed pleuritic right-sided chest pain and severe dyspnea at rest this morning. He denies headache, nausea, vomiting, or urinary symptoms. He has no recent travel history but reports a 40 pack-year smoking history. No known chronic medical conditions, takes no medications, and has no drug allergies.

Physical Examination

- General: Alert to voice, oriented to person and place only initially, improves to oriented times three after initial fluid resuscitation
- Head: Normocephalic, atraumatic
- Eyes: Sclera non-icteric, pupils equal and reactive
- Neck: Supple, full range of motion, trachea midline, no jugular venous distension
- Chest: Increased work of breathing, tenderness to palpation over right lower ribs, crackles bilaterally with diminished breath sounds at right base
- Cardiovascular: Regular rhythm, tachycardic, no murmurs, rubs, or gallops appreciated
- Abdomen: Soft, non-distended, normal bowel sounds, no tenderness or guarding
- Extremities: Cool and clammy, peripheral pulses weak but symmetric, no edema
- Neurological: Cranial nerves intact, moves all extremities equally, sensation grossly intact
- Skin: Mottling present on knees and elbows, diaphoretic

Diagnostic Studies

- CBC: WBC 18.5 (Neutrophils 90%, Bands 8%), Hgb 13.2, Plt 285
- BMP: Na 136, K 4.1, Cl 102, HCO_3 18, BUN 38, Cr 1.3, Glucose 142
- Coags: PT 12.8, INR 1.0, PTT 28
- LFTs: AST 28, ALT 31, Bilirubin 1.1

- Lactate: 4.2
- ABG: pH 7.32, PaCO2 32, PaO2 58 (RA) / 68 (NRB), HCO_3 16
- Chest X-ray: Dense RLL consolidation with air bronchograms, small right pleural effusion, no pneumothorax
- ECG: Sinus tachycardia at 128, normal intervals, no acute ischemic changes

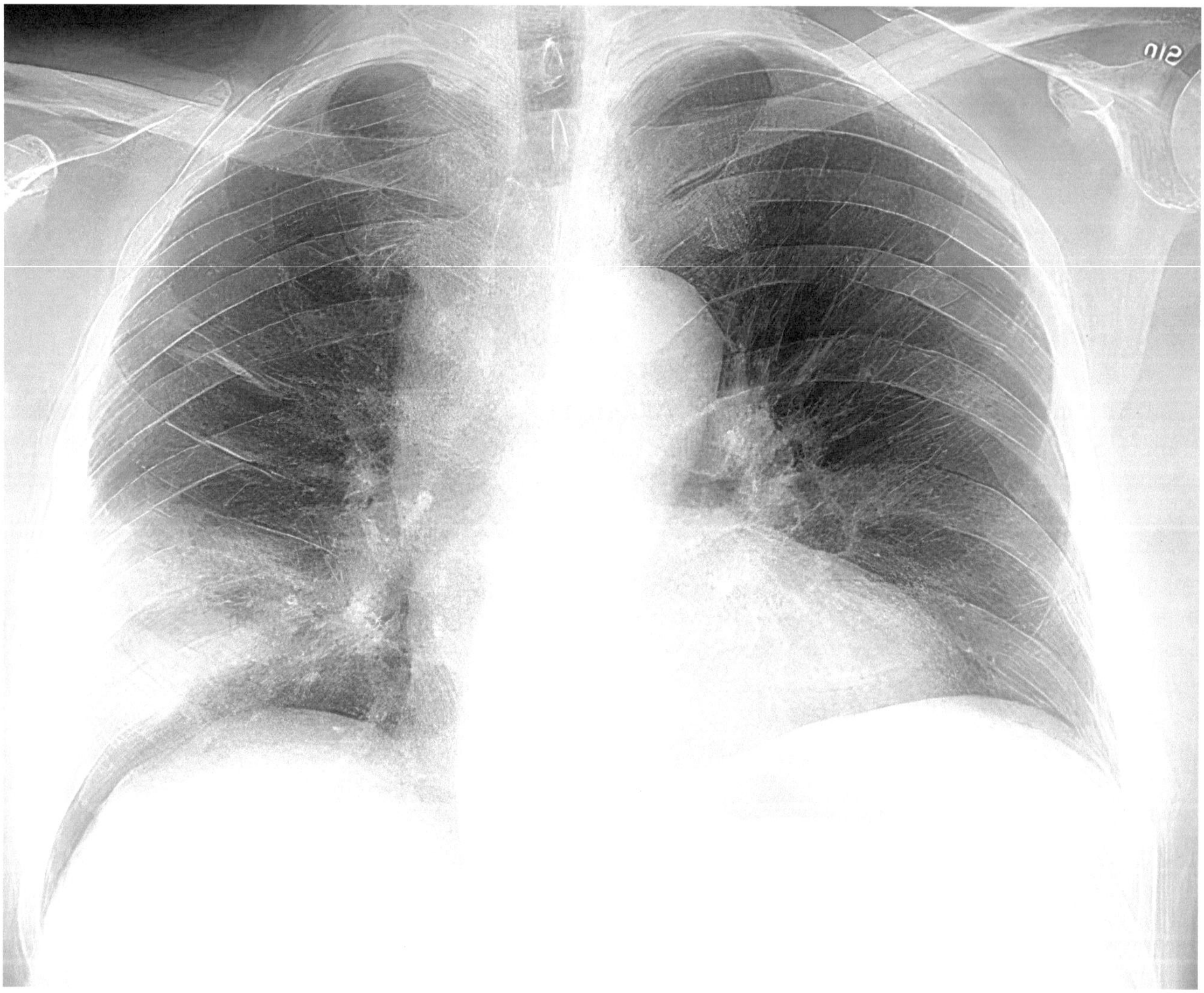

Reassessment

Following 2.5L NS over 90 minutes:

Vitals: BP 82/54 (minimal improvement), HR 124, RR 28, SpO_2 92% on NRB, Repeat lactate 3.8

Patient remains hypotensive with ongoing hypoperfusion despite adequate fluid resuscitation. Persistent septic shock requires vasopressor support.

Escalation of respiratory support to high flow nasal cannula or BIPAP.

Patient Communication

The patient becomes more alert and anxious. His wife arrives and asks about severity, prognosis, why ICU is needed, risks of intubation, and whether he can refuse interventions.

- Address concerns with empathy and clear communication
- Explain the life-threatening nature of septic shock and necessity of ICU-level monitoring

- Discuss potential need for possible future intubation based on respiratory status

Critical Actions

- Recognize septic shock immediately (hypotension, tachycardia, fever, altered mental status)
- Obtain blood cultures prior to antibiotics when possible without delaying treatment
- Initiate empiric antibiotics covering S. pneumoniae and atypical organisms within one hour
- Administer 30 mL/kg isotonic crystalloid and reassess hemodynamic response frequently
- Identify persistent septic shock requiring vasopressor support when hypotension continues despite fluid resuscitation
- Escalation of respiratory support.
- Obtain CXR to confirm pneumonia and identify complications (effusion, multilobar involvement)
- Communicate effectively with patient and family regarding severity, ICU necessity, and rationale for interventions including possible intubation
- Disposition to ICU based on hemodynamic instability and risk of deterioration
- Ongoing reassessment including lactate clearance, urine output, and mental status to guide resuscitation

Cardiac Arrest

Opening Scenario

You are the attending physician in a busy community emergency department. EMS arrives with a 68-year-old male complaining of crushing chest pain. Shortly after placement on the cardiac monitor, the patient becomes unresponsive and pulseless. Following successful resuscitation and return of spontaneous circulation, the patient remains hemodynamically unstable with recurrent ventricular arrhythmias. The patient's wife arrives with documented DNR/DNI advance directives, yet she becomes emotionally distressed and demands that you "do everything possible" to keep him alive, creating immediate conflict regarding treatment goals. The patient remains boarding in your department for over two hours awaiting interventional cardiology availability, requiring continuous reassessment and management of electrolyte disturbances and recurrent dysrhythmias.

Initial Assessment

- Age: 68 years
- Chief Complaint: Crushing substernal chest pain radiating to jaw and left arm
- History of Present Illness: Pain began 90 minutes ago while mowing lawn, associated with nausea, vomiting, and profuse diaphoresis
- Past Medical History: Hypertension, hyperlipidemia, type 2 diabetes mellitus
- Medications: Metformin, lisinopril, atorvastatin, aspirin (81 mg daily)

Vital Signs and Physical Examination

Initial Vital Signs (Pre-Arrest):

- Blood Pressure: 78/52 mmHg
- Heart Rate: 118 beats per minute
- Respiratory Rate: 26 breaths per minute
- Oxygen Saturation: 89 on room air
- T: 36.8°C

Physical Examination:

- General: Severe distress, diaphoretic, pale, clutching chest
- Cardiovascular: Tachycardic, regular rhythm, no murmurs appreciated, delayed capillary refill approximately 4 seconds
- Respiratory: Tachypneic, clear bilateral breath sounds, no accessory muscle use, no wheezes or rales
- Neurological: Alert and oriented, appropriate affect, anxious
- Skin: Cool, clammy extremities with ashen color

Diagnostic Studies

- 12-Lead ECG: Inferior STEMI with reciprocal ST depressions in leads I and aVL; frequent multifocal PVCs noted
- Chest X-ray: Mild pulmonary vascular congestion, cardiomegaly, no infiltrates
- BMP: Na 138, K 3.4, Cl 102, HCO_3 18, BUN 28, Cr 1.3
- Troponin: pending
- Bedside echocardiogram: Inferior wall hypokinesis, estimated EF 35, no pericardial effusion

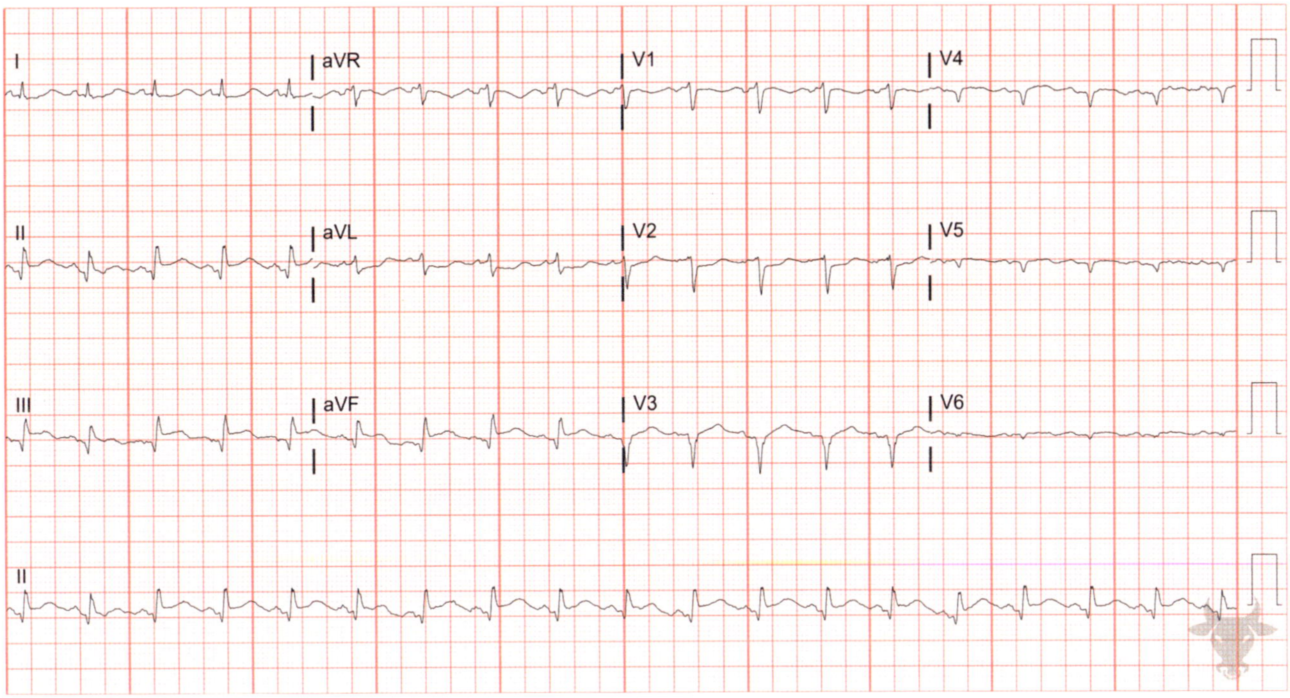

Reassessment

Phase 1: Cardiac Arrest and ACLS Management

- Minutes after arrival, the patient suddenly becomes unresponsive and pulseless. Monitor reveals ventricular fibrillation.
- Monitor reveals ventricular fibrillation (coarse)
- Immediate defibrillation performed at 360 J monophasic (or 200 J biphasic per manufacturer specifications)
- High-quality CPR initiated immediately with compressions at least 2 inches deep and rate of at least 100 per minute
- Compression-to-ventilation ratio maintained at 30:2 with ventilations delivered over 1 second sufficient to produce visible chest rise
- Chest compressions resumed immediately after shock delivery with minimal interruption for rhythm check
- Epinephrine 1 mg IV/IO administered every 3 to 5 minutes
- Amiodarone 300 mg IV/IO given after third defibrillation attempt over 1 minute
- Return of spontaneous circulation achieved after three cycles (6 minutes) with organized narrow complex rhythm at rate 92
- Post ROSC intubation while peripheral vasopressors are infused (if not patient arrests during intubation)

Phase 2: Managing Conflict

- Wife arrives 10 minutes post-ROSC with advance directive paperwork indicating DNR/DNI status signed 6 months prior
- She becomes emotionally distressed and states: “I know he signed those papers but I can’t let him die.”
- Requires empathetic negotiation regarding patient’s documented autonomous wishes versus surrogate decision-maker’s emotional response
- Discussion of prognosis following cardiac arrest with ongoing cardiogenic shock and inferior STEMI
- Exploration of goals of care including potential for temporary interventions versus comfort-focused care

- Addressing wife's need for information regarding what "doing everything" entails versus allowing natural death

Phase 3: Reassessment and Recurrent Deterioration

- Thirty minutes post-ROSC, during ongoing stabilization, patient develops sustained monomorphic ventricular tachycardia with palpable pulse but hypotension (BP 68/40 mmHg, HR 186)
- Patient remains unresponsive from post-anoxic status
- Immediate synchronized cardioversion performed at 100 J biphasic (or monophasic equivalent) with conversion to sinus tachycardia
- Amiodarone 150 mg IV bolus with scheduled infusion following bolus

Phase 4: Extended Boarding and Continuous Reassessment

- Patient remains in ED awaiting cardiac catheterization (cardiology enroute)
- Serial reassessment performed every 15 minutes including:
- Perfusion status and end-tidal CO2 monitoring (target > 20 mmHg to assess CPR quality and ROSC)
- Continuous cardiac monitoring for recurrent ectopy
- Hemodynamic parameters on norepinephrine infusion titrated to maintain MAP > 65 mmHg
- Neurological checks for seizure activity or improving mentation

Critical Actions

- Recognizes ventricular fibrillation as shockable rhythm requiring immediate defibrillation at appropriate energy levels without delay for prolonged pulse checks
- Demonstrates high-quality CPR technique with adequate depth (at least 2 inches), rate (at least 100 compressions per minute), complete chest recoil, and minimal interruptions in compressions for rhythm checks or medication administration
- Administers appropriate ACLS medications in correct sequence and dosing: epinephrine 1 mg IV/IO every 3 to 5 minutes, amiodarone 300 mg IV/IO for pulseless VT/VF followed by 150 mg infusion for recurrent ventricular arrhythmias with pulse
- Navigates conflict between advance directive documentation and surrogate decision-maker's emotional demands using principled negotiation, empathetic acknowledgment of grief, and clear explanation of patient autonomy versus surrogate authority
- Breaks bad news regarding cardiac arrest prognosis and potential outcomes using structured communication framework with attention to setting, invitation, knowledge, emotions, and strategy
- Performs synchronized cardioversion at 200 J biphasic for unstable monomorphic VT with pulse rather than delaying for medication trial
- Prioritizes interventions appropriately during conflicting demands, ensuring airway protection while managing hemodynamic collapse and malignant arrhythmias simultaneously
- Demonstrates understanding that drug timing is less critical than minimizing interruptions in chest compressions during active CPR

Lower Extremity Swelling Postoperative

Opening Scenario

A 52-year-old male arrives by private vehicle with three days of progressive left leg swelling and pain. Triaged to the hallway due to full capacity.

Initial Assessment

Vitals: BP 148/82, HR 96, RR 18, SpO_2 94% RA, T 37.1°C, Wt 95 kg

- Airway: Patent, speaking in full sentences
- Breathing: No respiratory distress, clear bilaterally
- Circulation: Warm skin, cap refill <2 seconds, pulses 2+ bilaterally
- General: Alert, oriented, moderate discomfort; left leg elevated

Immediate actions: Continuous monitoring, peripheral IV, CBC/BMP/coags/D-dimer, lower extremity duplex ultrasound.

History

- HPI: Three days of progressive left calf pain and swelling without trauma. Worsens with walking, improves with elevation. Subjective fever. Left knee arthroscopy ten days prior; eight-hour truck drive four days ago (long-haul driver). Denies chest pain, dyspnea, hemoptysis.
- PMHx: Hypertension, type 2 DM (A1c 7.2), Stage I prostate cancer (Gleason 6, active surveillance), no prior VTE
- Meds: Lisinopril 20 mg daily, metformin 1000 mg BID, apixaban 5 mg BID (missed last three doses due to cost/pharmacy delays)
- Allergies: NKDA

Physical Examination

- General: Alert, oriented, moderate discomfort; resting supine with left leg elevated on family member's jacket
- HEENT: Oropharynx clear, mucous membranes moist
- Cardiovascular: Regular rhythm, no murmurs, rubs, or gallops; peripheral pulses palpable bilaterally (2+ radial, dorsalis pedis)
- Respiratory: Clear to auscultation bilaterally, no wheezes, rales, or rhonchi; symmetric chest expansion
- Abdomen: Soft, non-distended, non-tender, normal active bowel sounds
- Left Lower Extremity: Calf circumference 42 cm (right calf 38 cm), mild pitting edema to ankle, erythema over posterior calf, warmth compared to contralateral side, tenderness to palpation along gastrocnemius and soleus, pain with passive dorsiflexion
- Right Lower Extremity: Normal examination, no edema or erythema
- Neuro: Sensation intact to light touch bilateral lower extremities, strength 5/5 all muscle groups

Diagnostic Studies

- CBC: WBC 9.2, Hgb 14.5, Plt 280
- BMP: Na 140, K 4.2, Cl 102, HCO_3 24, BUN 18, Cr 1.1, Glucose 156
- Coags: PT 12.5, PTT 32, INR 1.0
- D-Dimer: 3,450 (elevated)

- Left LE Duplex Ultrasound: Non-compressible left popliteal and peroneal veins, absent color flow. Acute DVT of the distal left lower extremity.

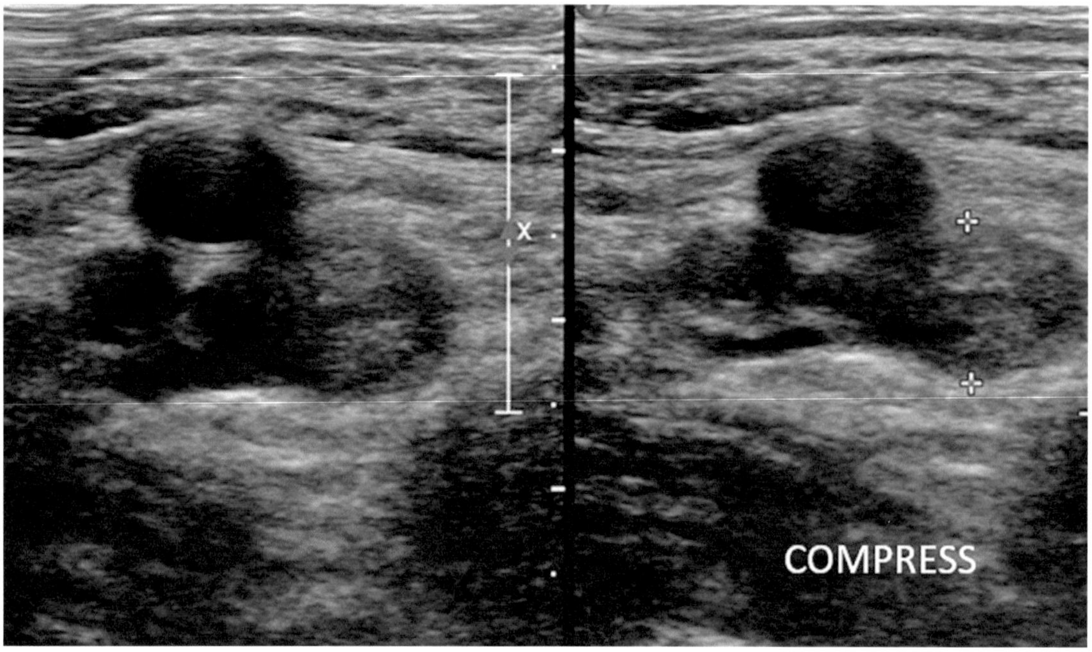

Management

Start subcutaneous enoxaparin 1 mg/kg q12h. Continue monitoring while boarding in ED.

Reassessment

90 minutes later, patient develops sudden left-sided pleuritic chest pain and dyspnea while using the bedside commode.

- New vitals: BP 142/88, HR 118, RR 22, T 37.2°C, SpO_2 89% RA
- Exam: Diaphoretic, tachypneic, decreased breath sounds left base
- CTPA: Acute PE with filling defect in left lower lobe subsegmental pulmonary artery
- ECG: Sinus tachycardia at 118, T wave inversions V1-V2, no S1Q3T3
- Troponin I: 0.08 (elevated), BNP: 280 pg/mL (elevated)

Recognize and presume the new diagnosis of a submassive PE (elevated troponin, tachycardia, no hypotension). Consult pulmonology and discuss possible thrombolysis but acknowledge her most recent arthroscopy.

Patient Communication

Patient anxious about bleeding from anticoagulation given recent knee surgery; asks whether you can stop the enoxaparin and just observe in the hospital instead.

Critical Actions

- Recognize multiple concurrent VTE risk factors (recent surgery, malignancy, prolonged immobilization, missed anticoagulant doses)
- Appropriate diagnostic approach: pre-test probability, D-dimer, duplex ultrasound
- Select weight-based parenteral anticoagulation with renal dose adjustment
- Immediately recognize clinical deterioration; obtain CTPA/ECG for suspected PE
- Risk-stratify PE as submassive; recognize thrombolysis contraindication

- Address adherence barriers and bleeding concerns with patient-centered communication
- Admit for submassive PE

Facial Swelling and Respiratory Distress

Opening Scenario

EMS calls ahead: 58-year-old male with progressive facial swelling, dyspnea at rest, and neck vein distension. Anxious, sitting upright, refusing to lie flat. ETA 10 minutes.

Initial Assessment

Vitals: BP 98/88, HR 112, RR 24, SpO_2 93% RA, T 37.2°C, Wt 82 kg

- Airway: Patent, speaking in short phrases, no stridor
- Breathing: Tachypneic, trachea midline, no cyanosis, supraclavicular fullness bilaterally
- Circulation: Warm, diaphoretic, cap refill <2 seconds, pulses 2+ bilaterally
- General: Anxious, sitting bolt upright, accessory muscle use, prominent JVD visible from across the room

Immediate actions: Continuous monitoring, O_2 2L NC (titrate SpO_2 >92%), large-bore IV in lower extremity (avoid upper extremities), 12-lead ECG, HOB elevated to 45 degrees, difficult airway cart at bedside.

History

- HPI: 58-year-old male with known Stage IIIA adenocarcinoma of the right lung (diagnosed 8 months prior, currently completing cycle 4 of carboplatin/paclitaxel). Reports 2-week progressive facial fullness and dyspnea on exertion, notably worse upon waking and improving after several hours upright. Today developed dyspnea at rest and new facial "tightness." Denies chest pain, hemoptysis, fever, chills, or syncope. No recent long travel or immobilization.
- Past Medical History: Lung adenocarcinoma, hypertension, hyperlipidemia
- Past Surgical History: Mediastinoscopy with lymph node sampling (8 months ago)
- Medications: Carboplatin/paclitaxel (last infusion 10 days ago), lisinopril, atorvastatin
- Allergies: No known drug allergies
- Social History: Former smoker with 30 pack-year history (quit 6 months ago), lives with spouse, works in construction management
- Family History: Non-contributory

Physical Examination

- General: Alert, anxious, uncomfortable but not in acute distress
- HEENT: Periorbital edema present, facial plethora/erythema, pupils equal and reactive, sclera non-icteric, oropharynx clear without edema
- Neck: Marked bilateral jugular venous distension extending to angle of jaw, no tracheal deviation, no palpable thyroid enlargement, no stridor
- Chest: Prominent dilated superficial collateral veins across anterior chest wall (SVC pattern), no deformity or tenderness to palpation
- Lungs: Clear to auscultation bilaterally, good air movement, no wheezes, rales, or rhonchi
- Cardiovascular: Tachycardic, regular rhythm, no murmurs, rubs, or gallops appreciated
- Abdomen: Soft, non-distended, non-tender, no guarding or rebound, no hepatomegaly, normal bowel sounds
- Extremities: 1+ pitting edema bilateral upper extremities, pulses intact, no cyanosis
- Neuro: Cranial nerves II through XII intact, gross motor strength 5/5 bilateral, sensation intact
- Skin: Warm, flushed, venous stasis changes noted on chest wall

Diagnostic Studies

- CBC: WBC 8.2, Hgb 14.8, Hct 44%, Plt 285
- BMP: Na 138, K 3.8, Cl 102, BUN 18, Cr 1.1, Glucose 112
- Coags: PT 11.5, aPTT 32, INR 1.0; D-dimer 850 (elevated)
- ABG: pH 7.46, pCO_2 44, pO_2 78 (RA)
- ECG: Sinus tachycardia, low voltage QRS in limb leads
- CXR: Widened mediastinum, right hilar mass, loss of azygoesophageal recess, prominent azygos vein
- CT Chest with IV Contrast: Large right mediastinal mass encasing and compressing SVC with extensive collateral circulation through azygos/hemiazygos systems

Management

- Position with head elevated to maximize venous drainage
- Gentle diuresis with furosemide 20 mg IV after confirming adequate BP
- Urgent Oncology consultation for admission and definitive therapy coordination
- IR consultation for SVC venography and potential endovascular stenting

Reassessment

20 minutes later: BP 102/84, HR 108, RR 20, SpO_2 98% on 2L NC. Improved dyspnea, speaking in full sentences, facial swelling slightly improved. Patient tearfully asks spouse, "Does this mean the chemo isn't working? Am I dying?" Refuses further interventions until he understands prognosis.

Patient Communication

Patient states: "If my head is filling with blood, does that mean the cancer has spread everywhere? Should I just stop treatment?"

- Acknowledge fear and validate emotional burden of living with cancer
- Explain SVC syndrome as mechanical compression, not necessarily metastatic spread or treatment failure
- Clarify this is a manageable complication; discuss treatment options (stenting, radiation)
- Assess decision-making capacity and desire to involve spouse
- Confirm understanding before proceeding

Critical Actions

- Recognize clinical triad of facial plethora, JVD, and upper extremity edema in a cancer patient as SVC syndrome
- Distinguish from anaphylaxis, angioedema, CHF, and constrictive pericarditis
- Prioritize non-invasive interventions (elevation, O_2) and obtain CT chest with contrast
- Avoid upper extremity IV access, central lines, and tight BP cuffs on arms
- Initiate gentle diuresis; consult Oncology and IR urgently
- Steroids reserved for airway compromise, not routine first-line
- Empathetic communication given patient's progressing malignancy

Headache with Vision Loss

Opening Scenario

A 44-year-old male presents with his spouse reporting severe right-sided headache and neck pain of sudden onset 6 hours ago, with two episodes of transient right eye "foggy vision" lasting 5-10 minutes each. Symptoms began 4 days after a high-speed MVC (restrained driver). Outside hospital cleared acute intracranial injury post-accident but no vascular imaging was performed.

Initial Assessment

Vitals: BP 156/94, HR 82, RR 16, SpO_2 98% RA, T 37.0°C

- Airway: Patent, speaking in full sentences
- Breathing: Non-labored, clear bilaterally
- Circulation: Warm, dry, cap refill <2 seconds, symmetric pulses
- General: Uncomfortable, holding right neck, eyes closed from photophobia, c-collar in place, anxious but alert

Immediate actions: Continuous monitoring, two large-bore IVs, O_2 2L NC, CBC/BMP/coags/type and screen, strict bed rest with c-spine precautions pending imaging.

History

- HPI: Frontal collision 4 days prior (vehicle struck concrete barrier at ~35 mph, seatbelt on, airbags deployed). Minor chest bruising, no LOC. Negative head CT at outside hospital, discharged with analgesics. This morning: sudden severe right temporal headache ("tearing" quality) radiating to right neck and jaw. Two episodes of transient right eye blurred vision, self-resolving. Denies nausea, vomiting, weakness, numbness, dysphasia. Pain 8/10.
- PMHx: Hypertension (poorly controlled), hyperlipidemia; PSHx: appendectomy
- Meds: Lisinopril (intermittent), atorvastatin
- Allergies: NKDA
- Social: Construction supervisor, former smoker (10 pack-years, quit 5 years ago), occasional alcohol
- FHx: Father with stroke at age 60

Physical Examination

- General: Alert and oriented to person, place, time, and situation. Mild distress due to pain.
- Head: Normocephalic, no scalp lacerations or hematomas. Temporal arteries non-tender.
- Eyes: Visual acuity 20/30 right eye, 20/20 left eye. Right upper eyelid ptosis present. Right pupil measured at 3 mm, left pupil at 5 mm in ambient light; both reactive to light and accommodation. Extraocular movements intact. No conjunctival injection. Fundoscopic examination reveals no papilledema or hemorrhages.
- Ears: Tympanic membranes clear bilaterally.
- Nose: No epistaxis or rhinorrhea.
- Neck: Right paraspinal muscle tenderness without midline cervical spine tenderness. A soft systolic bruit auscultated over the right carotid artery at the level of the thyroid cartilage. No jugular venous distension. Cervical collar in place.
- Cardiovascular: Regular rate and rhythm, no murmurs, rubs, or gallops. Peripheral pulses symmetric.
- Pulmonary: Clear to auscultation bilaterally, no wheezes, rales, or rhonchi.
- Abdomen: Soft, non-distended, non-tender, normal bowel sounds.

- Neurological: Alert, oriented. Cranial nerves II-XII intact except as noted with right Horner's syndrome (ptosis and miosis without anhidrosis). Motor strength 5/5 bilateral upper and lower extremities. Sensation intact to light touch and proprioception bilaterally. Finger-to-nose testing normal. Deep tendon reflexes 2+ and symmetric. Babinski sign negative bilaterally. Gait not tested due to cervical precautions.

Diagnostic Studies

- CBC: WBC 7.2, Hgb 14.8, Hct 43.2%, Plt 285
- BMP: Na 140, K 4.1, Cl 102, HCO_3 26, BUN 14, Cr 1.0, Glucose 112
- Coags: PT 12.4, PTT 28, INR 1.0
- ECG: Sinus rhythm at 82, normal intervals, no ST changes
- CT Brain (non-contrast): No hemorrhage, no midline shift. Hypodensity in right insular cortex and basal ganglia concerning for acute ischemic infarct.
- CTA Neck/Head: Intimal flap in right ICA from carotid bulb to petrous segment consistent with arterial dissection. Severe stenosis (>70) with diminished distal flow. No aneurysm or pseudoaneurysm.

Management

- Fentanyl 50 mcg IV for analgesia (avoid NSAIDs given suspected vascular pathology)
- Maintain c-spine immobilization
- Emergent neurology consultation for suspected cervical artery dissection
- Initiate weight-based unfractionated heparin infusion (bolus 80 units/kg, then 18 units/kg/hr) without thrombolytics. Do not give heparin if imaging shows intracranial extension or SAH.
- Vascular surgery consultation for possible endovascular stenting if medical therapy fails

Reassessment

45 minutes later, while awaiting radiology transport, patient reports headache now 10/10. New findings:

- Dysarthria and word-finding difficulty
- New left-sided facial droop
- Left arm drift
- BP 188/102 despite analgesia

Immediate neurologic reassessment required. Consider acute ischemic stroke versus hemorrhagic conversion; prepare for anticoagulation or neurosurgical intervention based on imaging.

Patient Communication

Discuss findings with patient and spouse: the neck injury from the accident tore the inner lining of the carotid artery, creating a flap blocking blood flow to the brain. Address concerns about anticoagulation after trauma; the greater immediate danger is stroke progression without treatment. Obtain informed consent for heparin.

Disposition

ICU admission for frequent neuro checks, BP control (goal SBP <140), monitoring for hemorrhagic transformation. Neurology admits to stroke service.

Critical Actions

- Recognize partial Horner's syndrome (ptosis, miosis without anhidrosis) plus recent neck trauma as pathognomonic for carotid artery dissection
- Prioritize neurovascular imaging (CTA/MRA) over simple c-spine radiographs
- Perform serial neurologic exams recognizing dynamic nature of dissection-related ischemia

- Obtain non-contrast head CT to exclude hemorrhage before initiating anticoagulation
- Communicate diagnosis balancing urgency of anticoagulation with patient anxiety about bleeding
- Initiate heparin for extracranial dissection without SAH; thrombolytics contraindicated
- Arrange neurology consultation and ICU admission

Syncope

Opening Scenario

A 67-year-old woman is brought by EMS after a witnessed syncopal episode at home 30 minutes ago. Reports feeling faint and weak for 48 hours. Husband present, anxious. Patient immediately expresses concern about cost, stating she lost insurance two months ago.

Initial Assessment

Vitals: BP 88/52 (MAP 64), HR 38, RR 18, SpO_2 97% RA, T 36.8°C

- General: Pale, lethargic but arousable, no respiratory distress
- Cardiovascular: Bradycardic, regular, no murmurs; well-healed left infraclavicular scar consistent with prior device implantation
- Extremities: Cool bilaterally, cap refill ~3 seconds, thready pulses, no edema

Immediate actions: Two large-bore IVs, continuous cardiac monitoring, transcutaneous pacing pads applied, atropine 0.5 mg IV, ECG/CBC/BMP/troponin/BNP/coags, CXR.

History

- HPI: Progressive fatigue and intermittent dizziness over two days. Brief LOC this morning (~30 seconds). Denies chest pain, palpitations, dyspnea, diaphoresis, headache, seizure activity, incontinence, or tongue biting.
- PMHx: Hypertension, type 2 DM, complete heart block s/p dual-chamber pacemaker (2 years prior), cholecystectomy
- Meds: Unable to afford lisinopril and metformin for 3 months; uncertain about cardiac meds/ anticoagulation
- Allergies: Penicillin (rash)
- Social: Lives with husband, retired teacher, uninsured, no tobacco/alcohol/substance use

Physical Examination

- General: Elderly female, pale, lethargic but arousable
- HEENT: PERRL, dry mucous membranes, no JVD
- Cardiovascular: Bradycardic, regular rhythm, no murmurs; left infraclavicular pacemaker scar
- Lungs: Clear bilaterally, symmetric
- Abdomen: Soft, non-tender, non-distended, no pulsatile masses
- Extremities: Cool, cap refill 3 seconds, no edema, thready pulses
- Neuro: A&Ox3, CN II-XII intact, no focal deficits, no meningeal signs

Diagnostic Studies

- CBC: WBC 7.2, Hgb 11.2, Hct 34.1%, Plt 245
- BMP: Na 141, K 4.1, Cl 103, HCO_3 24, BUN 22, Cr 1.4, Glucose 156
- Troponin I: <0.02; BNP: 145
- Coags: INR 0.9, PTT 32
- CXR: Cardiomegaly, left-sided pacemaker with intact-appearing leads, no pneumothorax
- ECG: Sinus bradycardia at 32 bpm, pacing spikes without evidence of capture, regular narrow complex

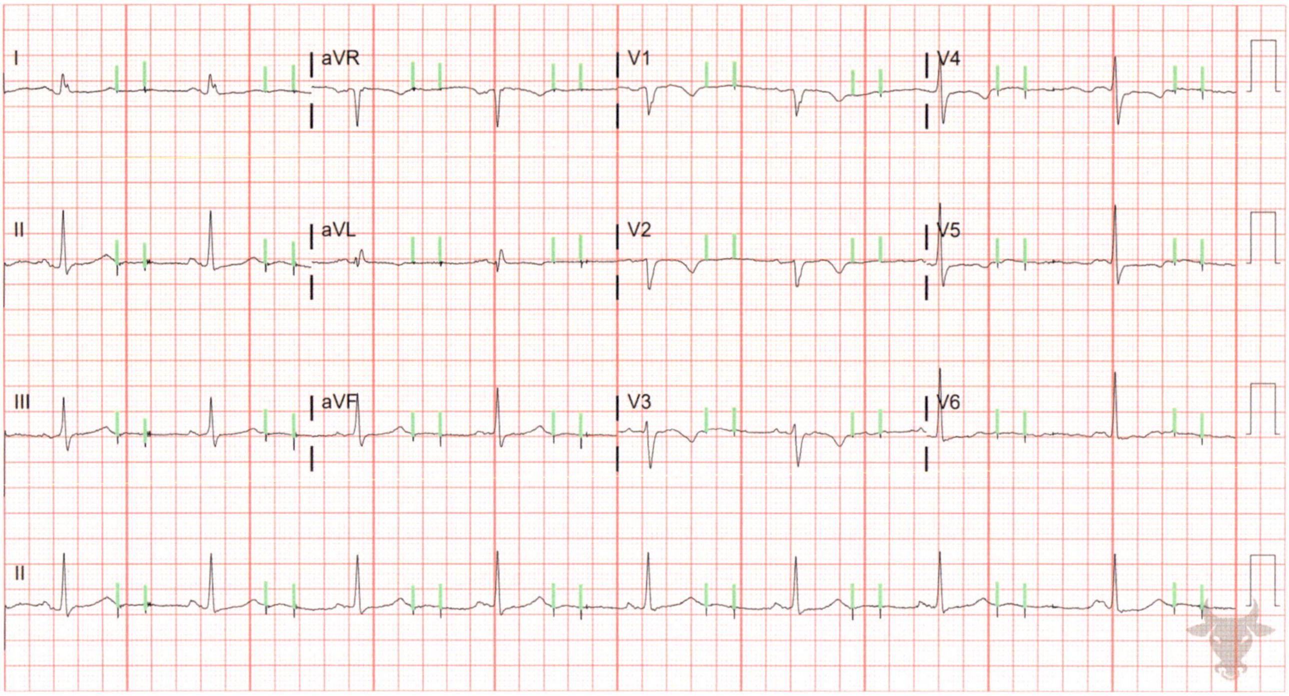

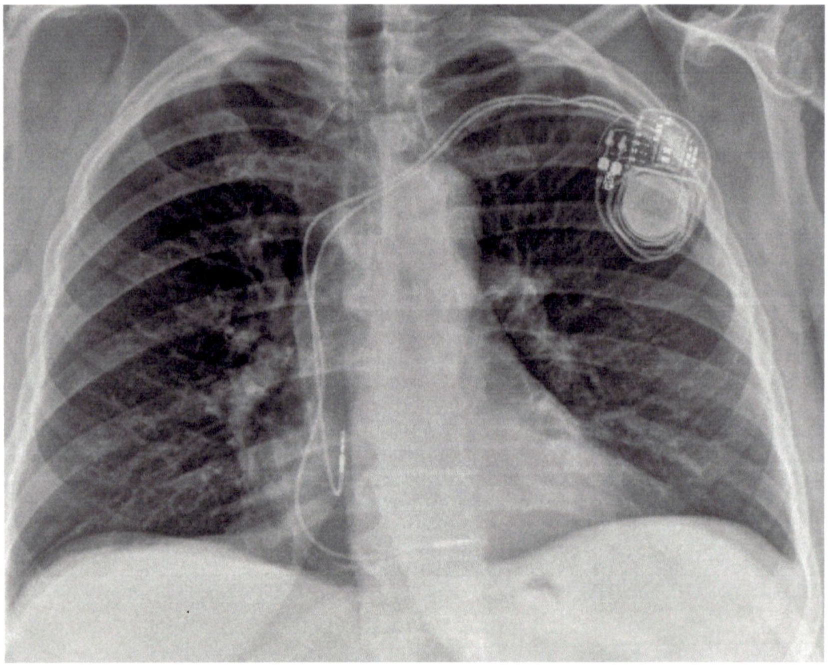

Management

- Atropine 0.5 mg IV: minimal heart rate response
- Patient initially refuses transcutaneous pacing due to possibility of pain and is also very concerned about the financial impact of this hospital stay. Address barriers with empathy while emphasizing life-threatening nature of condition; discuss charity care and hospital financial assistance. Also administer pain medication and discuss anxiolysis with benzodiazepines administration while pacing.
- Following counseling and consent, initiate transcutaneous pacing at 70 bpm with confirmed electrical and mechanical capture
- Urgent cardiology consultation for device interrogation and temporary transvenous pacing

Reassessment

30 minutes after transcutaneous pacing and fluid resuscitation: BP 102/68, warm extremities, cap refill <2 seconds, dizziness resolved. Remains on external pacing pending cardiology.

Critical Actions

- Recognize pacemaker on chest exam and identify symptomatic bradycardia with hemodynamic compromise
- Administer atropine per ACLS while preparing transcutaneous pacing
- Address insurance/financial barriers with empathy while emphasizing medical necessity; explore charity care
- Apply transcutaneous pacing; verify both electrical and mechanical capture
- Apply magnet to differentiate failure modes from battery depletion/lead fracture
- Urgent cardiology consultation for device interrogation
- Reassess vitals, perfusion, and mentation after interventions
- Discuss medication adherence and outpatient follow-up despite financial constraints

Alcohol Intoxication

Opening Scenario

A 52-year-old male with known alcohol use disorder is brought in by his sister, who found him confused and unsteady at home this morning. Sister waiting to speak with you. EMS witnessed a brief shaking episode (~30 seconds) at scene.

Initial Assessment

Vitals: BP 138/84, HR 94, RR 18, SpO_2 97% RA, T 36.9°C, Wt 74 kg

- Airway: Patent, speaking incoherently but protecting airway
- Breathing: No distress, clear bilaterally
- Circulation: Pale, warm, pulses equal bilaterally
- Disability: GCS 13 (E3 V4 M6), PERRL
- General: Disheveled, urine-soaked clothing, confused to time and place

Immediate actions: O_2 via NC, two large-bore IVs, POC glucose (78), thiamine 100 mg IV, D50 25 g IV push, naloxone 0.4 mg IV (no response).

Diagnostic Studies

- CBC: WBC 6.2, Hgb 13.8, Plt 185
- BMP: Na 115, K 3.0, Cl 80, HCO_3 25, BUN 14, Cr 0.8, Glucose 82
- LFTs: AST 75, ALT 48, Alk Phos 165, T Bili 1.1, Albumin 3.8
- Coags: PT 12.8, INR 1.0
- Ethanol: 108; Serum Osmolality: 262 mOsm/kg; Urine Osmolality: 58 mOsm/kg
- Urine tox screen: Negative; Ammonia: 28 μmol/L (normal)
- ECG: Sinus rhythm at 94, normal intervals, no QTc prolongation
- CXR: Clear, no aspiration
- CT Head (non-contrast): No hemorrhage, no mass effect, mild sulcal effacement suggestive of cerebral edema

Patient Communication

Sister expresses frustration, states he has been hospitalized twice for "being drunk," asks if he can receive fluids and "go home to sleep it off." Explain that AMS is out of proportion to ethanol level, indicating dangerous metabolic derangement – not simple intoxication.

Reassessment

While discussing with sister, patient develops GTC seizure lasting ~90 seconds. Post-ictal GCS 10 (E2 V2 M6).

- Repeat vitals: BP 148/92, HR 112, RR 22, SpO_2 96% on NC
- Repeat sodium: 114

Management

- 3% Hypertonic saline 100 mL IV bolus (may repeat up to 3 times; goal: raise Na by 2-3 acutely)
- Continuous cardiac monitoring for QTc
- Strict I&O monitoring
- Neurosurgery consultation for cerebral edema

- ICU admission; nephrology consultation

After 3 hours: Repeat Na 118 (correcting ~1/hr). Patient alert to person and place, follows commands, no further seizures, no focal deficits. Limit total correction to 6-8 in first 24 hours to prevent osmotic demyelination.

Critical Actions

- Recognize AMS out of proportion to ethanol level, indicating metabolic cause beyond intoxication
- Identify severe hypo-osmolar hyponatremia (Na 115, Osm 262) as cause of cerebral edema and seizure
- Distinguish beer potomania from SIADH by low solute intake pattern with low urine osmolality (58 mOsm/kg)
- Treat seizure with 3% hypertonic saline; limit correction to 6-8 in 24 hours to prevent osmotic demyelination
- Reassess electrolytes every 2-4 hours to avoid over-correction
- Admit to ICU for controlled sodium correction and neurologic monitoring

Constipation in an Elderly Patient

Opening Scenario

A 72-year-old female is brought in by her daughter with one week of progressive confusion, refusal to eat, and severe constipation despite OTC laxatives. This morning, found attempting to leave the house dressed inappropriately and speaking to her deceased husband. Requires ADL assistance.

Initial Assessment

Vitals: BP 166/92, HR 56, RR 18, SpO_2 95% RA, T 98.6°F

- Airway: Patent, speaking but confused
- Breathing: No distress, breath sounds present bilaterally
- Circulation: Warm, dry, cap refill ~3 seconds, bradycardic pulses, no edema

History

- HPI: One week of progressive lethargy and confusion (disorientation, visual hallucinations of deceased relatives, decreased oral intake). Constipation for five days despite laxatives. Diffuse bony pain (lower back and hips), polyuria, polydipsia. Increasing weakness requiring assistance to ambulate for three days.
- PMHx: Hypertension, osteoporosis, osteoarthritis; PSHx: total hysterectomy (age 45)
- Meds: Hydrochlorothiazide, calcium carbonate with vitamin D, acetaminophen PRN, multivitamin
- Allergies: NKDA
- Social: Former smoker (30 pack-years, quit 10 years ago), lives with daughter, retired teacher, no alcohol/drugs
- FHx: Mother with breast cancer, father with lung cancer

Physical Examination

- General: Cachectic, disheveled elderly female, oriented only to self, attempting to remove hospital gown
- Head: Normocephalic, atraumatic, dry mucous membranes
- Eyes: Extraocular movements intact, pupils equal and reactive to light, conjunctivae pale
- Ears: Normal tympanic membranes, no cerumen impaction
- Neck: Full range of motion, no jugular venous distension, no thyromegaly, no cervical lymphadenopathy
- Cardiovascular: Regular bradycardia at 56 bpm, no murmurs, rubs, or gallops appreciated
- Lungs: Clear to auscultation bilaterally, breath sounds somewhat distant, no wheezes or crackles
- Abdomen: Distended, hypoactive bowel sounds, soft with diffuse mild tenderness to palpation particularly in the lower quadrants, no rebound tenderness or guarding, no palpable masses
- Musculoskeletal: Generalized muscle weakness, tenderness to palpation over the thoracic and lumbar spine as well as bilateral rib cages, no joint swelling or deformities
- Neurological: Confused and agitated, inappropriate responses to orientation questions, cranial nerves II-XII intact, motor strength 4/5 in lower extremities and 5/5 in upper extremities, sensation intact to light touch, normal gait not tested due to weakness
- Skin: Warm, dry, poor skin turgor with tenting, no rashes or lesions

Diagnostic Studies

- CBC: WBC 7.1, Hgb 10.8, Hct 33%, Plt 295

- BMP: Na 139, K 2.8, Cl 104, HCO_3 26, BUN 32, Cr 2.3, Glucose 92
- Calcium: Total 14.2, Ionized 1.85; Mg 0.6; Phos 1.8; Albumin 2.8
- Alk Phos 145, Lipase 28, T Bili 0.7
- ECG: Sinus bradycardia at 56, shortened QTc (380 ms), widened T waves, no ST changes
- CXR: Left upper lobe spiculated mass ~3.5 cm with hilar lymphadenopathy and possible left pleural effusion

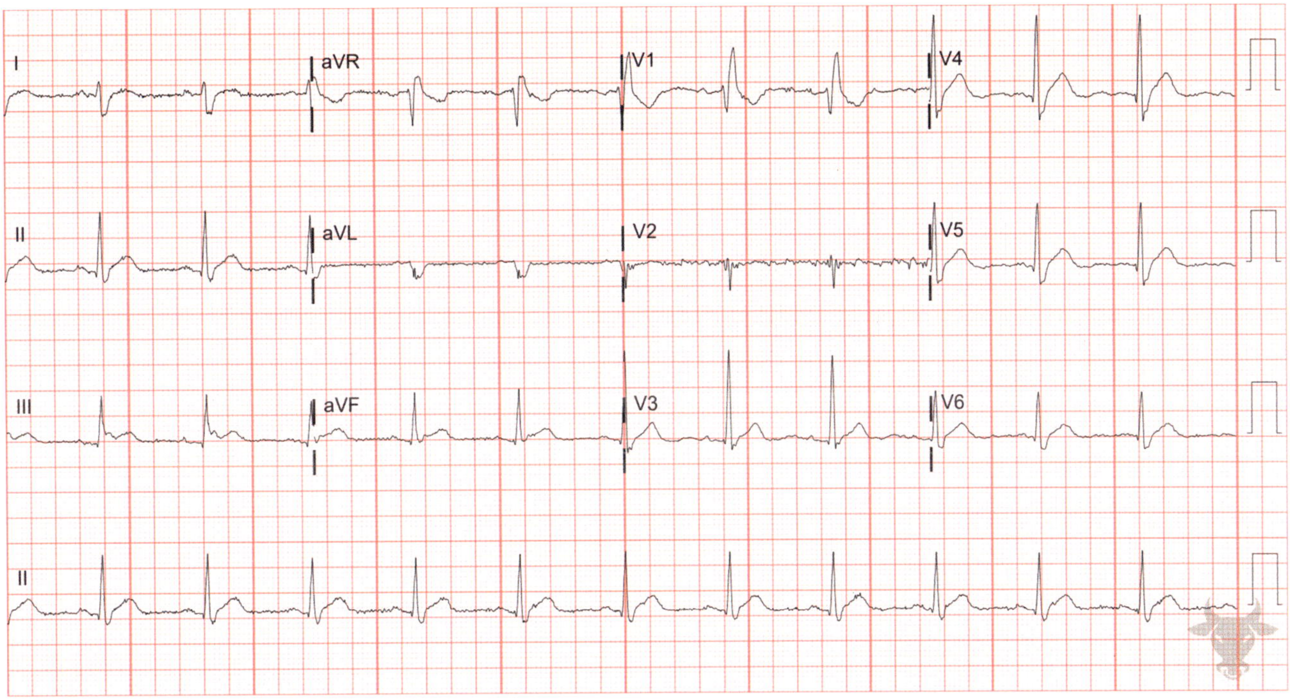

Management

- Aggressive IV NS resuscitation to restore volume and promote calciuresis
- Avoid loop diuretics until adequate hydration and urine output established
- Bisphosphonate therapy (zoledronic acid 4 mg IV or pamidronate 90 mg IV) only after hydration and UOP confirmed
- Consider calcitonin if neurologic symptoms worsen or cardiac instability
- Potassium and magnesium repletion
- Continuous telemetry

Reassessment

After 2L NS over 2 hours: BP 152/84, HR 64, UOP 100 mL/hr. Patient oriented to place, recognizes daughter. At 4 hours: Repeat Ca 11.0. A&Ox3, no hallucinations, conversing appropriately. QTc normalizing to 420 ms. Pain improved 7/10 to 3/10.

Patient Communication

Meet with daughter privately:

- Explain confusion and hallucinations are reversible manifestations of severe hypercalcemia, not dementia
- Discuss CXR findings suggestive of malignancy with sensitivity; validate daughter's decision to bring patient today
- Explain need for ICU admission, oncology consultation, goals of care and code status discussion

- Prepare family for likely need for SNF given functional decline

Disposition

ICU admission for bisphosphonate infusion, cardiac monitoring, oncology consultation, possible thoracentesis.

Critical Actions

- Recognize classic hypercalcemia presentation ("stones, bones, moans, groans") in setting of malignancy
- Prioritize aggressive IV NS resuscitation before other therapies
- Interpret shortened QTc as pathognomonic for hypercalcemia
- Identify pulmonary mass as likely source of paraneoplastic hypercalcemia (PTHrP, squamous cell)
- Order ionized calcium to confirm true hypercalcemia in hypoalbuminemia
- Add bisphosphonate only after adequate hydration/urine output
- Empathetic communication with caregiver about reversible delirium and new malignancy
- Admit to ICU regardless of initial stabilization; monitor for treatment complications

Arm Pain in a Child

Opening Scenario

A 3-year-old boy is sitting on his mother's lap, cradling his left arm close to his chest. His brother was swinging him by the arms at the playground twenty minutes ago, and now he refuses to move his arm and screams when it is touched.

Initial Assessment

Vitals: BP 88/52, HR 122, RR 26, T 37.4°C, SpO_2 100% RA, Weight 15 kg

Chief complaint: Acute left arm pain and refusal to move the arm following playground play.

History

- Child was in his usual state of health this morning with normal activity level
- While at the playground, the patient's 7-year-old brother lifted him by the wrists and swung him in a circular motion between two children
- The patient immediately cried out and ceased playing, refusing to use the left arm
- No witnessed falls, direct blows to the elbow, or axial loading injuries occurred
- No associated fever, vomiting, or recent upper respiratory illness
- No prior episodes of similar arm pain or injury
- PMHx: Full-term vaginal delivery, mild atopic dermatitis. No prior orthopedic injuries or surgeries.
- Medications: Hydrocortisone cream PRN for eczema
- Allergies: Amoxicillin (urticarial rash)
- Social: Lives with both parents and one older sibling. Immunizations current for age.

Physical Examination

- General: Alert and interactive when undisturbed, crying intensely when left arm is manipulated, sitting with left elbow held in approximately 20 degrees of flexion and forearm pronated against his body
- Airway: Patent, phonating appropriately with vigorous crying
- Breathing: No increased work of breathing, symmetric chest rise, lungs clear to auscultation bilaterally, no cyanosis
- Circulation: Radial pulses equal and strong bilaterally, capillary refill less than 2 seconds in all extremities, warm and well-perfused distal extremities
- Head, Eyes, Ears, Nose, and Throat: Pupils equal, round, and reactive to light; moist oral mucosa; oropharynx clear without erythema; tympanic membranes translucent without bulging or erythema bilaterally; no scalp hematomas or lacerations
- Neck: Supple, no midline cervical spine tenderness, no lymphadenopathy
- Chest and Cardiovascular: No chest wall tenderness or bruising, normal heart sounds without murmurs, rubs, or gallops
- Abdomen: Soft and non-tender, no distention or bruising
- Extremities:
- Left upper extremity held in guarded position with the elbow slightly flexed and the forearm pronated
- No gross deformity, significant swelling, or ecchymosis appreciated
- Localized tenderness over the anterolateral aspect of the radial head
- Passive range of motion full at the shoulder and wrist, but the patient screams with attempted supination or extension of the elbow

- Refuses to use the left hand to grasp objects or reach for toys
- Right upper extremity and bilateral lower extremities demonstrate full range of motion, no tenderness, normal strength, and intact neurovascular status
- Neurologic: Age-appropriate behavior and interaction; sensation intact to light touch in all extremities; grips normally with the right hand; refuses to grasp with the left hand

Diagnostic Studies

- Left elbow radiograph (AP and lateral): No fracture or dislocation; anterior humeral line bisects middle third of capitellum; normal fat pads; no joint effusion; normal bone mineralization for age

Differential: Radial head subluxation (nursemaid's elbow), occult supracondylar fracture, radial head fracture. Normal radiographs support clinical diagnosis of radial head subluxation.

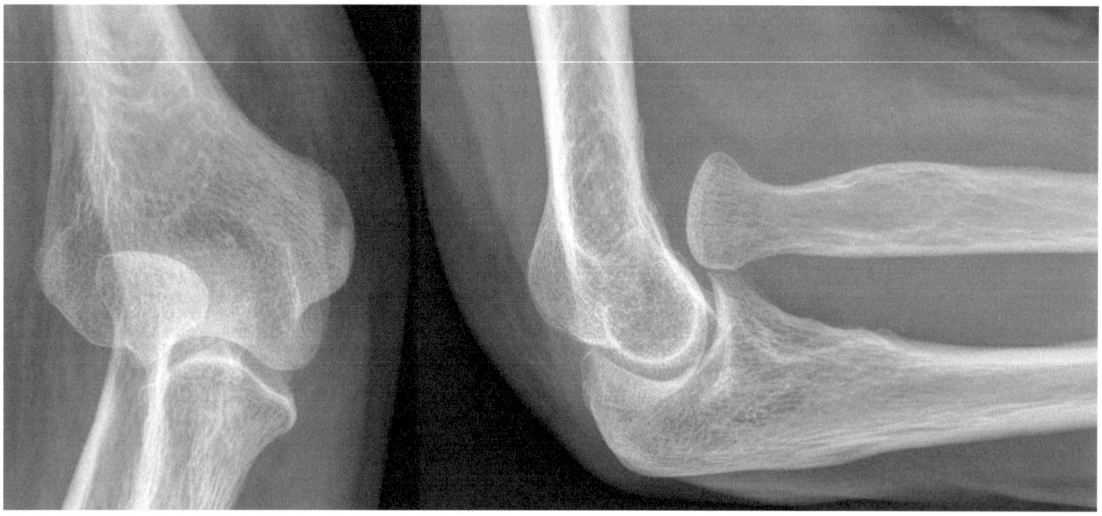

Management

Reduction using either hyperpronation (forearm pronation with pressure over radial head) or supination-flexion method, elbow at 90 degrees of flexion, thumb over radial head for counter-pressure.

Patient Communication

- Explain nursemaid's elbow in clear, non-technical language; normalize as a common toddler injury
- Address mother's guilt by reassuring this is an extremely common mechanism
- Obtain informed consent for reduction: explain steps, expected sensation, and high likelihood of immediate resolution
- Engage the child directly using age-appropriate language and distraction techniques
- Provide discharge instructions with activity restrictions, prevention strategies, and return precautions

Reassessment

- Observe for spontaneous arm use and return of normal ROM within 5-10 minutes post-reduction
- Allow 15-30 minute observation period to confirm sustained recovery

Critical Actions

- Identify radial head subluxation based on classic history (axial traction on pronated forearm) and characteristic positioning (slight flexion, pronation, refusal to supinate)

- Perform appropriate reduction technique and confirm success by documenting normal arm use within 5-10 minutes
- Demonstrate empathy toward mother's concerns while maintaining clinical efficiency
- Provide anticipatory guidance: future occurrences are common and preventable by avoiding traction on child's arms when lifting or playing
- Recognize indications for orthopedic consultation: failure of reduction after two attempts, significant swelling or deformity, neurovascular abnormalities, or suspicion for fracture/infection

Found Down at Home

Opening Scenario

EMS brings in an 89-year-old female found by her daughter on the bedroom floor after failing to answer her phone for 24 hours. She lives alone with hired daily caregiver assistance. Found incontinent of urine and stool with dried feces on sacrum and heels. Confused but able to state her name. EMS started IV and gave 500 mL NS en route.

Initial Assessment

Vitals: BP 112/58, HR 118, RR 14, T 36.4°C (97.5°F), SpO_2 97% RA, Fingerstick glucose 92

- Airway: Patent, speaking in short phrases
- Breathing: No increased work of breathing, clear bilaterally
- Circulation: Tachycardic, weak peripheral pulses, capillary refill 3 seconds, cool extremities
- Disability: Confused to time and situation, moves all extremities, no focal deficits
- Exposure: Cachectic, frail, poor hygiene, malodorous. Sacral and bilateral heel ulcers with necrotic tissue. Ecchymosis in "grab mark" pattern on bilateral upper arms.

Immediate actions: Continuous cardiac monitor and SpO_2, two large-bore IVs, warmed isotonic crystalloid 1L bolus, point-of-care glucose. Labs: CBC, CMP, coags, type and screen, lactate, troponin, CPK, UA. 12-lead ECG. Foley catheter for urine output monitoring. Pressure injury prevention protocol.

History

- HPI: 89-year-old female with moderate dementia and hypertension found down at home for unknown duration. Daughter states hired caregiver was supposed to visit daily but has been "unreliable" recently. Patient unable to provide clear history due to confusion. No witnesses to fall. Unknown last time she ate or drank. Daughter reports patient was "fine" when she visited one week ago.
- PMHx: Dementia (moderate stage), hypertension, osteoarthritis
- PSHx: Right hip replacement (2019)
- Allergies: No known drug allergies
- Medications: Donepezil, amlodipine, acetaminophen as needed (exact list unknown, daughter bringing medication bag from home)
- Social: Widowed, lives alone independently, daughter visits weekly, daily caregiver assistance (supposedly) for meals and hygiene
- FHx: Non-contributory

Physical Examination

- General: Alert, confused to details, cachectic, poor hygiene, strong odor of urine
- HEENT: Sunken eyes, dry mucous membranes, poor dentition, tongue furrowed
- Neck: Supple, no jugular venous distension, no stridor
- Chest: Clear to auscultation bilaterally, no retractions, symmetric expansion
- Cardiovascular: Regular rhythm, tachycardic, no murmurs, rubs, or gallops
- Abdomen: Soft, non-distended, normal bowel sounds, no tenderness, no guarding
- Musculoskeletal: No deformities, full passive range of motion, tenderness to palpation over sacrum and bilateral heels
- Neurological: Confused to time and place, follows simple commands, cranial nerves II through XII grossly intact, strength 4/5 bilateral lower extremities, sensation intact to light touch

- Skin: Stage III decubitus ulcer (4 cm diameter) over sacrum with necrotic base and surrounding erythema, bilateral heel ulcers (Stage II) with eschar, poor skin turgor, multiple fingerprint-pattern ecchymoses on bilateral upper arms consistent with grasping injuries
- Lymph: No lymphadenopathy

Reassessment

After 1L NS bolus (30 minutes): BP 124/72, HR 98, RR 16, SpO_2 98% RA. Foley catheter placed with 80 mL dark amber urine returned. ECG shows sinus tachycardia rate 98, no ST changes, normal intervals. Patient more alert, asking for water. Daughter requesting to speak regarding discharge plans.

After 2L total crystalloid (60 minutes): BP 128/76, HR 88, RR 14, T 36.6°C, SpO_2 98% RA. Mental status improved — oriented to person and place but confused regarding date and events. States she is hungry and thirsty. Urine output 180 mL over the past hour (dark yellow). Repeat POC glucose 110. Skin remains cool, mucous membranes slightly less dry, capillary refill improved to 2 seconds. Patient expresses fear about returning home and mentions the caregiver "hurts my arms when she moves me."

Diagnostic Studies

- CBC: WBC 8.2, Hgb 11.2 (low), Hct 34.8%, Plt 285
- BMP: Na 152 (high), K 4.8, Cl 110, HCO_3 24, BUN 62, Cr 2.4 (elevated), Glucose 108
- Lactate: 2.2 (borderline), CPK: 245 (elevated), Troponin I: <0.04 (negative)
- Urinalysis: SG >1.030, 2+ ketones, trace protein, negative nitrites, negative LE
- ECG: Sinus tachycardia rate 98, no ST changes, normal intervals
- Chest X-ray: No acute infiltrate, mild cardiomegaly, no pulmonary edema
- CT Head (non-contrast): No acute intracranial hemorrhage, age-appropriate atrophy, no mass effect

Difficult Conversations and Managing Conflict

The daughter approaches you in the hallway demanding to take her mother home immediately, stating "she's fine, just needs a good meal and her own bed." She becomes defensive when questioned about the caregiver's absence, stating she "can't afford better help" and "did her best given her own work schedule." She insists her mother has "always been independent" and refuses to consider nursing home placement. You must navigate this conflict while explaining the medical necessity of admission and the mandatory reporting requirements. Additionally, you must speak with the patient regarding her statement about the caregiver causing pain, using appropriate sensitivity given her cognitive impairment.

Disposition

- Schedule repeat BMPs to monitor sodium correction
- Admit to internal medicine service for acute kidney injury, hypernatremic dehydration, and wound care
- Mandatory report to Adult Protective Services regarding suspected elder neglect and possible physical abuse
- Social work consultation for capacity assessment and safe discharge planning
- Wound care consultation for decubitus ulcer management
- Photography of injuries with patient consent for documentation
- Notify hospital risk management regarding potential abuse indicators

Critical Actions

- Recognition of elder neglect and potential physical abuse based on physical findings including hypernatremic dehydration, multiple Stage II-III decubitus ulcers, poor hygiene, and patterned ecchymosis consistent with grasping injuries

- Appropriate initial resuscitation with isotonic crystalloids while monitoring for rapid correction of hypernatremia (no more than 10mEq per day)
- Complete skin examination and documentation of all injuries, including locations and characteristics suggestive of abuse
- Mandatory reporting of suspected elder abuse/neglect to Adult Protective Services as required by state law regardless of family objections
- Reassessment of mental status, vital signs, and urine output after fluid resuscitation to guide ongoing management
- Recognition of acute kidney injury (BUN:Cr ratio >20:1, hypernatremia) secondary to prerenal azotemia from dehydration
- Assessment of decision-making capacity and determination that patient cannot safely return to prior living situation due to medical needs and unsafe environment
- Effective management of conflict with family member using empathetic communication, clear explanation of medical necessity for admission, and firm boundaries regarding discharge to unsafe conditions
- Patient-centered communication with a cognitively impaired patient regarding sensitive allegations of abuse, using simple language and validation of feelings
- Appropriate admission for intravenous antibiotics (if wounds infected), continued hydration, wound care, and social work evaluation rather than discharge to unsafe environment

Fever and Altered Mental Status

Opening Scenario

A 67-year-old male with known decompensated cirrhosis is brought in by his daughter. He has been increasingly confused and febrile over 24 hours with worsening abdominal discomfort. He is irritable, stating he "just wants to go home and sleep."

Initial Assessment

Vitals: BP 88/58, HR 112, RR 20, T 38.9°C (102.0°F), SpO_2 96% RA, Fingerstick glucose 94

- Airway: Patent, speaking in short sentences
- Breathing: No increased work of breathing, clear bilaterally
- Circulation: Tachycardic, hypotensive, weak peripheral pulses, capillary refill ~3 seconds
- Disability: GCS 14 (E4 V4 M6), asterixis present on wrist extension
- Exposure: Cachectic, jaundiced, spider angiomata on chest, palmar erythema

History

The patient is reluctant to provide history, stating "I already told my daughter everything, just fix my stomach ache." He minimizes his symptoms and smells of alcohol despite claiming six months of sobriety.

- History of Present Illness: 67-year-old male with decompensated cirrhosis secondary to alcohol use disorder. Over the past 48 hours, he has developed diffuse abdominal pain described as constant and 7/10 severity, worsened by movement. Associated with fever, rigors, and progressive somnolence. Daughter notes he was difficult to arouse this morning and nearly fell when attempting to walk. Denies vomiting, diarrhea, or hematemesis. No recent travel or sick contacts.
- Past Medical History: Cirrhosis (Child-Pugh Class C), prior hepatic encephalopathy, esophageal varices (banded 2 years ago), chronic kidney disease stage 3, hypertension
- Past Surgical History: Esophageal variceal banding, umbilical hernia repair
- Medications: Lactulose (taking sporadically), rifaximin (non-compliant), furosemide, spironolactone, propranolol
- Allergies: No known drug allergies
- Social History: Lives with daughter. Remote alcohol use disorder (claims last drink 6 months ago), tobacco 20 pack-years (quit 5 years ago), no IV drug use. Currently unemployed.
- Family History: Non-contributory

Physical Examination

- General: Alert, confused, cachectic male in moderate distress, fetor hepaticus present
- HEENT: Scleral icterus, dry mucous membranes, poor dentition
- Cardiovascular: Tachycardic, regular rhythm, no murmurs appreciated, capillary refill 3 seconds peripherally
- Respiratory: Clear to auscultation bilaterally, no wheezes, rales, or rhonchi
- Abdomen: Markedly distended with shifting dullness, diffuse tenderness to palpation without rebound or guarding, positive fluid wave, hepatosplenomegaly appreciated, no abdominal wall ecchymosis, no surgical scars except midline below umbilicus
- Extremities: 2+ pitting edema to mid-shins, no clubbing, no cyanosis
- Neurological: Alert but confused to time and situation, cranial nerves II-XII intact, asterixis present with arm extension, normal motor strength

- Skin: Jaundiced, warm, multiple spider angiomas on upper chest, palmar erythema

Diagnostic Studies

- CBC: WBC 15.5, Hgb 11.2, Hct 33.8%, Plt 95 (low)
- BMP: Na 132, K 4.8, Cl 108, HCO_3 22, BUN 42, Cr 2.8 (elevated), Glucose 94
- LFTs: AST 110, ALT 145, ALP 180, T.Bili 5.8, D.Bili 4.2, Albumin 2.0
- Coags: PT 18.2, INR 1.8, PTT 38
- Lactate: 3.1, Ammonia: 135 (elevated)
- Blood cultures: Drawn prior to antibiotics, pending
- Urinalysis: SG 1.025, trace protein, no WBCs, no nitrites, bilirubin positive
- Bedside Ultrasound: Nodular liver consistent with cirrhosis, massive ascites with particulate matter, no free air, no biliary dilation, plethoric IVC with minimal respiratory variation

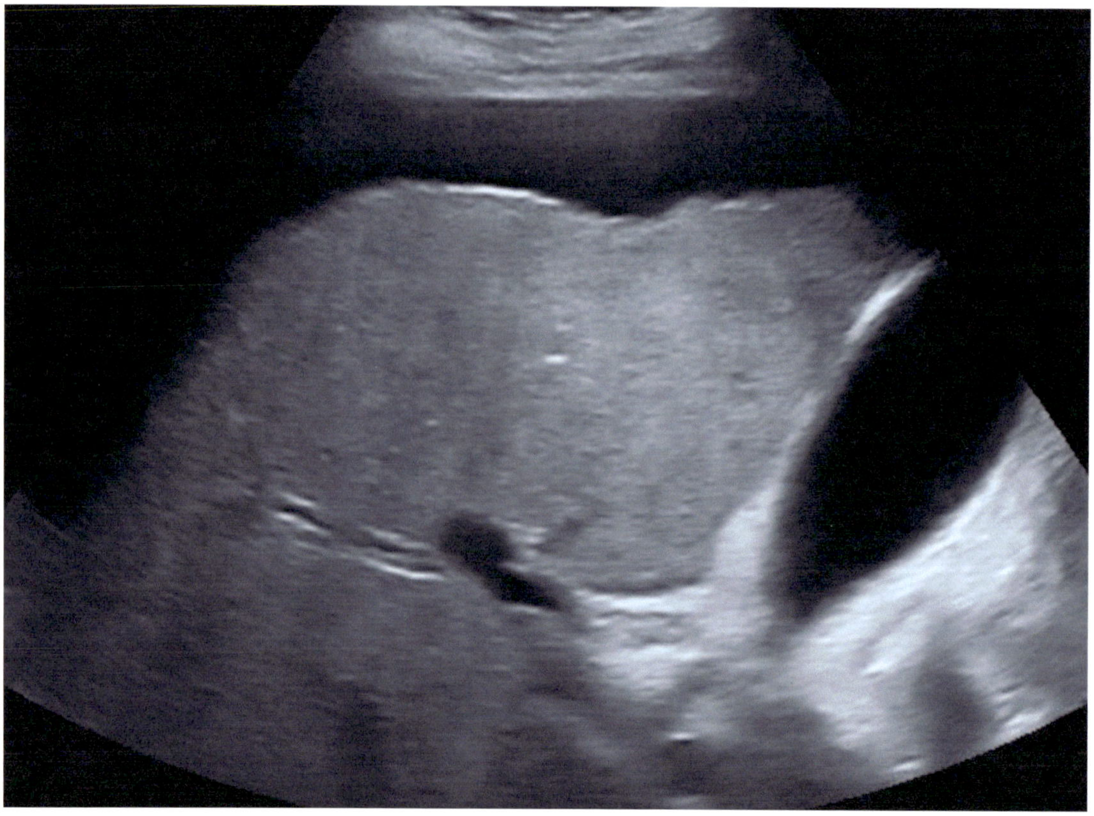

- Chest X-ray: No acute infiltrates, small right pleural effusion, elevated right hemidiaphragm

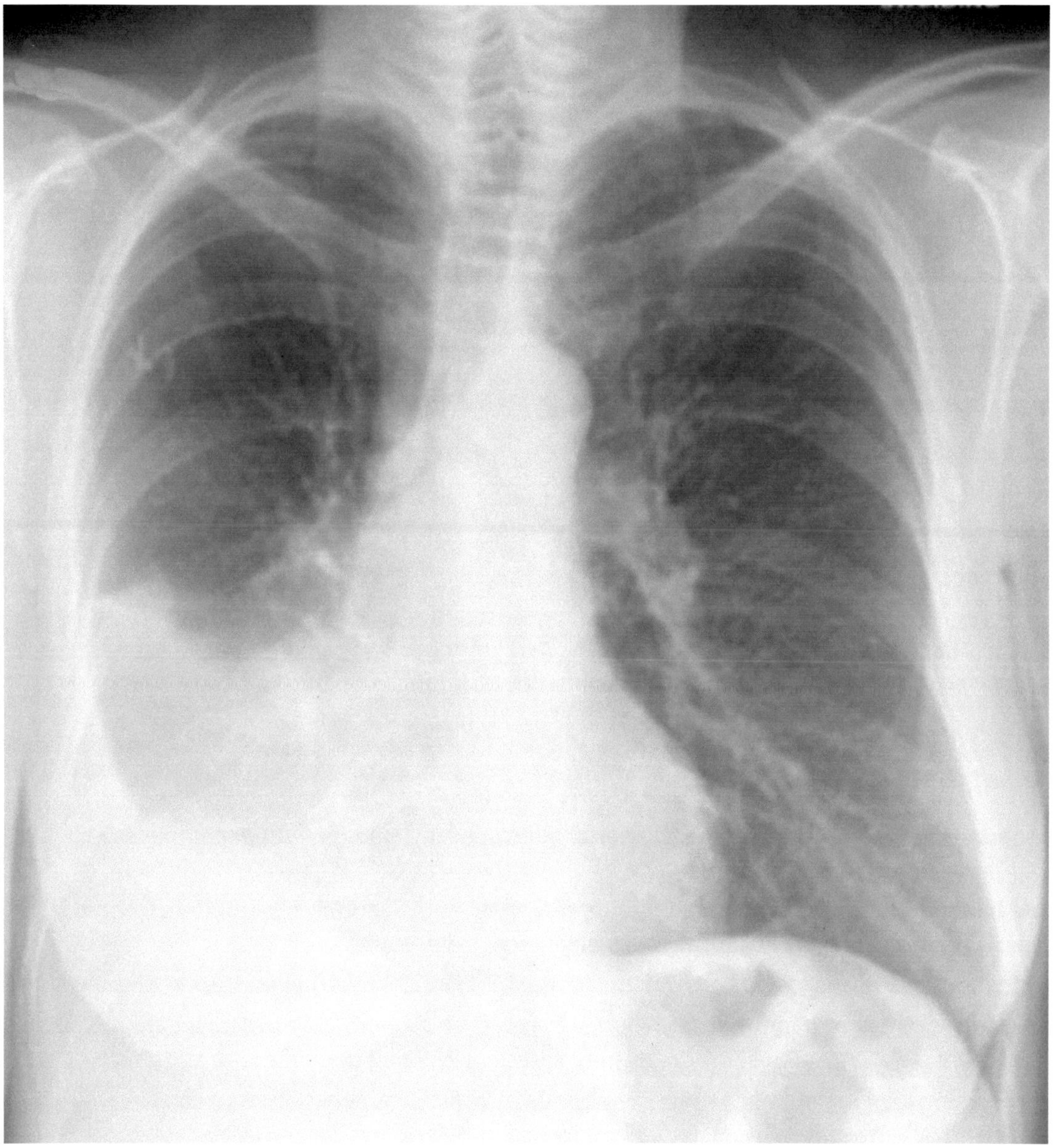

Managing Conflict

The patient attempts to remove his IV line, stating: "I feel fine, just tired. My daughter overreacts to everything. I want to go home now." The daughter insists: "He was almost comatose this morning. If you let him leave, he'll die at home." The patient responds: "It's my life, not yours. I don't want to be here." He refuses further blood draws and asks to sign out AMA. After back and forth with patient and family at bedside, the patient agrees to have antibiotics and stay for management but only if his daughter stays in the room during the procedure.

Management

- Two large-bore peripheral IVs established
- 1L lactated Ringer's bolus
- Blood cultures drawn prior to antibiotics
- Empiric ceftriaxone 2g IV (covering typical SBP organisms)
- Lactulose 30mL orally for encephalopathy
- Diagnostic paracentesis under ultrasound guidance

Paracentesis Results:

- Appearance: Cloudy, straw-colored fluid
- Cell count: 380 nucleated cells/μL with 85 polymorphonuclear leukocytes
- Total protein: 0.6
- SAAG: 1.4
- Gram stain: No organisms seen
- Culture: Pending (inoculated into blood culture bottles at bedside)

Reassessment

Time Elapsed: 90 minutes

Updated Vital Signs:

- Blood Pressure: 102/64 mmHg
- Heart Rate: 98 beats per minute
- Respiratory Rate: 18 breaths per minute
- T: 38.4°C (101.1°F)
- Oxygen Saturation: 98 on room air

Clinical Status: Patient remains mildly confused but is less somnolent and more conversant. Capillary refill improved to 2 seconds. Abdominal pain persists but patient is less guarded. Patient continues to express desire to leave but is less agitated. Daughter reports he seems "more like himself" compared to earlier.

New Information: Blood culture preliminary Gram stain shows gram-negative rods.

Critical Actions

- Recognize sepsis secondary to spontaneous bacterial peritonitis in a patient with decompensated cirrhosis
- Demonstrate immediate resuscitation with IV fluids and early empiric antibiotics (third-generation cephalosporin) without waiting for culture results or paracentesis results
- Obtain diagnostic paracentesis to confirm SBP (ascitic fluid PMN >250 cells/μL) and guide therapy
- Employ patient-centered communication techniques to establish rapport, acknowledge patient's autonomy concerns, and explain the life-threatening nature of SBP and need for admission
- Navigate conflict between patient and family member using principled negotiation to achieve mutual understanding and patient-centered outcome (voluntary admission)
- Reassess hemodynamic and mental status after fluid resuscitation and antibiotic administration, recognizing improvement in perfusion but persistent infection
- Admit to monitored setting for continued IV antibiotics, monitoring for hepatorenal syndrome, and hepatic encephalopathy management
- Recognize that non-compliance with lactulose/rifaximin contributed to encephalopathy presentation without being judgmental
- Consider need for albumin administration to prevent hepatorenal syndrome in high-risk SBP patients
- Ensure appropriate disposition to inpatient service rather than observation or discharge

Massive Hematemesis in a Cirrhotic

Opening Scenario

A 58-year-old male with known alcoholic cirrhosis is brought by EMS after vomiting a large volume of bright red blood at home. His wife called 911 after he filled a mixing bowl with bloody emesis. EMS reports two additional episodes of hematemesis in transit. He is pale, diaphoretic, and confused.

Initial Assessment

Vitals: BP 74/42, HR 132, RR 28, T 36.2°C, SpO_2 94% RA, Fingerstick glucose 68

- Airway: Patent but at risk — ongoing hematemesis, blood pooling in oropharynx
- Breathing: Tachypneic, clear bilaterally
- Circulation: Pale, diaphoretic, cool extremities, cap refill 5 seconds, thready radial pulses
- Disability: GCS 13 (E3, V4, M6), confused and agitated
- Exposure: Jaundiced, spider angiomata on chest, abdominal distension, caput medusae

Immediate actions: Two large-bore IVs (14- or 16-gauge), activate massive transfusion protocol suction at bedside, type and crossmatch, prepare equipment for possible intubation.

History

- HPI: 58-year-old male with known alcoholic cirrhosis (Child-Pugh C, MELD 28) and history of esophageal varices (banded twice, last EGD 8 months ago). He has been non-compliant with nadolol and lactulose for the past 3 weeks after running out of medication. Tonight he developed sudden-onset nausea followed by large-volume hematemesis of bright red blood with clots. Wife estimates total volume >1 liter across three episodes. No melena prior to today. No recent NSAID use, anticoagulants, or alcohol use (sober 6 months per wife). No recent fever, abdominal pain, or illness.
- PMHx: Alcoholic cirrhosis (Child-Pugh C), esophageal varices (grade III), prior variceal banding x2, portal hypertensive gastropathy, ascites, hepatic encephalopathy (prior episodes)
- Meds: Nadolol 40 mg daily (non-compliant), lactulose (non-compliant), spironolactone, furosemide
- Allergies: NKDA
- Social: Former heavy alcohol use (quit 6 months ago per family), no tobacco, lives with wife

Physical Examination

- General: Pale, diaphoretic, confused, actively retching with bloody emesis
- HEENT: Icteric sclerae, blood in oropharynx, dry mucous membranes
- Cardiovascular: Tachycardic, regular rhythm, no murmurs
- Pulmonary: Clear bilaterally, tachypneic
- Abdomen: Distended with ascites, non-tender, no peritoneal signs, caput medusae visible
- Extremities: Cool, pale, trace pedal edema, no clubbing
- Neurologic: Confused, follows simple commands, no focal deficits, mild asterixis

Diagnostic Studies

- CBC: WBC 12.4, Hgb 4.2 (critically low), Plt 62
- BMP: Na 131, K 4.8, Cl 100, HCO_3 18, BUN 48, Cr 2.4 (elevated, likely hepatorenal syndrome or prerenal from hemorrhage), Glucose 68
- INR 2.2, PT 26, PTT 42, Fibrinogen 128 (low)
- Lactate: 6.8 (severely elevated — hemorrhagic shock)

- T.Bili 6.4, AST 88, ALT 52, Albumin 2.1, Ammonia 112
- Type and Screen: O-positive, crossmatch sent
- ABG: pH 7.28, pCO_2 32, pO_2 88, HCO_3 16 (metabolic acidosis with respiratory compensation)

Management

Simultaneous resuscitation and source control:

Resuscitation: - Massive transfusion protocol: Initiate with 2 units pRBCs immediately, followed by 1:1:1 ratio (pRBCs:FFP:platelets). Target Hgb >7 (avoid over-transfusion in varices — excessive volume increases portal pressure and rebleeding risk) - Correct coagulopathy: FFP for INR >1.5 with active bleeding, consider 4-factor PCC if massive hemorrhage; cryoprecipitate if fibrinogen <150 - Calcium replacement with massive transfusion (citrate chelation) - Vasopressors (norepinephrine) if hypotension persists after initial volume resuscitation

Variceal-specific therapy (start immediately, do not wait for endoscopy): - Octreotide 50 mcg IV bolus, then 50 mcg/hour continuous infusion (reduces splanchnic blood flow and portal pressure) - Pantoprazole 80 mg IV bolus, then 8 mg/hour infusion (adjunct, though primary pathology is variceal not ulcer) - Ceftriaxone 1 g IV (prophylactic antibiotics reduce mortality in cirrhotic GI bleeding — SBP develops in up to 20% of variceal hemorrhage episodes) - Erythromycin 250 mg IV (prokinetic to clear gastric blood prior to endoscopy)

Airway protection: - With ongoing hematemesis and altered mental status, this patient requires endotracheal intubation before endoscopy - RSI with hemodynamic-sparing agents: ketamine or etomidate for induction, avoid propofol in hemorrhagic shock - Suction available, large-bore orogastric tube to decompress stomach and evacuate blood

Emergent GI consult for endoscopic variceal band ligation.

Reassessment

30 minutes after MTP activation, intubation, octreotide, and antibiotics:

- 4 units pRBCs, 2 units FFP, 1 unit platelets transfused
- Vitals: BP 92/58 (improved from 74/42), HR 112, SpO_2 98% on ventilator
- OG tube draining dark blood, slowing in volume
- Lactate repeat: 4.2 (improving)
- Repeat Hgb: 8.1

GI arrives for emergent endoscopy. EGD reveals three columns of grade III esophageal varices with active spurting from one varix. Band ligation applied to the actively bleeding varix and two additional varices. Bleeding controlled after banding.

If endoscopy fails or is unavailable: place Blakemore (Sengstaken-Blakemore) tube as temporizing measure. Inflate gastric balloon first (250 mL air, confirm position with X-ray), apply 2 kg traction. Inflate esophageal balloon only if gastric balloon fails to control hemorrhage. Maximum esophageal balloon time: 24 hours (risk of esophageal necrosis). Xray below confirms Blakemore tube insufflation in stomach.

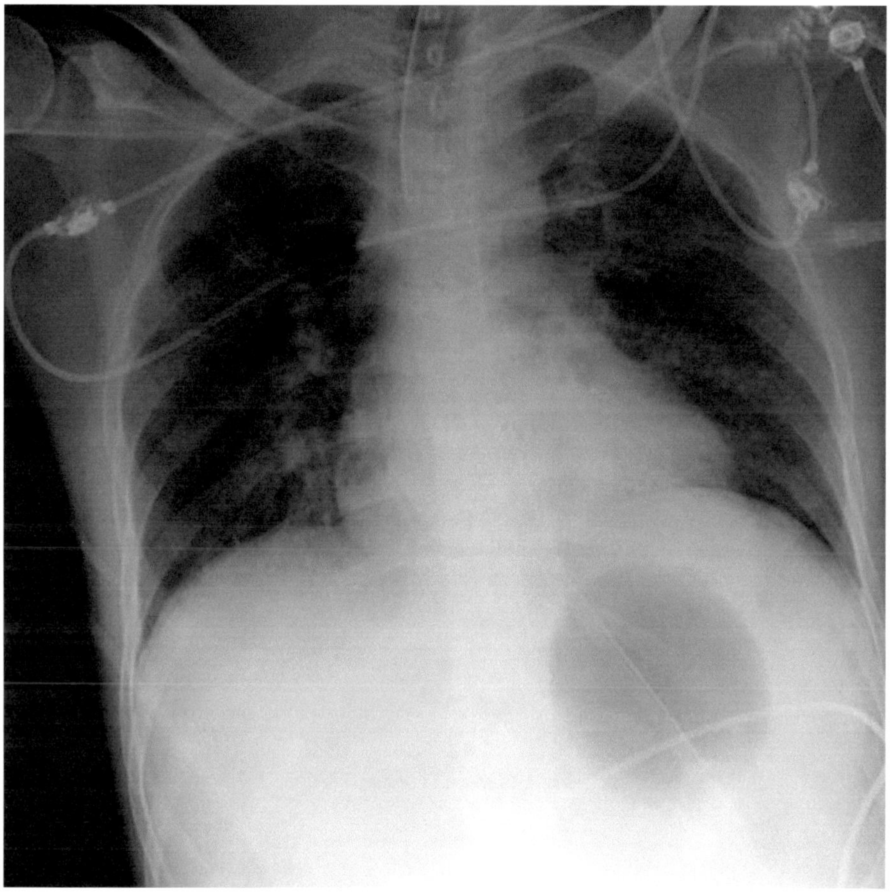

Patient Communication

The patient's wife and adult son arrive. The son states: "We want everything done. Don't give up on him." The wife is crying and asks: "Is he going to die tonight?"

- Acknowledge the severity of the situation honestly: "Your husband is critically ill. He has had a large amount of bleeding from blood vessels in his esophagus related to his liver disease. We are giving him blood transfusions and medication, and the GI specialist is working to stop the bleeding."
- Address the family's request for "everything done" while providing honest prognostication: with advanced cirrhosis (MELD 28), each variceal bleed carries significant mortality (15-20% at 6 weeks). Frame the conversation around goals rather than interventions.
- If the patient stabilizes, discuss the need for ICU admission, potential for rebleeding, and long-term prognosis with advanced liver disease. Introduce the concept of hepatology referral and transplant evaluation if appropriate.
- If the patient is not a transplant candidate, this is an opportunity to discuss realistic goals of care without withdrawing hope. Offer palliative care consult alongside aggressive medical management.

Disposition

- ICU admission on mechanical ventilation

Critical Actions

- Recognize massive upper GI hemorrhage in a cirrhotic as variceal bleeding until proven otherwise and initiate variceal-specific therapy immediately (octreotide, antibiotics)

- Activate massive transfusion protocol for hemorrhagic shock; avoid over-resuscitation (target Hgb 7-8 in variceal bleeding to avoid increasing portal pressure)
- Protect the airway with endotracheal intubation before endoscopy in a patient with ongoing hematemesis and altered mental status
- Administer prophylactic antibiotics (ceftriaxone) — this is a mortality-reducing intervention in cirrhotic GI bleeding, not optional
- Obtain emergent GI consult for endoscopic band ligation as definitive therapy
- Know the rescue pathway: Blakemore tube as temporizing measure if endoscopy unavailable
- Correct coagulopathy with blood products guided by lab values and clinical response
- Navigate a complex goals-of-care conversation with family members who want "everything done" in the setting of advanced liver disease

Hypotension During Dialysis

Opening Scenario

A 58-year-old female with SLE and ESRD is brought from her outpatient dialysis center with acute dyspnea, anxiety, and dizziness that developed during treatment. She became progressively hypotensive over the final 30 minutes of therapy. Arrives with peripheral IV and fluid bolus running.

Initial Assessment

Vitals: BP 84/42, HR 132, RR 24, T 36.8°C, SpO_2 96% RA, Glucose 142

- Airway: Patent, speaking in full sentences
- Breathing: Tachypneic, clear bilaterally, no accessory muscle use, trachea midline
- Circulation: Cool, pale extremities, capillary refill 3 seconds, prominent JVD at 45 degrees
- Anxious, cachectic female with mild respiratory distress

Immediate actions: Continuous cardiac monitoring and SpO_2, two large-bore IVs (16 gauge or larger), 1L NS bolus wide open, 12-lead ECG, supplemental O2 via NC titrated to SpO_2 >94%. Labs: CBC, BMP, coags, type and screen, lactate, troponin.

History

- HPI: Patient was undergoing routine hemodialysis via her left arm AV fistula when she developed sudden anxiety and a sense of impending doom approximately 2.5 hours into her 3-hour session. Progressive shortness of breath and lightheadedness. Dialysis technician observed declining BP and stopped ultrafiltration. Denies chest pain, palpitations, fever, cough, or recent illness. Reports lupus has been "flaring" recently with increased joint pain and fatigue.
- PMHx: SLE (diagnosed 15 years ago), lupus nephritis with progression to ESRD (on hemodialysis 3 years), hypertension, prior acute pericarditis requiring hospitalization (3 years ago), anemia of chronic disease
- Medications: Hydroxychloroquine 200 mg BID, prednisone 10 mg daily, amlodipine 5 mg daily (held today due to low BP), sevelamer 800 mg with meals, aspirin 81 mg daily
- Social: Lives with adult daughter, retired teacher, former smoker (10 pack-years, quit 10 years ago), no alcohol or illicit drugs
- FHx: Autoimmune disease (mother with rheumatoid arthritis)

Physical Examination

- General: Alert and oriented to person, place, and time; anxious affect; mild respiratory distress with tachypnea
- Head: Normocephalic, atraumatic
- Eyes: Extraocular movements intact, pupils equal and reactive to light, no scleral icterus
- Cardiovascular: Tachycardic, regular rhythm, distant heart sounds with muffled S1 and S2, no pericardial rub appreciated, no murmurs; prominent JVD
- Pulmonary: Clear to auscultation bilaterally, no wheezes, rales, or rhonchi; good air entry; no chest wall tenderness
- Abdomen: Soft, non-tender, non-distended, normal bowel sounds; no hepatosplenomegaly appreciated
- Extremities: No peripheral edema; thready radial pulses; AV fistula in left upper extremity with palpable thrill and no signs of infection
- Skin: Faint malar rash across cheeks and nasal bridge; no cyanosis or diaphoresis

- Neurological: Cranial nerves II-XII intact; normal strength and sensation in all extremities; no focal deficits

Reassessment

Nurse reports: "The liter bolus is complete. Blood pressure initially improved to 100/68, but it's trending down again and she's working harder to breathe."

Updated Vital Signs:

- Blood Pressure: 92/58 mmHg (narrow pulse pressure)
- Heart Rate: 124 beats per minute
- Respiratory Rate: 28 breaths per minute
- Oxygen Saturation: 94 on 2 liters nasal cannula

Updated Physical Examination:

- Pulsus paradoxus now clearly present (systolic blood pressure drop >12 mmHg during inspiration)
- Increased jugular venous distension despite sitting upright
- Patient reports worsening dyspnea, describing a sensation of "drowning" or suffocating
- Cool, clammy skin with mottling of extremities

Diagnostic Studies

Bedside Echocardiography (Point-of-Care Ultrasound):

- Large circumferential pericardial effusion present
- Right ventricular diastolic collapse
- Right atrial systolic collapse

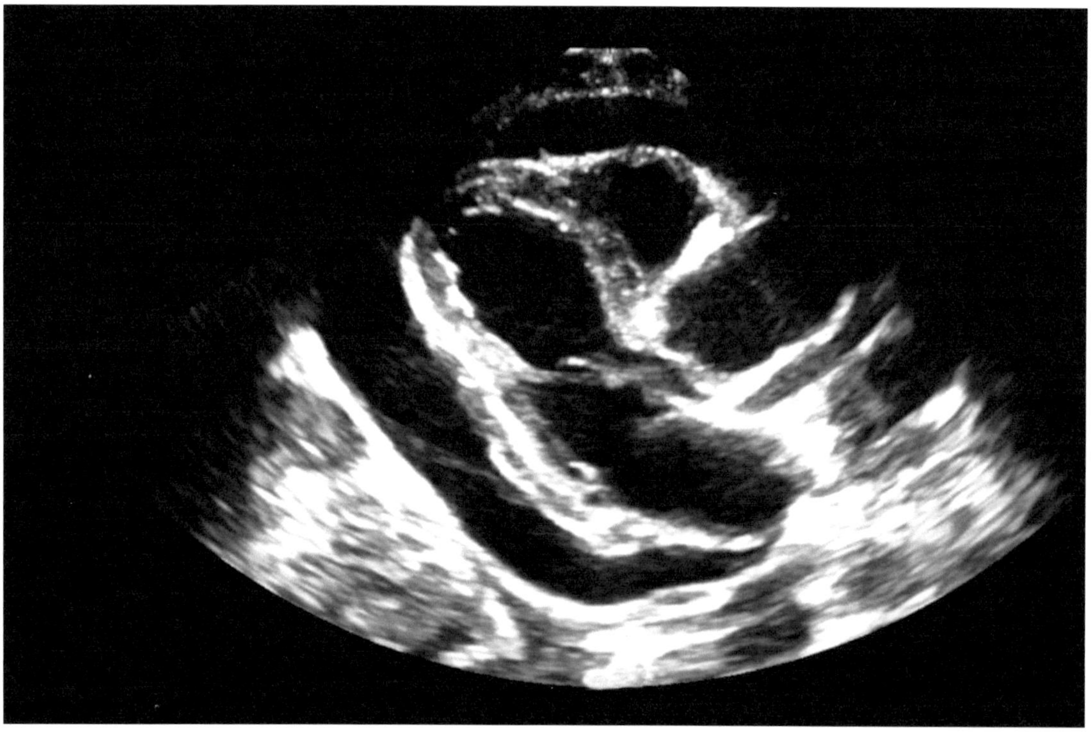

Chest X-Ray:

- Enlarged cardiac silhouette with "water bottle" configuration
- Clear lung fields without evidence of pulmonary edema or effusion

- 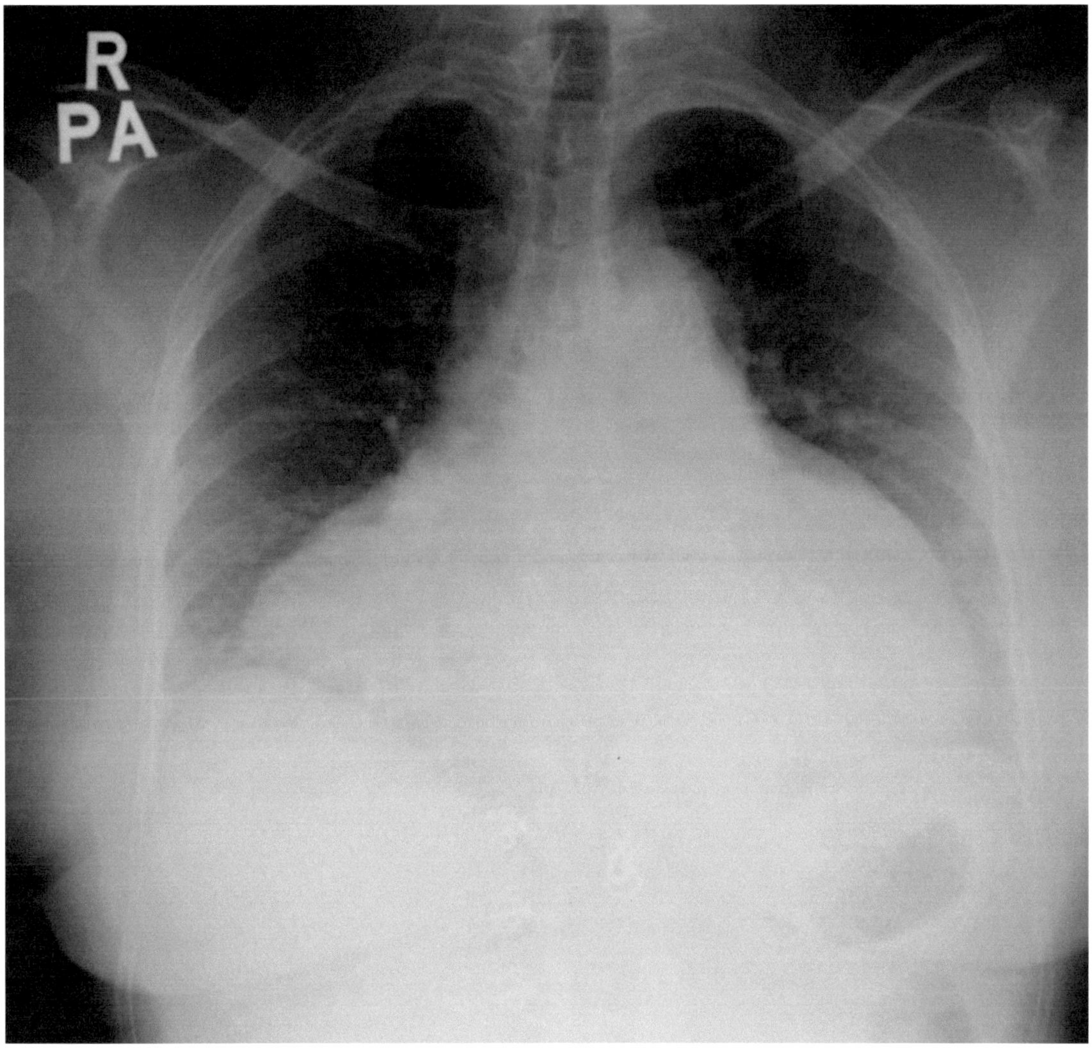

12-Lead ECG:

- Sinus tachycardia at 128 beats per minute
- Low voltage QRS complexes (<5 mm in limb leads)
- Electrical alternans (beat-to-beat variation in QRS amplitude)
- No ST-segment elevation or depression suggesting acute ischemia

Patient Communication

Daughter asks: "Is my mother having a heart attack? She had fluid around her heart before—will she need surgery? Is she going to die?"

Acknowledge anxiety. Explain cardiac tamponade in accessible terms (fluid compressing the heart, preventing proper pumping). Distinguish from myocardial infarction. Explain urgency and need for immediate intervention. Discuss treatment options: emergent pericardiocentesis as temporizing measure vs. definitive surgical pericardial window. Address underlying lupus as the likely cause. Obtain informed consent for emergency procedures.

Reassessment

Nurse reports: "Her pressure is dropping despite the fluids, and she's becoming less responsive."

Updated Vital Signs (15 minutes later):

- Blood Pressure: 68/44 mmHg

- Heart Rate: 142 beats per minute
- Respiratory Rate: 32 breaths per minute
- Oxygen Saturation: 90 on non-rebreather mask
- T: 36.5°C

Clinical Status:

- Altered mental status (drowsy but arousable to painful stimuli)
- Profound pulsus paradoxus (>20 mmHg)
- Mottled extremities with delayed capillary refill
- Patient is unable to speak in full sentences due to respiratory distress

Management

- Emergent bedside pericardiocentesis under ultrasound guidance (subxiphoid approach)
- Cautious fluid resuscitation with 250 mL boluses (avoid fluid overload in ESRD)
- Vasopressor support (dopamine or norepinephrine) for inotropic support
- Activate cardiothoracic surgery for urgent pericardial window procedure
- Type and crossmatch given thrombocytopenia and potential operative intervention
- Stress-dose steroids if concern for adrenal suppression from chronic prednisone use

Diagnostic Studies

- CBC: WBC 6.8, Hgb 9.8, Hct 29.4%, Plt 82 (low)
- BMP: Na 138, K 4.2, Cl 103, HCO_3 19, BUN 52, Cr 7.8, Glucose 168
- Coags: PT 13.5, PTT 29, INR 1.2
- Troponin I: 0.03 (negative), BNP: 520 (elevated)
- Inflammatory markers: ESR 58, CRP 12 (elevated)
- Lactate: 3.8

Critical Actions

- Recognized hemodynamic instability and initiated immediate resuscitation with large-bore IV access and isotonic fluid bolus
- Identified the clinical triad of cardiac tamponade (Beck's triad): hypotension, jugular venous distension, and distant/muffled heart sounds
- Performed or ordered timely bedside echocardiography demonstrating pericardial effusion with right ventricular diastolic collapse
- Recognized pulsus paradoxus and narrow pulse pressure as key diagnostic physical examination findings
- Demonstrated appropriate reassessment after initial fluid bolus, recognizing transient improvement followed by clinical deterioration indicating the need for definitive intervention
- Communicated effectively with family regarding the diagnosis of cardiac tamponade, distinguishing it from myocardial infarction, and explaining the urgency of procedural intervention
- Ordered appropriate definitive therapy including emergent pericardiocentesis or immediate cardiothoracic surgery consultation for pericardial window
- Avoided harmful interventions such as thrombolytics, excessive fluid resuscitation beyond initial bolus, or delaying diagnosis with unnecessary CT imaging
- Recognized underlying etiology (lupus-related pericardial effusion in a dialysis patient) and adjusted management accordingly (consideration of steroid stress dosing, platelet transfusion given low count before procedure)

- Demonstrated understanding that pericardiocentesis is temporizing while pericardial window is definitive therapy for recurrent effusion

Pediatric Trauma

Opening Scenario

You are the attending physician in a busy community emergency department. A 4-year-old male is brought in by his mother and her partner with complaints of abdominal pain following a reported fall. The child appears uncomfortable and is clinging to his mother. The triage nurse notifies you that the mechanism seems unclear and the mother appears anxious while her partner is pacing and demanding to be seen immediately.

Initial Assessment

- Vital Signs: BP 108/72 mmHg, HR 148 bpm, RR 26 breaths/min, Temperature 37.0°C (98.6°F), SpO_2 100% on room air, Weight 18 kg
- General Appearance: Alert, anxious, crying intermittently, holding abdomen with both hands, avoiding eye contact with the male companion

Primary Survey

- Airway: Patent, crying with adequate air movement, speaking in short phrases
- Breathing: Unlabored, no cyanosis, breath sounds bilaterally clear and equal
- Circulation: Capillary refill less than 2 seconds, skin warm and pink, radial pulses palpable and strong
- Disability: Moving all extremities spontaneously, GCS 15, pupils equal and reactive to light

History

- History of Present Illness: Mother reports the child "fell off the bunk bed ladder" approximately 3 hours ago while playing in his bedroom. She states he cried immediately, then took a nap. He awoke complaining of "tummy pain" and has refused dinner. When questioned separately, the child becomes silent and looks toward the mother's partner. The mother denies witnessing the event, stating she was downstairs while her partner was "watching the kids." The partner interjects frequently, stating "it was just an accident, kids fall all the time." The child denies vomiting but rates pain as "really bad" when asked using the Faces scale.
- Past Medical History: Healthy, immunizations up to date, no previous surgeries
- Social History: Lives with mother, 18-month-old sibling, and mother's new partner of 6 months. Recently moved in together. No pets. Mother works double shifts frequently.
- Medications/Allergies: None known

Physical Examination

- General: Irritable but consolable by mother, moderate distress with any abdominal palpation, flinches when partner approaches
- Head: Normal inspection, no scalp hematomas, notable bilateral periorbital ecchymosis (raccoon eyes)
- Eyes: No obvious subconjunctival hemorrhage on initial inspection, pupils reactive
- Neck: Supple, no midline tenderness, no ligature marks
- Chest: Clear to auscultation, no tenderness to palpation, no crepitus
- Cardiovascular: Tachycardic, regular rhythm, no murmurs appreciated
- Abdomen: Diffuse tenderness to palpation with voluntary guarding, most pronounced in left upper quadrant and epigastrium, bowel sounds present, no visible distension initially, no seatbelt sign
- Back: Multiple bruises of varying ages (yellow, purple, and fresh) over lower back and buttocks, no spinal step-offs or midline tenderness

- Extremities: Scattered bruises on upper arms (bilateral, circumferential) and inner thighs, no deformities, full range of motion, healing abrasions on knuckles
- Skin: Patterned bruising on right forearm consistent with finger marks

Diagnostic Studies

- All labs delayed due to lab power failure (hospital on internal disaster)
- FAST Exam: Negative for free fluid in Morrison's pouch, splenorenal recess, pelvis, or pericardium
- CT Abdomen/Pelvis with IV Contrast: Grade II splenic laceration with perisplenic hematoma, no active extravasation, moderate hemoperitoneum in left paracolic gutter and pelvis

Difficult Conversations

- The physician must sensitively discuss with the mother that the injury pattern is inconsistent with the reported mechanism and that mandatory reporting to child protective services is required by law
- Explain the medical findings (splenic injury, anemia, bruising patterns) without using accusatory language, using statements such as "The injuries we see don't match the story of a simple fall"
- Address the mother's emotional distress while maintaining professional boundaries, acknowledging her fear while ensuring the child's safety

Managing Conflict

- Navigate the partner's increasingly aggressive and defensive behavior when questioned about the incident
- Set clear boundaries regarding intimidation tactics, involving security if the partner becomes threatening or refuses to allow separate interviewing
- [Maintain focus on patient care while de-escalating tension, stating "I understand you're upset, but I need to focus on [child's name] medical care right now"]
- Negotiate with both adults regarding the need for further evaluation (skeletal survey, ophthalmology consult) despite resistance

Patient Communication

- Engage the child using age-appropriate language and positioning at eye level to establish trust before painful examinations
- Explain procedures to both child and parent in understandable terms, offering choices when possible to give the child autonomy
- Validate the child's emotions and pain experience without leading questions that could compromise potential forensic investigation
- Communicate clearly with mother regarding treatment plan, admission necessity, and the role of social services

Reassessment (45 Minutes Later)

- Vital Signs: BP 95/60 mmHg (decreased from 108/72), HR 165 bpm, RR 30, SpO_2 98% on room air
- Clinical Status: Child becomes increasingly lethargic and difficult to arouse despite weight-based pain medication. Abdomen more distended and rigid on examination. Capillary refill now 4 seconds. Mucous membranes dry.
- Interventions: Patient receives fluid bolus of 20 mL/kg normal saline. Type and crossmatch obtained. Pediatric surgery and blood bank notified.
- Repeat Laboratory Studies:
- Hemoglobin: 8.4 (decreased from 9.8)

- Hematocrit: 26.1

Critical Actions

- Recognize pattern of injuries inconsistent with reported mechanism (bilateral periorbital ecchymosis, buttock/back bruising in various stages of healing, circumferential arm bruising, patterned bruising)
- Obtain contrast-enhanced CT imaging for suspected intra-abdominal injury in hemodynamically stable pediatric patient with abdominal tenderness and guarding
- Initiate mandatory reporting to child protective services and law enforcement based on clinical suspicion of nonaccidental trauma before discharge or transfer
- Consult pediatric surgery urgently for splenic injury management with hemodynamic instability and dropping hemoglobin
- Perform comprehensive secondary survey documenting all injuries with precise measurements, locations, and descriptions using body diagrams or photography when available
- Recognize worsening clinical status requiring immediate fluid resuscitation and potential blood transfusion (Type O-negative if unstable)
- Demonstrate ability to deliver difficult news regarding suspected abuse using empathetic, non-accusatory communication while fulfilling legal reporting obligations
- Effectively manage conflict with confrontational family members by setting boundaries, ensuring safety, and maintaining focus on patient care
- Order skeletal survey to identify occult fractures and dating of previous injuries
- Maintain patient-centered approach when communicating with the pediatric patient, using developmentally appropriate language and trauma-informed care principles

Penetrating Chest Trauma in the Agitated Patient

Opening Scenario

You enter the resuscitation bay to evaluate a 34-year-old male construction worker brought in by EMS following an altercation at a job site. The paramedic reports the patient was stabbed in the left anterior chest with what witnesses describe as a box cutter approximately 15 minutes prior to arrival. The patient is reportedly anxious, complaining of severe chest pain and difficulty breathing, and has attempted to remove his oxygen cannula en route.

Initial Assessment

- Vital Signs: BP 88/42 mmHg, HR 124 bpm, RR 32 breaths/min, Temperature 36.9°C (98.4°F), SpO_2 91% on room air
- General Appearance: Diaphoretic, anxious-appearing male in moderate respiratory distress, speaking in short phrases, preferential positioning sitting upright

Primary Survey

- Airway: Patent, speaking in short phrases, no stridor
- Breathing: Tachypneic with accessory muscle use, diminished breath sounds over left hemithorax,
- Circulation: Tachycardic with weak peripheral pulses, capillary refill 3 seconds, skin cool and clammy

Patient Communication

The patient is agitated and states, "I don't want any tubes. Just stitch this up and let me go. I can't afford to miss work and I don't trust hospitals." He attempts to remove his oxygen cannula and refuses IV placement. You must address:

- His immediate safety concerns while acknowledging his anxiety
- The life-threatening nature of tension pneumothorax using clear, jargon-free language
- The necessity of immediate decompression to prevent cardiac arrest
- His financial/work concerns with empathy while emphasizing that stabilization must precede discharge planning
- Obtaining informed consent for procedures despite initial refusal

Initial Actions

- Place patient on 15 L/min non-rebreather mask
- Establish two large-bore peripheral IVs (14- or 16-gauge) after explaining necessity
- Draw blood for CBC, comprehensive metabolic panel, PT/PTT, type and crossmatch (4 units PRBC given hemodynamic instability)
- eFast Ultrasound: negative for intraabdominal free fluid
- Prepare for immediate needle decompression of left hemithorax
- Administer analgesia (fentanyl 50 mcg IV or morphine 4 mg IV) to facilitate cooperation

Critical Decision Point

If candidate performs immediate needle decompression:

- Proceed to reassessment section

If candidate delays for imaging (CXR/CT) or attempts to complete full secondary survey first:

- Patient deteriorates within 3 minutes: BP drops to 72/30, HR 145, RR 40, SpO_2 85%

- Patient becomes confused and lethargic
- Prompt from examiner: "The patient is becoming unresponsive. What is your next step?"

Reassessment

Following Needle Decompression (2nd intercostal space, mid-clavicular line or 4th-5th intercostal space, anterior axillary line):

- Vital Signs: BP 106/68 mmHg, HR 96 bpm, RR 20 breaths/min, SpO_2 98% on 15L NRB
- Patient Report: States breathing is "much easier," chest pressure decreased significantly
- Physical Exam: Breath sounds improved but still diminished on left, trachea now midline, JVD resolved
- Required Actions:
- Proceed immediately to tube thoracostomy (chest tube placement) as definitive management
- Place left chest tube to water seal (anticipate air leak and possible hemothorax given penetrating mechanism)

If No Decompression Performed:

- Vital Signs: BP 64/24 mmHg, HR 158 bpm, RR 44 breaths/min, SpO_2 79%
- Patient Status: Obtunded, profound respiratory distress, hypotension refractory to 2L crystalloid
- Cardiac Status: Patient develops pulseless electrical activity (PEA) arrest requiring ACLS protocol and emergent bilateral needle decompression and the patient has ROSC. If no decompression the case ends.

Physical Examination

- Head: Normocephalic, no signs of trauma
- Neck: Trachea midline (post-decompression), no subcutaneous emphysema
- Chest: 2.5 cm laceration over left 4th intercostal space at mid-clavicular line; chest tube placed to water seal with air leak and 300 mL immediate blood return
- Cardiovascular: Regular rhythm, no murmurs, pulses equal bilaterally, warm extremities after resuscitation
- Abdomen: Soft, non-tender, no distension, normal bowel sounds
- Extremities: No deformities, distal pulses intact, full range of motion
- Neurologic: Alert and oriented, moving all extremities, sensation intact
- Skin: Cool extremities improving to warm after resuscitation, no other lacerations noted

Diagnostic Studies

- Labs pending

- Xray (post chest tube on left) - bent chest tube (requires withdrawal to straighten) - if not acknowledge and adjusted patient begins to develop hypotension

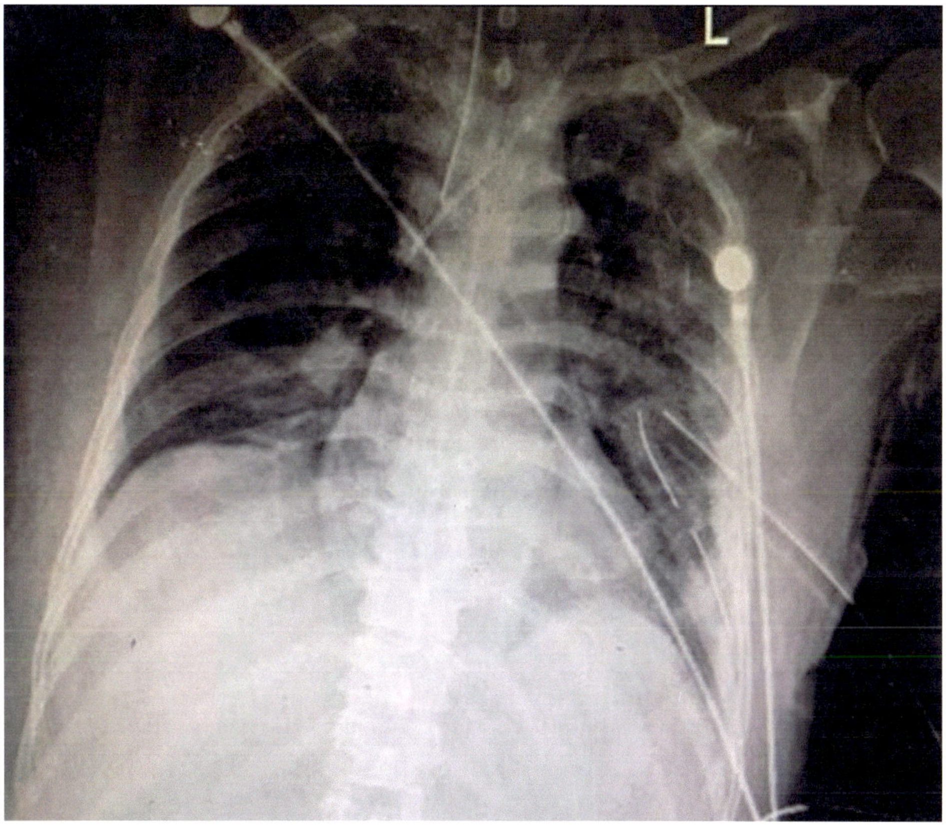

Disposition

- Immediate consultation with Trauma Surgery for admission
- Reassessment of chest tube function with confirmation on repeat xray and evaluation with pleurovac tidaling
- Tetanus prophylaxis and broad-spectrum antibiotics per trauma protocol
-

Critical Actions

- Recognize tension pneumothorax clinically based on the constellation of hypotension, tachycardia, unilateral absent breath sounds (utilizes bedside ultrasound to asses for absence of lung sliding)
- Evaluates poorly positioned chest tube and describes steps to adjust by withdrawing and getting repeat Xray.
- Demonstrate immediate needle decompression followed by definitive tube thoracostomy without delaying for imaging in the unstable patient
- Exhibit patient-centered communication by addressing the patient's refusal of treatment, acknowledging his socioeconomic concerns, explaining the immediate life threat using understandable language, and obtaining informed consent
- Perform reassessment after intervention to confirm hemodynamic improvement, resolution of mediastinal shift, and need for chest tube placement
- Evaluate for concomitant hemothorax given penetrating mechanism and initial hemodynamic instability (anticipate blood return with tube placement)

- Identify need for surgical consultation and admission for monitoring
- Avoid delaying critical interventions to complete full secondary survey or obtain definitive imaging in the hemodynamically unstable patient with suspected tension physiology

Left Lower Quadrant Pain

Opening Scenario

A 58-year-old male arrives via private vehicle with his spouse, clutching his lower abdomen. He demands to be seen immediately because he has a critical business meeting in three hours. He is pacing while talking on his cell phone.

Initial Assessment

Vitals: BP 146/92, HR 106, RR 22, T 38.7°C, SpO_2 97% RA, Fingerstick glucose 142

- Airway: Patent, speaking without stridor
- Breathing: Non-labored, no cyanosis
- Circulation: Warm, dry skin, capillary refill <2 seconds, peripheral pulses intact
- Uncomfortable, diaphoretic, restless, pauses conversation to clutch left lower abdomen

Immediate actions: Two large-bore IVs, 1L NS bolus, continuous cardiac monitoring, analgesia (morphine sulfate). Labs: CBC with differential, CMP, LFTs, coags, UA, lipase, lactate, type and screen.

History

- Chief Complaint: Severe left lower quadrant abdominal pain for 36 hours
- History of Present Illness: The patient reports constant, sharp pain localized to the left lower quadrant that has progressively worsened. He notes nausea without vomiting, subjective fever and chills, and constipation over the past two days. He denies urinary symptoms, hematochezia, melena, or prior similar episodes. Pain does not radiate.
- Past Medical History: Hypertension, Type 2 diabetes mellitus
- Past Surgical History: Appendectomy (age 12)
- Medications: Lisinopril, Metformin
- Allergies: No known drug allergies
- Social History: Financial executive, high-stress occupation, denies tobacco or illicit drug use, occasional alcohol consumption. Currently agitated about missing an important client presentation.
- Family History: Non-contributory

Physical Examination

- General: Alert and oriented to person, place, and time; moderate distress; persistent time-checking behavior
- Head: Normocephalic, atraumatic
- Eyes: PERRL, EOMI
- Cardiovascular: Tachycardic, regular rhythm, no murmurs, rubs, or gallops
- Respiratory: Clear to auscultation bilaterally, no wheezes, rales, or rhonchi
- Abdomen: Soft, nondistended, normal active bowel sounds, focal tenderness and voluntary guarding at left lower quadrant, no rebound tenderness, negative Murphy sign, nontender at McBurney point, no palpable masses or hernias
- Genitourinary: Normal external genitalia, no suprapubic tenderness
- Rectal: Normal sphincter tone, brown stool, hemoccult negative
- Extremities: No edema, normal pulses
- Neurological: Cranial nerves II-XII intact, motor strength 5/5 bilateral, sensation intact
- Skin: Warm, diaphoretic

Managing Conflict

The patient states: "I need to leave now. This pain is manageable, and I cannot miss this meeting. It's a career-defining presentation. Just write me a prescription for antibiotics and I'll see my primary doctor tomorrow."

Acknowledge professional obligations. Explain concern for acute diverticulitis with risk of perforation or abscess. Discuss consequences of leaving AMA including sepsis and emergency surgery. Negotiate alternatives (postponing meeting, teleconference, medical excuse letter). Assess decision-making capacity. Offer expedited workup if he agrees to remain.

Difficult Conversations

The patient asks: "How serious is this really? Can't this wait?"

Deliver clear diagnosis: "You have an infection in your colon called diverticulitis." Explain severity: risk of bowel wall weakening, abscess formation, or perforation. Discuss treatment necessity: IV antibiotics, possible admission, monitoring for complications. Express empathy regarding the professional conflict while maintaining firm recommendation against departure. Patient can be persuaded to get a CT if risks are explained well.

Diagnostic Studies

- CBC: WBC 17.5, Hgb 13.8, Hct 41.2%, Plt 289
- BMP: Na 136, K 4.1, Cl 102, HCO_3 28, BUN 18, Cr 1.0, Glucose 156
- LFTs: AST 28, ALT 31, ALP 78, T.Bili 0.9
- Lipase: 42 (normal)
- Urinalysis: Yellow, SG 1.018, pH 6.0, LE negative, nitrites negative, blood negative
- CT abdomen/pelvis with IV contrast: Sigmoid diverticulosis with focal wall thickening, pericolonic fat stranding, and 2.5 cm pericolonic fluid collection consistent with moderate sized abscess and free air.

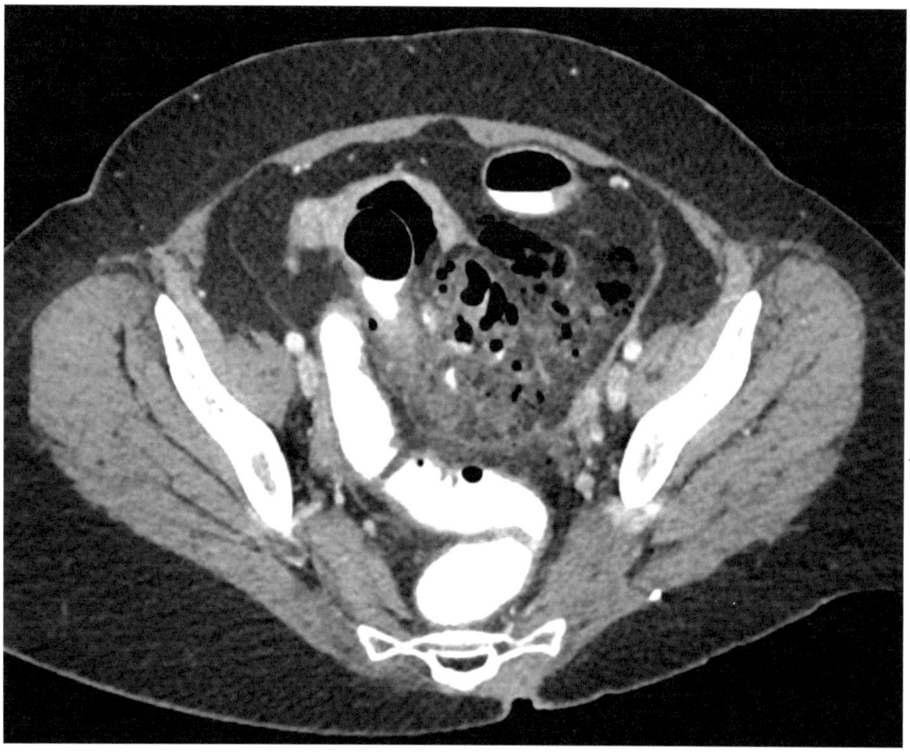

Reassessment

Two hours after initial presentation, while awaiting surgical consultation and inpatient bed assignment, the patient develops rigors and increased distress.

Updated Vital Signs:

- Blood Pressure: 108/68 mmHg (decreased from 146/92)
- Heart Rate: 124 beats per minute
- T: 39.4°C
- Respiratory Rate: 24 breaths per minute
- Oxygen Saturation: 95 on room air

Patient appears increasingly ill, skin cool and clammy, worsening abdominal pain despite analgesia. States: "I think something is really wrong."

Recognize clinical deterioration suggesting sepsis. Administer additional fluid bolus (30 mL/kg). Initiate broad-spectrum antibiotics immediately (piperacillin-tazobactam or ceftriaxone + metronidazole + vancomycin). Reassess need for urgent surgical intervention vs. IR drainage. Update patient regarding change in condition. Expedite admission to monitored setting.

Disposition

- General surgery consultation for complicated diverticulitis with small abscess
- Appropriate antibiotic coverage
- Admission to medical-surgical unit; if hemodynamically unstable, ICU
- Abscess management: IR drainage if abscess >3 cm or failure to improve; current 2.5 cm may be managed with antibiotics alone
- NPO initially, advance as clinical improvement allows

Critical Actions

- Demonstrates structured approach to undifferentiated abdominal pain with appropriate differential diagnosis (diverticulitis, colitis, ischemic bowel, nephrolithiasis, urinary tract infection)
- Performs conflict resolution by acknowledging patient's concerns while clearly communicating medical risks and negotiating acceptable alternatives
- Utilizes empathetic communication techniques when breaking bad news regarding severity of illness and necessity of admission
- Recognizes sepsis on reassessment with appropriate hemodynamic resuscitation and antibiotic escalation
- Orders appropriate diagnostic imaging (CT with contrast) to confirm complicated diverticulitis
- Selects appropriate antibiotic regimen covering gram-negative and anaerobic organisms
- Makes appropriate disposition decision (admission vs. discharge) based on clinical findings and patient stability
- Maintains patient safety as priority while respecting professional autonomy through shared decision-making

Blunt Abdominal Trauma

Opening Scenario

EMS brings in a 58-year-old male following a high-speed motorcycle collision. He was thrown approximately 20 feet, is on spinal precautions, and complains of severe abdominal pain and dizziness. Helmeted, no reported LOC.

Initial Assessment

Vitals: BP 88/56, HR 128, RR 24, T 36.0°C, SpO_2 97% RA, Fingerstick glucose 142

- Airway: Patent, speaking in short sentences
- Breathing: Tachypneic, breath sounds present bilaterally, no accessory muscle use
- Circulation: Cool, clammy skin, capillary refill >3 seconds, weak peripheral pulses
- Disability: GCS 15 (E4 V5 M6), PERRL
- Exposure: Horizontal abrasion across epigastrium, no active external hemorrhage

Immediate actions: High-flow O2 via NRB at 15 L/min, two large-bore IVs (14-16 gauge), 1L NS bolus, cardiac monitoring and continuous SpO_2. Type and crossmatch 4 units PRBC (increased due to suspected anticoagulation). Labs: CBC, CMP, coags (PT/INR/PTT), lactate, blood alcohol, type and screen.

History

- HPI: 58-year-old male with history of atrial fibrillation on warfarin and hypertension. Patient was the operator of a motorcycle involved in a collision with a passenger vehicle at approximately 40 mph, thrown approximately 20 feet from the vehicle. Patient was wearing a DOT-approved helmet. Denies loss of consciousness. Complains of severe epigastric and left upper quadrant pain radiating to the left shoulder (Kehr sign). Denies chest pain, shortness of breath, or headache.
- PMHx: Atrial fibrillation (on warfarin), hypertension
- Medications: Warfarin 5 mg daily (last dose taken yesterday evening), metoprolol
- Allergies: No known drug allergies
- Social history: Former smoker (quit 10 years ago), occasional alcohol use, lives with wife, works as accountant
- Family history: Non-contributory

Reassessment

- Blood pressure: 92/64 mmHg (transient response)
- Heart rate: 118 beats per minute
- Patient reports worsening abdominal pain and increasing anxiety
- Nurse notes increasing abdominal distension

Physical Examination

- General: Alert, oriented to person, place, and time; moderate distress; diaphoretic
- Head: Normocephalic, atraumatic, helmet hair present, no lacerations or contusions
- Eyes: Extraocular movements intact, pupils equal and reactive to light and accommodation
- Ears: Normal tympanic membranes, no hemotympanum
- Nose: No discharge or epistaxis
- Neck: C-collar in place, no step-offs or deformity, no jugular venous distension
- Chest: Tenderness to palpation over left lower lateral ribs (ribs 9-11), nontender sternum, no crepitus

- Lungs: Clear to auscultation bilaterally, no wheezes or rales
- Heart: Tachycardic, regular rhythm, no murmurs, rubs, or gallops appreciated
- Abdomen: Distended, diffuse tenderness with guarding and rebound tenderness in left upper quadrant and epigastrium, positive Grey Turner sign (ecchymosis of left flank), bowel sounds absent, no palpable masses
- Pelvis: Stable on compression and distraction, no tenderness
- Genitourinary: Normal external genitalia, no blood at urethral meatus
- Rectal: Normal tone, brown stool, occult blood negative, normal prostate
- Extremities: Full range of motion, no deformities, pulses palpable but weak (2+)
- Back: No tenderness to palpation on log roll, no step-offs
- Neurologic: Cranial nerves II-XII intact, normal sensation and strength in all extremities, no focal deficits
- Skin: Cool and clammy

Diagnostic Studies

- FAST examination: Positive for free fluid in hepatorenal space, splenorenal space, and pelvis (complex free fluid)
- Chest X-ray: No pneumothorax or hemothorax, fractures of left ribs 9, 10, and 11 noted
- Pelvic X-ray: No fractures or diastasis of pubic symphysis
- ECG: Atrial fibrillation with rapid ventricular response, rate 118, no ST-segment elevations
- CBC: WBC 12.4, Hgb 9.8 (low), Hct 29.4%, Plt 285
- Coags: INR 3.2 (supratherapeutic), PT 28.5, PTT 42
- Lactate: 5.8 (elevated)
- Cr 1.2, AST 45, ALT 38, Amylase 65, Lipase 35
- Urinalysis: SG 1.025, pH 6.0, negative for blood/protein/glucose
- Type and Screen: O positive, antibody negative

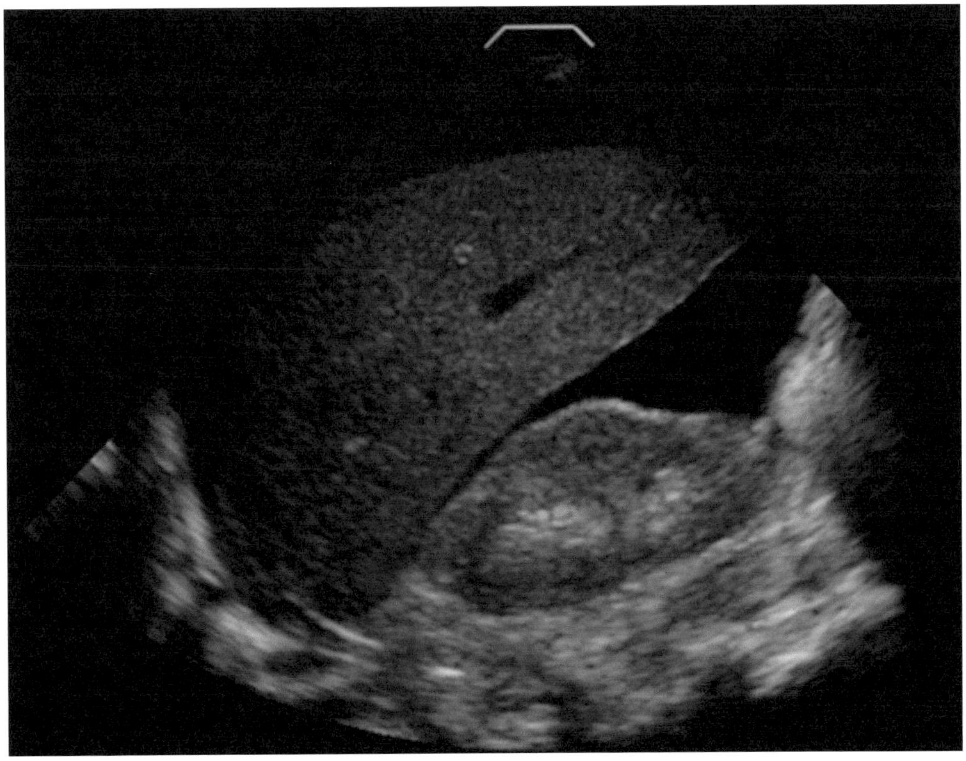

Management

- Recognize hemorrhagic shock (tachycardia, hypotension, cool clammy skin, elevated lactate) with positive FAST indicating hemoperitoneum
- Reverse anticoagulation immediately with 4-factor PCC 50 units/kg (do not wait for vitamin K alone)
- Activate massive transfusion protocol anticipating ongoing blood loss
- Hemodynamic instability precludes conservative management or angioembolization as primary therapy

Patient Communication

The patient states: "I don't want to die, but I'm terrified of surgery. Can't you just watch me for a while?"

Acknowledge and validate fear. Explain the life-threatening nature of splenic rupture and ongoing internal bleeding in clear, jargon-free language. Discuss risks of non-operative management in the setting of anticoagulation and hemodynamic instability. Use teach-back method to confirm understanding. Address questions about recovery and long-term prognosis (vaccination considerations, activity restrictions). Obtain informed consent for surgical intervention.

Managing Conflict

The trauma surgery fellow suggests observation in ICU with serial hemoglobin checks and possible splenic artery embolization rather than immediate OR.

Advocate firmly: present objective data (persistent hypotension despite 2L crystalloid, tachycardia, INR 3.2, positive FAST with deterioration). Reference trauma guidelines: hemodynamically unstable patients with positive FAST require operative intervention. Suggest they reconsider and go to the OR. Offer to involve the trauma attending if disagreement persists. Maintain professional demeanor while being persistent.

Reassessment

Forty-five minutes after initial presentation, despite administration of 2 liters normal saline, 2 units packed red blood cells, and reversal of anticoagulation:

- Blood pressure: 72/48 mmHg
- Heart rate: 142 beats per minute
- Respiratory rate: 28 breaths per minute
- Oxygen saturation: 94 on 15L non-rebreather mask
- T: 35.8°C (developing hypothermia)
- Patient becomes confused and agitated (GCS drops to 13: E3 V4 M6)
- Abdomen becomes increasingly distended, rigid, and diffusely tender
- Repeat FAST shows increased free fluid

Immediate actions required:

- Recognition of decompensating hemorrhagic shock with development of lethal triad (hypothermia, coagulopathy, acidosis)
- Continuation of massive transfusion protocol with 1:1:1 ratio of packed red blood cells, fresh frozen plasma, and platelets
- Re-emphasis on emergent surgical intervention as the only life-saving option
- Notification of blood bank for additional products
- Preparation for immediate transport to operating room
- Brief update to family regarding critical status and immediate surgical necessity

Critical Actions

- Immediate recognition of hemodynamic instability and need for aggressive resuscitation

- Appropriate primary survey with attention to airway protection, ventilatory status, and circulatory compromise
- Recognition of the impact of therapeutic anticoagulation on trauma outcomes and immediate reversal with appropriate agents (PCC preferred over FFP for warfarin reversal in acute bleeding)
- Correct interpretation of positive FAST examination in the context of blunt abdominal trauma
- Activation of massive transfusion protocol based on hemodynamic status and mechanism of injury
- Effective patient-centered communication regarding the life-threatening nature of the injury and the necessity of surgical intervention, including informed consent
- Demonstration of conflict management skills when advocating for operative intervention with a reluctant consultant, using objective data and professional persistence
- Timely reassessment of patient condition and recognition of clinical deterioration despite initial resuscitative efforts
- Understanding that hemodynamically unstable patients with intra-abdominal hemorrhage require definitive operative hemostasis regardless of imaging findings or temporary response to resuscitation
- Recognition and prevention/management of the lethal triad (hypothermia, acidosis, coagulopathy) through appropriate blood product resuscitation and warming measures

Neonatal Hematochezia

Opening Scenario

A 24-day-old male infant is brought by parents with bloody stools and increasing fussiness. Born prematurely at 28 weeks gestation, discharged from NICU 10 days ago. Parents report poor feeding for 18 hours, increasing sleepiness, and bright red blood with mucus in stool.

Initial Assessment

Vitals: BP 62/38 (MAP 46), HR 178, RR 62, T 36.8°C (axillary), SpO_2 94% RA, Weight 2450 g

- Airway: Patent, weak cry
- Breathing: Mild subcostal retractions, breath sounds equal bilaterally, no cyanosis
- Circulation: Delayed capillary refill (4 seconds), mottled skin, weak brachial pulses
- Disability: Lethargic but arousable, sunken fontanelle
- Exposure: Abdominal distension noted, no rashes or bruising

History

- HPI: Former 28-week premature infant discharged home 10 days ago after 8-week NICU stay. Started on standard term formula 4 days ago after previously tolerating breast milk with formula supplements. Over the past 18 hours, increasing irritability followed by lethargy, refusal of feeds, and abdominal bloating. Two diapers with bright red blood and mucoid material. No vomiting or fever at home.
- Birth history: Birth weight 1100 g (2.2lbs) treated 48 hours with phototherapy for hyperbilirubinemia
- Medications: vitamin D
- Allergies: No known drug allergies
- Social: Lives with both parents, no tobacco or drug exposure, no sick contacts
- Family history: Non-contributory

Physical Examination

- General: Lethargic, ill-appearing infant in moderate distress
- Head: Anterior fontanelle sunken, posterior fontanelle flat, no cephalohematoma
- Eyes: Sunken, dry mucous membranes
- Neck: Supple, no masses
- Chest: Mild intercostal retractions, clear bilaterally
- Cardiovascular: Tachycardic, regular rhythm, no murmur, weak peripheral pulses
- Abdomen: Markedly distended, shiny appearance, diffuse tenderness with guarding, absent bowel sounds, liver edge palpable 2 cm below costal margin
- Genitourinary: Normal male genitalia, testes descended
- Rectal: Patent anus, no fissures, guaiac positive
- Extremities: Pale, cool, delayed capillary refill
- Skin: Poor turgor, mottled appearance
- Neurologic: Decreased tone, weak suck reflex, withdraws to pain

Diagnostic Studies

Abdominal radiograph: Dilated loops of bowel, pneumatosis intestinalis, no free air on upright view

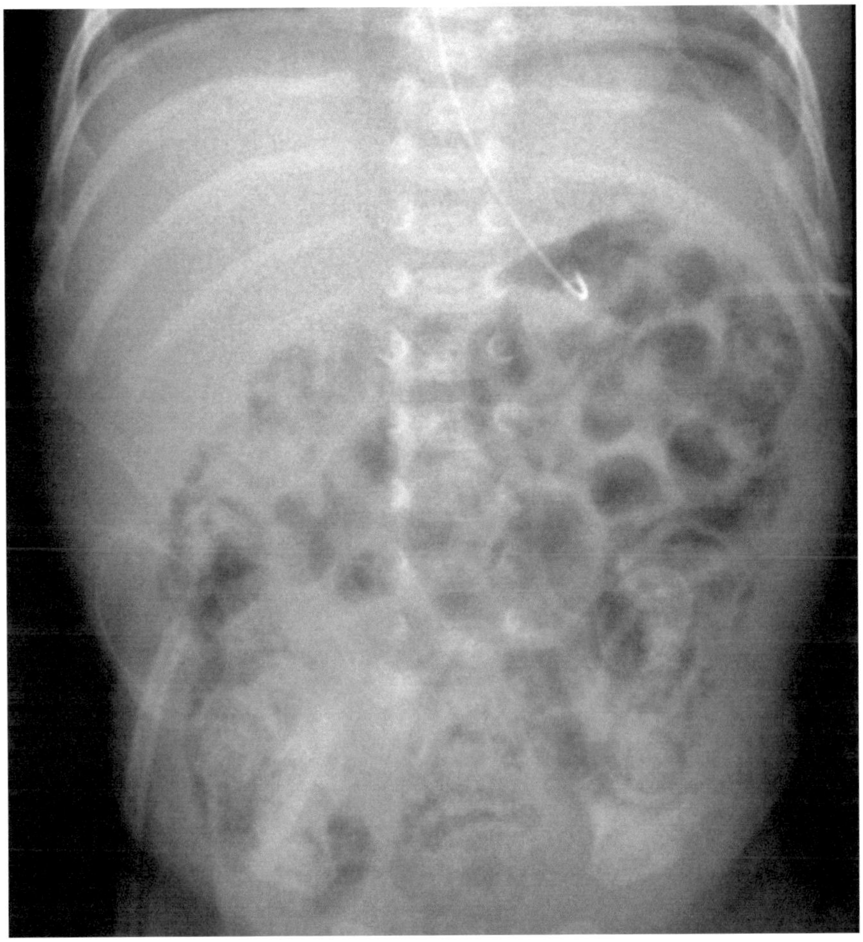

Point-of-care ultrasound: Poor cardiac contractility, collapsible IVC

- WBC 4.2 (low), Hgb 11.2, Hct 34%, Plt 89 (thrombocytopenia)
- Na 136, K 5.8 (elevated), Cl 102, HCO_3 16 (acidosis), BUN 28 (elevated), Cr 1.1, Glucose 45 (hypoglycemia)
- Lactate 6.2 (elevated); VBG pH 7.28, base deficit -8

Management

- Place in radiant warmer; blow-by oxygen to maintain SpO_2 >95%
- Peripheral IV access (24-gauge); NPO status; NG tube to low intermittent suction
- Fluid resuscitation: 20 mL/kg NS bolus
- Recognize NEC in this premature infant with classic triad of hematochezia, abdominal distension, and systemic illness
- Despite being 24 days old, corrected gestational age is approximately 32 weeks — still at risk
- Switch from breast milk to formula may have precipitated the episode
- Thrombocytopenia, metabolic acidosis, and elevated potassium indicate severe disease (Bell stage II progressing to III)
- Early surgical consultation despite initial hemodynamic improvement; neonatal hypotension is a late sign of shock
- Anticipate need for vasopressors and blood products

Reassessment

After initial fluid bolus: BP 68/42 (improved but still hypotensive), HR 156, capillary refill 3 seconds. Infant remains lethargic. Abdominal girth increased by 2 cm. NG tube returns 15 mL bilious fluid.

Two hours after arrival, despite fluids and antibiotics, the infant deteriorates: BP 52/30 (MAP 37), HR 190, RR 70 with apneic periods, SpO_2 88%, T 35.9°C. Abdominal girth increased by additional 3 cm with wall erythema. Repeat x-ray: pneumoperitoneum indicating perforation.

- Recognize intestinal perforation with septic shock
- Emergent intubation and mechanical ventilation
- Additional IV access or intraosseous line
- Fluid boluses; dopamine or epinephrine for refractory hypotension
- Urgent pediatric surgery notification for emergent laparotomy
- Blood products (PRBCs, platelets, FFP)
- Update parents regarding critical change and need for surgery

Patient Communication

The parents express guilt about switching from breast milk to formula. The mother asks, "Is this my fault?" The father demands to know why the NICU never warned them.

- Sit at eye level, acknowledge distress with empathic statements
- Explain NEC in lay terms as intestinal inflammation that can happen in premature babies, not caused by anything they did
- Address the feeding change: breast milk is protective, but formula alone does not cause NEC
- Provide clear information about the treatment plan and what to expect
- If the infant decompensates in front of parents, be honest about severity without being overly pessimistic
- Discuss potential outcomes including stomas and long-term nutritional issues, while emphasizing many babies recover fully

Managing Conflict

The on-call pediatric surgery fellow recommends observation in the pediatric ward, deferring surgical evaluation until morning.

- Advocate by communicating severity: thrombocytopenia, metabolic acidosis, pneumatosis intestinalis, peritoneal signs
- Express concern about perforation risk given clinical trajectory
- If fellow remains reluctant, escalate to attending or arrange transfer to tertiary center
- Maintain composure while emphasizing this is a time-sensitive surgical emergency

Critical Actions

- Immediate recognition of NEC in a premature infant with hematochezia, abdominal distension, and systemic illness
- Appropriate stabilization: NPO, gastric decompression, fluid resuscitation, broad-spectrum antibiotics covering gut flora including anaerobes
- Recognition of severity markers (thrombocytopenia, metabolic acidosis, hyponatremia) indicating Bell stage II-III disease
- Early surgical consultation for NEC with pneumatosis intestinalis, even if initially hemodynamically stable
- Effective communication addressing parental guilt with empathy and clear explanations

- Management of conflict with reluctant consultants using objective data and appropriate escalation
- Timely reassessment leading to recognition of deterioration and intestinal perforation (pneumoperitoneum)
- Appropriate interventions for neonatal septic shock: airway management, vasoactive support, blood products
- NEC is a surgical emergency once perforation occurs or despite maximal medical therapy with deterioration

Intentional Overdose

Opening Scenario

A 42-year-old male is brought by his partner after disclosing he took a large quantity of pain medication in a suicide attempt the previous evening. He has been despondent since sustaining a painful fracture earlier in the week. His partner is anxious and present in the room.

Initial Assessment

Vitals: BP 118/72, HR 88, RR 14, T 36.8°C, SpO_2 98% RA, Weight 70 kg

Thin-appearing male sitting quietly on stretcher with right forearm in fiberglass splint. Minimal eye contact, withdrawn, flat affect. Alert, no respiratory distress or cyanosis.

- Airway: Patent, speaking in full sentences
- Breathing: Clear breath sounds bilaterally, no cyanosis
- Circulation: Warm, dry skin, normal capillary refill, radial pulses 2+
- Disability: Alert and oriented, GCS 15

History

- HPI: Right distal radius fracture five days ago from motorcycle collision. Struggling with immobility and chronic pain with worsening depression. Ten hours ago, while drinking whiskey alone, intentionally consumed 35 tablets of hydrocodone/acetaminophen (5/325 mg) with suicidal intent. Went to sleep expecting not to awaken. Woke with nausea and disclosed ingestion to partner. Denies co-ingestion. Reports daily alcohol use, no prior suicide attempts or psychiatric history. Currently denies active suicidal ideation but expresses intense shame and guilt.
- PMHx: None reported
- Medications: None
- Allergies: NKDA
- Social: Daily alcohol use

Physical Examination

- General: Alert, appropriate but tearful, gaze averted, cooperative
- Eyes: Pupils pinpoint bilaterally (3 mm), EOMI, sclera anicteric
- Neck: Full ROM, no JVD, no lymphadenopathy
- Cardiovascular: Regular rate and rhythm, no murmurs
- Respiratory: Clear bilaterally, no wheezes or crackles
- Abdomen: Soft, non-distended, mild epigastric tenderness without guarding or rebound; normal bowel sounds
- Extremities: Right forearm in fiberglass splint, distal neurovascular intact; no edema
- Neurological: CN II-XII intact, normal sensation and strength, normal reflexes
- Skin: Warm and dry, no track marks or bruising

Diagnostic Studies

- Acetaminophen level 145 mcg/mL (toxic), Ethanol 220, Salicylate <5
- AST 48 (elevated), ALT 35, Alk Phos 65, T Bili 1.2, INR 1.0
- Cr 1.0, BUN 14, Glucose 108
- WBC 6.2, Hct 42%, Plt 280

- Urine toxicology negative; ABG pH 7.40, PCO2 40, PO2 95, HCO_3 24
- ECG: NSR at 88, normal intervals, no ischemic changes
- Total ingested dose: approximately 11.4 g acetaminophen (162 mg/kg), well above 140 mg/kg toxic threshold

Management

- Two large-bore peripheral IV lines; cardiac and pulse oximetry monitoring
- Calculate total ingested dose and plot acetaminophen level on Rumack-Matthew nomogram (145 mcg/mL at 10 hours is above treatment line)
- Initiate N-acetylcysteine (NAC) immediately without delaying for hepatic enzyme elevation
- Screen for co-ingestions: salicylates, urine drug screen
- Contact Poison Control Center
- Initiate suicide precautions: one-to-one observation, remove personal belongings
- Activated charcoal is not indicated given 10-hour delay since ingestion

Reassessment

At 90 minutes, patient reports increasing nausea and right upper quadrant discomfort. Vitals: BP 122/78, HR 92, RR 16, T 37.1°C. Exam now reveals mild RUQ tenderness. Rising transaminases confirm developing hepatic injury requiring continued monitoring and full NAC course.

Difficult Conversations

- Address the patient privately regarding circumstances of the overdose with non-judgmental, empathetic tone
- Explore current suicidal ideation and protective factors
- Communicate the risk of fulminant hepatic failure without treatment to patient and partner
- Discuss need for psychiatric hospitalization and medical admission, addressing fears about losing autonomy
- Navigate resistance to psychiatric evaluation by emphasizing medical stabilization first while validating emotional distress

Patient Communication

- Acknowledge pain and frustration regarding injury and loss of function
- Use open-ended questions to understand emotional context leading to overdose
- Explain NAC therapy including side effects and 21-hour treatment course
- Emphasize that early treatment significantly improves outcomes
- Invite partner to participate with patient's consent

Disposition

- Admit to inpatient medical floor for full NAC protocol (21-hour IV infusion) with concurrent psychiatric evaluation and continuous observation
- Consult Poison Control and psychiatry for combined medical-psychiatric admission

Critical Actions

- Calculate total acetaminophen dose (162 mg/kg or 11.4 g), recognizing this exceeds the 140 mg/kg toxic threshold

- Initiate NAC immediately based on toxic level plotted on Rumack-Matthew nomogram, without delaying for hepatic enzyme elevation
- Screen for co-ingestions including salicylates and other toxins
- Comprehensive suicide risk assessment with direct questioning about ideation, plan, and protective factors; immediate suicide precautions
- Empathetic, non-judgmental conversation regarding suicide attempt while maintaining safety boundaries
- Communicate with partner regarding prognosis, treatment course, and need for combined medical-psychiatric admission
- Reassess at 60-90 minutes for early hepatic injury signs (RUQ pain, nausea, rising transaminases)
- Recognize that activated charcoal is not indicated given 10-hour delay
- Consult Poison Control and psychiatry; arrange inpatient admission for NAC completion with psychiatric evaluation

Neurologic Deficits

Opening Scenario

A 58-year-old female is brought by EMS with acute onset left-sided weakness and slurred speech. Last seen normal at 11:00 PM; found at 7:00 AM on bedroom floor unable to move her left side. Positive Cincinnati Prehospital Stroke Scale. History of hypertension and tobacco use, no prior stroke.

Initial Assessment

Vitals: BP 198/112, HR 78, RR 16, T 36.8°C, SpO_2 97% RA, Fingerstick glucose 94

Awake and alert but anxious. Obvious left facial droop and dysarthria. No respiratory distress.

- Airway: Patent, slurred speech, no stridor
- Breathing: Non-labored, symmetric chest rise, clear bilaterally
- Circulation: Warm, well-perfused, capillary refill <2 seconds, no edema

History

- HPI: 58-year-old female with hypertension. Went to bed at 11:00 PM in normal condition. Found at 7:00 AM with complete left-sided weakness and slurred speech. Denies headache, chest pain, SOB, or seizure. Reports transient right arm weakness five days ago that resolved after ten minutes without evaluation (possible TIA). No trauma.
- PMHx: Hypertension (medication non-adherent), hyperlipidemia
- PSHx: Laparoscopic cholecystectomy
- Allergies: NKDA
- Medications: Lisinopril (taken intermittently), atorvastatin (recently stopped due to cost)
- Social: 30 pack-year smoking history, denies alcohol or illicit drug use, lives with husband
- Family: Father with ischemic stroke at 62, mother with MI at 70

Physical Examination

- General: Alert and oriented to person, place, and time; mild psychological distress; cooperative with examination
- Head: Normocephalic, atraumatic; left central facial droop with forehead sparing
- Eyes: Extraocular movements intact, pupils equal and reactive to light, no visual field cut appreciated on confrontation
- Ears: Tympanic membranes clear bilaterally
- Neck: Supple, no nuchal rigidity, no carotid bruits auscultated, no jugular venous distension
- Cardiovascular: Regular rate and rhythm, no murmurs, rubs, or gallops; peripheral pulses 2+ bilaterally
- Pulmonary: Clear to auscultation bilaterally, no wheezes, rales, or rhonchi
- Abdomen: Soft, non-tender, non-distended, normal bowel sounds
- Extremities: No clubbing, cyanosis, or edema; left arm and leg flaccid with no voluntary movement
- Neurological:
  - Mental status: Alert, follows commands, fluent but dysarthric, inattention to left-sided space
  - Cranial Nerves: Left lower facial weakness (central seventh), dysarthria, otherwise intact
  - Motor: 0/5 left upper and lower extremities; 5/5 right
  - Sensory: Decreased light touch and pinprick on left face, arm, and leg

- Neglect: Extinction to double simultaneous stimulation on left, anosognosia, left hemineglect on clock drawing (numbers 1-6 only)
- Cerebellar: Unable to test left; finger-to-nose intact on right

Diagnostic Studies

- WBC 7.2, Hgb 13.8, Plt 285
- Na 140, K 4.1, Cl 102, HCO_3 26, BUN 18, Cr 0.9, Glucose 108
- PT 11.5, PTT 28.0, INR 1.0; Troponin <0.04
- ECG: Sinus rhythm at 72, no ST changes, LVH by voltage criteria, no atrial fibrillation
- Head CT (non-contrast): No hemorrhage; early ischemic changes in right MCA territory; hyperdense right MCA sign (thrombus); no midline shift

Management

- Continuous pulse oximetry and cardiac monitoring; two large-bore IVs
- Supplemental oxygen to maintain SpO_2 >94%
- Immediate non-contrast head CT within 25 minutes of arrival
- Establish last known well time (11:00 PM — >8 hours ago)
- "Wake-up stroke" with unknown onset excludes standard IV tPA (0-4.5 hour window) unless advanced imaging suggests salvageable penumbra
- BP management: treat SBP >220 or DBP >120 with IV agents; avoid precipitous drops
- Aspirin 325 mg once hemorrhage excluded
- Early stroke team/neurology consultation; evaluate for mechanical thrombectomy given large vessel occlusion

Reassessment

At 90 minutes: BP 232/136 despite labetalol 10 mg IV x2, HR 68. Patient becomes somnolent, opens eyes only to voice, new severe headache (8/10), vomits once. New right pupil 5 mm with sluggish reaction (left 3 mm, brisk) — Cushing response from uncal herniation compressing right CN III.

- Immediate repeat non-contrast head CT for hemorrhagic conversion or malignant cerebral edema
- IV nicardipine drip for BP control (goal SBP 140-160)
- Elevate HOB to 30 degrees
- Urgent neurosurgery and stroke team notification
- Consider mannitol or hypertonic saline for herniation signs
- Prepare for possible decompressive craniectomy if malignant MCA syndrome confirmed

Patient Communication

- Explain imaging confirms ischemic stroke affecting the right brain, causing left-sided weakness and spatial inattention
- Unknown time of onset (last known well >8 hours) prevents IV tPA due to unacceptable hemorrhage risk
- Recovery possible with rehabilitation but may require weeks to months
- Provide clear instructions regarding NPO status, frequent neuro checks, and consultations

Difficult Conversations

- Inform husband of significant right MCA stroke with substantial motor deficits and left-sided neglect impacting safety and independence

- Some recovery expected but extent uncertain; may require extended care facility and intensive rehabilitation
- Initiate code status and surrogate decision-making discussion given new profound disability

Managing Conflict

The husband insists on thrombolytic therapy: "You have to give her the clot-buster drug."

- Acknowledge distress, validate desire for aggressive treatment
- Explain that the medication can only be given within 4.5 hours of onset; unknown timing creates unacceptable bleeding risk
- Offer alternatives: aspirin, BP optimization, evaluation for mechanical thrombectomy
- Provide written stroke education materials; offer chaplaincy or social work

Critical Actions

- Establish exact time last known well for thrombolytic eligibility
- Immediate fingerstick glucose to exclude hypoglycemia mimicking stroke
- Non-contrast head CT within 25 minutes to exclude hemorrhage before antiplatelet therapy
- Recognition that wake-up stroke excludes standard IV tPA unless advanced imaging qualifies
- BP management: treat SBP >220 or DBP >120; avoid precipitous drops
- Recognition of right MCA syndrome: left hemiplegia, sensory loss, neglect (extinction, anosognosia), central CN VII palsy
- Aspirin 325 mg within 24-48 hours once hemorrhage excluded
- Reassessment recognizing deterioration with emergent repeat imaging
- Effective communication regarding tPA exclusion with clear reasoning and empathy
- Early stroke team consultation and consideration of endovascular therapy for large vessel occlusion

Pelvic Trauma

Opening Scenario

A 64-year-old male pedestrian struck by an SUV at 25-30 mph, thrown approximately 10 feet, landing on his left side. Trauma surgery en route (ETA 15 minutes). Patient has obvious lower extremity deformities and complains of severe pelvic and left thigh pain. Immobilized on backboard with cervical collar.

Initial Assessment

Vitals: BP 118/76, HR 112, RR 24, T 36.8°C, SpO_2 97% RA, Glucose 142

Alert, moderate distress, lying supine on backboard. Pale, diaphoretic skin.

- Airway: Patent, speaking in full sentences
- Breathing: Tachypneic but non-labored, clear bilaterally, no cyanosis
- Circulation: Peripheral pulses thready, capillary refill 3 seconds, cool and pale skin
- Disability: GCS 15, obvious shortening and external rotation of left lower extremity, abrasions to left flank and thigh

History

- HPI: Crossing street when struck by SUV. Recalls impact and being thrown. Landed on left side with immediate severe pelvic and left leg pain. Denies LOC, headache, neck pain, chest pain, or SOB. Reports taking "blood thinner medication" but unsure of name. Last meal 2 hours ago.
- PMHx: Atrial fibrillation, hypertension, osteoarthritis
- PSHx: Right total knee replacement
- Allergies: Penicillin (rash)
- Medications: Warfarin 5 mg daily, metoprolol, lisinopril
- Social: Lives with spouse, retired, denies tobacco or illicit drug use, occasional alcohol

Physical Examination

- General: Alert and oriented x4, anxious but cooperative
- Head: No lacerations or step-offs, left temporal contusion
- Eyes: PERRL, EOMI
- Neck: No midline tenderness, ROM limited by collar
- Chest: TTP over left ribs (8-10), no crepitus or paradoxical movement
- Lungs: Clear bilaterally
- Heart: Tachycardic, regular rhythm, no murmurs
- Abdomen: Soft, mildly distended, suprapubic tenderness, no guarding or rebound
- Pelvis: Unstable on compression and distraction, 3 cm diastasis, severe tenderness over symphysis and bilateral SI joints
- GU: No blood at urethral meatus, Foley with clear urine
- Rectal: Normal tone, guaiac negative
- Left LE: Shortened and externally rotated, mid-shaft femur tenderness, 2 cm open wound lateral thigh, weak distal pulses, capillary refill 4 seconds
- Right LE: Non-tender, neurovascular intact
- Back: No step-offs, abrasions over left flank
- Neurological: GCS 15, CN II-XII intact, 5/5 strength UE and right LE, limited by pain on left

- Skin: Pale, cool, diaphoretic

Diagnostic Studies

- WBC 12.5, Hgb 9.2, Hct 28%, Plt 225
- PT 22.5, INR 2.8 (elevated), PTT 42
- Na 138, K 4.1, Cl 105, HCO_3 22, BUN 18, Cr 1.1, Glucose 156
- Lactate 4.2 (elevated); Type: O positive, antibody negative
- CXR: No pneumothorax/hemothorax; left rib fractures (8-10); normal mediastinal width
- AP Pelvis: Open-book fracture, 4 cm symphyseal diastasis
- Left Femur: Mid-shaft fracture with mild displacement
- FAST: Negative for free fluid

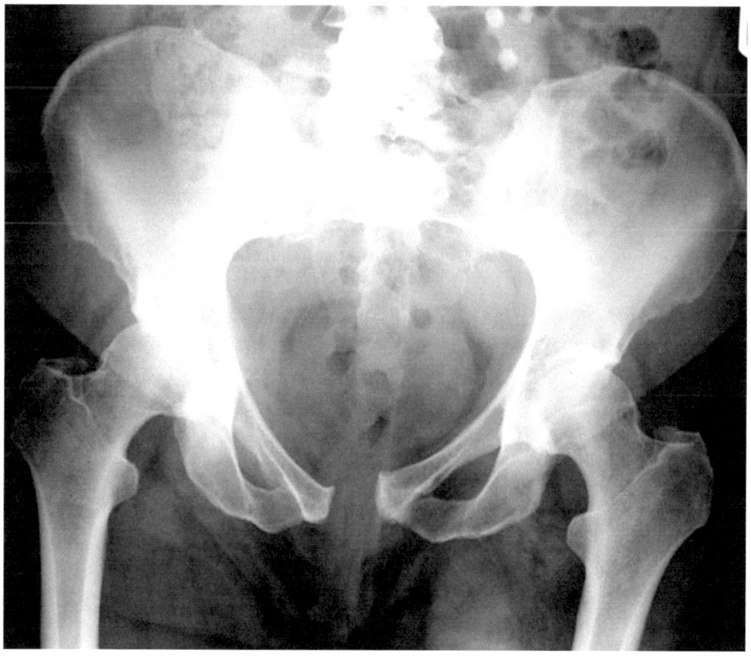

Management

- Supplemental O2 via NRB at 15 L/min; two large-bore IVs (16-gauge)
- Trauma labs: CBC, BMP, coags, type and crossmatch for 4 units PRBCs
- Warmed NS bolus; cardiac monitoring; Foley (after inspecting for urethral blood)

Reassessment

Nurse update after initial NS bolus: BP 94/58, HR 128, RR 26, SpO_2 99% on NRB. Increasing pelvic pressure and dizziness. POC Hct 30%.

At 15 minutes: BP 72/44, HR 145, RR 32, SpO_2 96% on NRB. Increasingly confused and restless. Skin cold/clammy with LE mottling. UOP <20 mL.

- Activate massive transfusion protocol
- Apply pelvic binder to reduce volume and stabilize fracture
- 2 units O-negative PRBCs immediately
- Reverse anticoagulation: 4-factor PCC 50 units/kg and Vitamin K 10 mg IV
- Consult IR for emergent pelvic angiography and embolization
- Consult orthopedic surgery for external fixation

- Calcium chloride 1 g IV with blood products

Patient Communication

- Explain critical condition and need for emergent IR angiography to stop internal bleeding
- Discuss procedure risks: contrast nephropathy, vascular injury, potential need for open surgery
- Provide analgesia (fentanyl 100 mcg IV) while monitoring hemodynamics

Difficult Conversations

Family demands CT scan before any procedures and questions why surgery is not being performed.

- Escort family to private area; acknowledge concerns
- Explain hemodynamic instability and pelvic hemorrhage worsened by anticoagulation
- CT is currently not possible as patient is not stable: transporting an actively hemorrhaging patient risks arrest
- Embolization is standard of care, and orthopedic surgery will also come and explain as well

Critical Actions

- Recognition of hemodynamic instability secondary to pelvic fracture with retroperitoneal hemorrhage
- Appropriate prioritization of pelvic stabilization (binder/sheet application) before definitive imaging or fracture management
- Early activation of massive transfusion protocol and blood products rather than excessive crystalloid resuscitation
- Recognition of warfarin anticoagulation and appropriate reversal with PCC and Vitamin K prior to or concurrent with invasive procedures
- Decision to proceed with emergent angiography without awaiting CT given hemodynamic instability (damage control resuscitation)
- Effective reassessment recognizing clinical deterioration despite initial interventions
- Clear communication with patient regarding critical condition and informed consent for high-risk procedure
- Skillful management of family conflict using empathy while maintaining firm direction toward life-saving therapy
- Appropriate consultation with IR, trauma surgery, and orthopedic surgery
- Recognition that open femur fracture is secondary priority to life-threatening pelvic hemorrhage

Elderly Patient with Dementia

Opening Scenario

EMS brings a 78-year-old male from an assisted living facility with fever and altered mental status. His daughter (healthcare proxy) is in the waiting room requesting to speak with you urgently.

Initial Assessment

Vitals: BP 94/58, HR 118, RR 28, SpO_2 90% RA, T 39.1C, glucose 142

- Cachectic male, lethargic but arousable to voice, pale, diaphoretic, mottled distal extremities, accessory muscle use
- Airway: Patent, speaking in short phrases but confused
- Breathing: Tachypneic, coarse breath sounds bilaterally
- Circulation: Weak radial pulses, cap refill ~3 seconds, cool and clammy
- Disability: Eyes open to voice, confused to time/place, moves all extremities to command

History

- HPI: At baseline yesterday. Found confused and febrile to 103F this morning. Cloudy urine in Foley bag over past 24 hours.
- PMHx: Alzheimer dementia, type 2 DM, HTN, BPH
- Meds: Metformin, lisinopril, donepezil, tamsulosin
- Allergies: NKDA
- Social: Assisted living, widowed, daughter is healthcare proxy

Physical Examination

- General: Cachectic, pale, diaphoretic, confused
- HEENT: PERRL, EOM intact
- Neck: Supple, no JVD
- Cardiovascular: Tachycardic, regular, no murmurs
- Pulmonary: Bilateral crackles at bases, accessory muscle use, no wheezes
- Abdomen: Soft, non-distended, suprapubic tenderness, no rebound or guarding
- GU: Foley with cloudy, foul-smelling urine
- Extremities: Cool with mottling of lower extremities, weak pulses
- Neurological: Confused to time/place/situation, follows simple commands, CN II-XII intact, no focal deficits

Diagnostic Studies

- CBC: WBC 19.4 (12% bands), Hgb 11.8, Plt 128
- BMP: Na 142, K 3.9, HCO_3 18, BUN 42, Cr 2.6 (baseline 1.0)
- Lactate: 5.2
- UA: Positive LE, positive nitrites, >100 WBCs/hpf
- ECG: Sinus tachycardia 108, no acute ST changes
- CXR: Mild vascular congestion, no focal consolidation
- IVC US: > 75% collapsibility

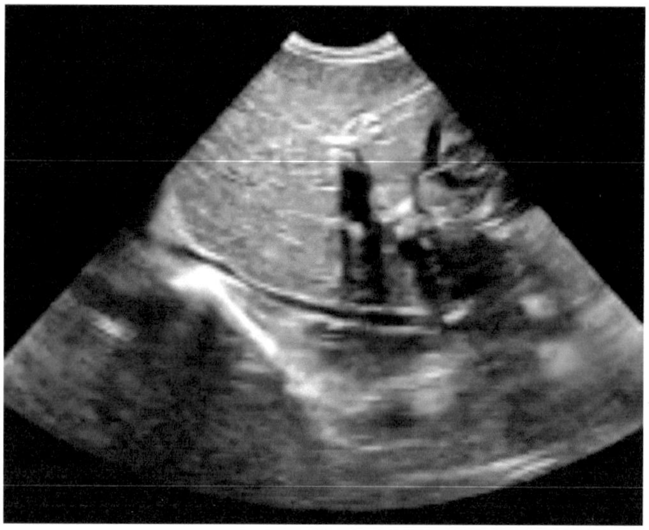

Management

- Continuous monitoring, O2 via NC to SpO_2 >94%, two large-bore IVs
- 30 mL/kg crystalloid resuscitation
- Blood/urine cultures, then broad-spectrum antibiotics within one hour (ceftriaxone or piperacillin-tazobactam; add vancomycin if MRSA risk)

Reassessment

45 minutes later: BP 78/52 (despite 2L crystalloid), HR 128, RR 32, T 39.4C. Worsening despite initial resuscitation. Perform IVC ultrasound to asses for fluid responsiveness and start vasopressors. Repeat IVC ultrasound shows minimal collapsibility of IVC so no additional fluids will be beneficial.

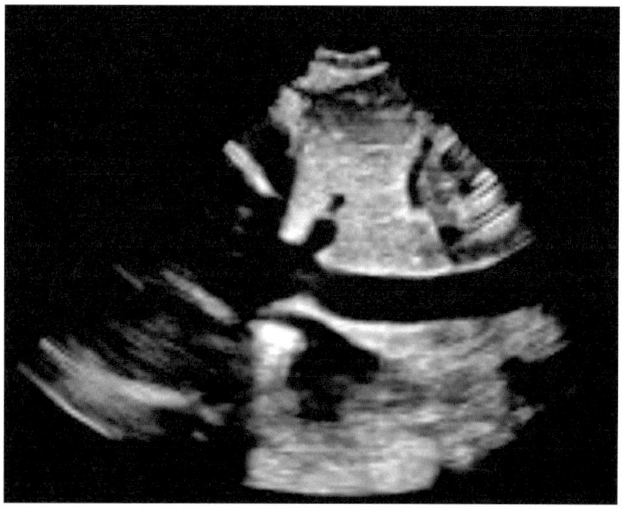

Difficult Conversations

Daughter approaches, distressed: "He has dementia and we never talked about what he'd want if he was really sick. I don't want him to suffer." Discuss goals of care and code status with empathetic communication (SPIKES protocol). Assess patient's previously expressed wishes.

Disposition

- ICU admission for vasopressor support given refractory hypotension
- Evaluate for additional infection sources

Critical Actions

- Recognize septic shock secondary to complicated UTI/pyelonephritis
- Initiate 30 mL/kg crystalloid and broad-spectrum antibiotics within one hour
- Utilize IVC ultrasound for initial and subsequent volume assessments.
- Obtain cultures before antibiotics when feasible
- Identify deterioration despite resuscitation; escalate to ICU with vasopressors
- Engage surrogate decision-maker in goals-of-care discussion
- Reassess hemodynamic status after interventions

Acute Back Pain

Opening Scenario

A 38-year-old male construction worker arrives with his wife, reporting severe lower back pain radiating down both legs, inability to urinate for 8 hours, new groin numbness, and bilateral leg weakness after lifting heavy equipment 3 days ago.

Initial Assessment

Vitals: BP 156/94, HR 108, RR 18, SpO_2 99% RA, T 37.2C

- Diaphoretic, moderate distress, prefers supine with knees flexed
- Airway: Patent, speaking in full sentences
- Breathing: Clear bilaterally
- Circulation: Warm, cap refill <2 seconds, symmetric radial pulses
- Disability: A&O x3, GCS 15

History

- HPI: Sudden severe lumbar pain 3 days ago lifting construction materials. Progressed to bilateral buttock/posterior thigh radiation. Past 24 hours: perineal numbness (saddle anesthesia), bilateral foot weakness, unable to void for 8 hours with one incontinence episode. Afebrile.
- PMHx: HTN (poorly controlled), chronic low back pain
- PSHx: Appendectomy
- Meds: Lisinopril (irregular), ibuprofen 800mg TID x3 days
- Allergies: NKDA
- Social: Former smoker, occasional alcohol

Physical Examination

- Back: Severe tenderness over L4-L5, painful limited ROM
- Neurologic: Decreased perineal sensation (S2-S4), decreased rectal tone, 3/5 left ankle dorsiflexion, 4/5 right ankle dorsiflexion, 5/5 bilateral knee extension, absent bilateral Achilles reflexes, positive crossed SLR on left
- Abdomen: Suprapubic fullness with palpable bladder dome ~4 cm above symphysis, dullness to percussion

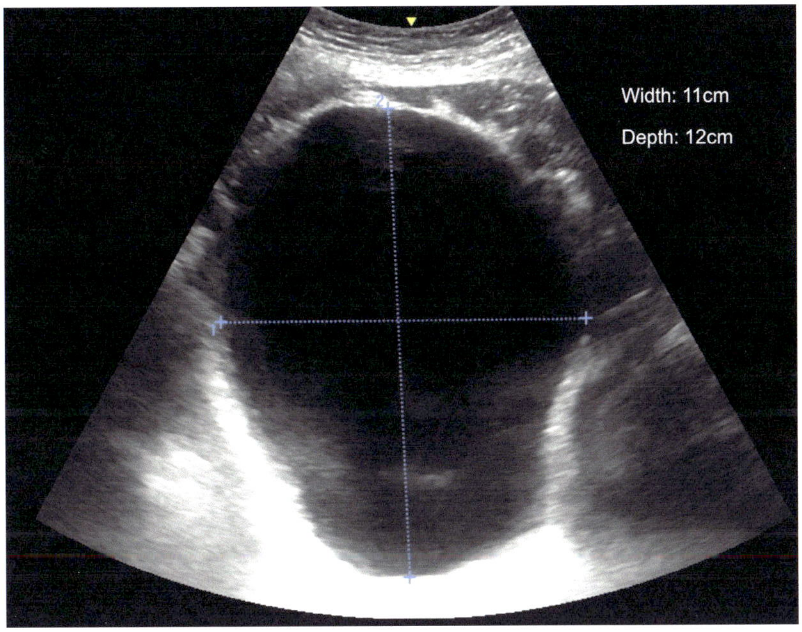

Diagnostic Studies

- CBC: WBC 11.2, Hgb 14.8, Plt 285
- BMP: Na 138, K 4.2, Cl 102, HCO_3 24, BUN 48, Cr 1.4 (baseline 0.9), glucose 112
- UA: Normal
- CT lumbar spine: Large central disc herniation at L4-L5 with severe central canal stenosis

Management

- Two large-bore IVs, CBC/BMP/coags/type and screen
- Analgesia: ketorolac 30mg IV and morphine 4mg IV
- Foley catheter for urinary retention (800 mL returned)
- Emergent MRI

Patient Communication

Patient expresses severe claustrophobia and refuses MRI, requesting discharge with oral pain meds. Explain surgical emergency nature of cauda equina syndrome, risk of permanent paralysis/incontinence/sexual dysfunction without urgent decompression. Offer anxiolytic pre-medication or open MRI. Involve wife in shared decision-making. After successful negotiation, patient consents.

- MRI lumbar spine: Confirms large central L4-L5 disc herniation with mass effect on thecal sac and bilateral traversing nerve roots consistent with cauda equina syndrome

Reassessment

- Post-analgesia: Pain 5/10, HR 92, tolerates supine for imaging
- Post-MRI: No change in neurologic exam (stable weakness, persistent saddle anesthesia)

Disposition

- Urgent neurosurgery consult for emergent L4-L5 discectomy and decompression
- Admit to ICU

Critical Actions

- Recognize red flags for cauda equina syndrome (urinary retention, saddle anesthesia, bilateral leg symptoms, decreased rectal tone)
- Perform focused neurologic exam including perianal sensation, rectal tone, and L5/S1 motor testing
- Order emergent MRI
- Address claustrophobia barrier to care with patient-centered communication
- Recognize urinary retention on ultrasound and perform catheterization
- Consult neurosurgery urgently

Seizing and Altered

Opening Scenario

A 48-year-old man is brought by EMS after a witnessed generalized tonic-clonic seizure lasting ~90 seconds that terminated prior to arrival. Currently confused but following commands. Wife reports fatigue, myalgias, fevers for one week, and new bruising on arms and legs over two days.

Initial Assessment

Vitals: BP 124/82, HR 114, RR 20, T 38.7C, SpO_2 97% RA

- Middle-aged male, drowsy but arousable, pale
- Airway: Patent, handling secretions
- Breathing: Clear bilaterally
- Circulation: Warm, dry, cap refill <2 seconds

History

- HPI: No prior seizure history. One week of fatigue, myalgias, subjective fevers. New bruising on arms/legs x2 days. No head trauma with seizure. Denies headache, neck stiffness, chest pain, or dyspnea.
- PMHx: HTN, hyperlipidemia
- Meds: Amlodipine, atorvastatin
- Allergies: NKDA
- Social: Accountant, occasional alcohol, no tobacco/drugs

Physical Examination

- General: Alert and oriented x3, mild distress
- HEENT: Pale conjunctivae, dry mucous membranes
- Skin: Diffuse petechiae on bilateral lower extremities and forearms; ecchymoses on trunk and back; no active bleeding
- Neurological: CN intact, no focal motor deficits, sensation intact
- Cardiovascular: Regular rhythm, no murmurs
- Abdomen: Soft, mild epigastric tenderness, no rebound or guarding

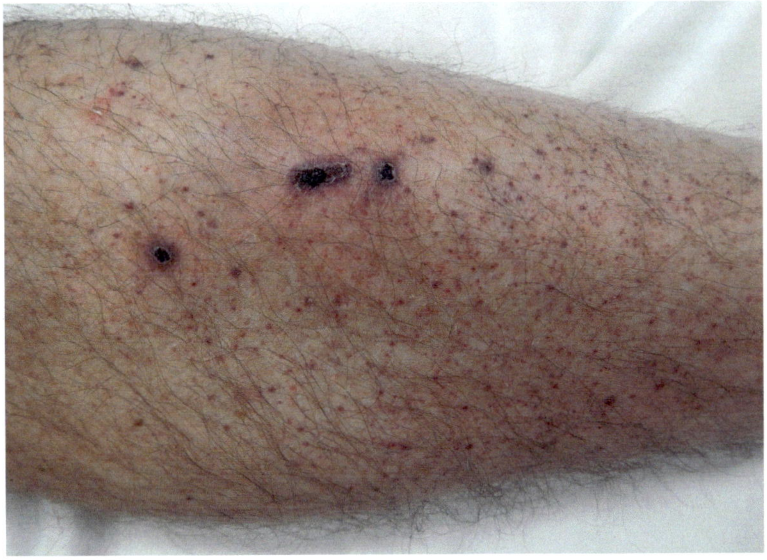

Diagnostic Studies

- CBC: WBC 10.8, Hgb 6.2, Hct 21.3%, Plt 10
- BMP: Na 139, K 4.3, Cl 104, HCO_3 24, BUN 28, Cr 2.1, glucose 94
- LFTs: AST 45, ALT 22, T.Bili 1.8, D.Bili 0.6, LDH elevated
- Coags: PT 12.8, PTT 31, INR 0.9
- Peripheral smear: Numerous schistocytes, helmet cells, fragmented RBCs; decreased platelets
- CT head: No acute hemorrhage, no mass effect

Management

- Continuous monitoring, two large-bore IVs, 1L NS bolus, ECG
- CT head without contrast
- Peripheral blood smear
- Acetaminophen for fever

Patient Communication

Wife states: "Can you just give him seizure medicine and let us go home? We have a flight tomorrow for our anniversary trip." Explain serious diagnosis requiring immediate hospitalization. Seizure medication alone is insufficient; the underlying blood disorder is life-threatening.

Reassessment

45 minutes later: Worsening headache, visual disturbances ("seeing spots"), BP 168/98, HR 106. New epistaxis and oozing from IV sites. Urine output 30 mL/hour.

- Hematology consult for concern for TTP
- Arrange emergent therapeutic plasma exchange with hematology and nephrology
- Avoid platelet transfusion unless life-threatening hemorrhage
- Nephrology consult for AKI
- ICU admission

Critical Actions

- Recognize classic TTP features (fever, MAHA, thrombocytopenia, renal impairment, neurologic symptoms)
- Order peripheral smear showing schistocytes
- Identify contraindication of platelet transfusion in TTP
- Initiate emergent plasma exchange
- Communicate with patient/family regarding serious diagnosis
- Reassess and recognize clinical deterioration
- Consult hematology/nephrology; admit to ICU

Burn

Opening Scenario

EMS arrives with a 28-year-old male involved in a combustible dust explosion in a poorly ventilated warehouse 45 minutes ago. Short sleeves, no facial protection. Ambulatory at scene, severe pain to face and arms. O2 via NC and single IV started by EMS.

Initial Assessment

Vitals: BP 142/88, HR 118, RR 24, T 37.8C, SpO_2 96% RA (100% on 15L NRB)

Physical Examination

- General: Alert, moderate distress due to pain, facial soot noted
- HEENT: Soot in nares and oropharynx, singed nasal area, blistering burns to face and lips, voice hoarse
- Neck: Anterior neck burns with soft tissue edema, no stridor currently
- Chest: Anterior chest wall with blistering burns, breath sounds clear bilaterally
- Extremities: Circumferential full-thickness burn to right upper extremity (white, leathery, insensate), radial pulse diminished, delayed capillary refill (>3 seconds)
- Remainder of physical examination normal

History

- HPI: Spray-painting metal shelving when flash fire from combustible dust. Shielded face with right arm. No LOC.
- PMHx: None
- Meds: None
- Allergies: NKDA
- Social: 1 ppd smoker, occasional alcohol

Diagnostic Studies

- CBC: WBC 16.2, Hgb 14.8, Hct 44%, Plt 312
- BMP: Na 140, K 4.0, Cl 103, HCO_3 20, BUN 28, Cr 1.4, glucose 110
- Coags: PT 12.8, PTT 32, INR 1.0
- Carboxyhemoglobin: 8.2
- Lactate: 3.8
- ECG: Sinus tachycardia, no ischemic changes
- CXR: Clear lung fields

Management

- Recognize high-risk inhalation injury (facial burns, soot, hoarseness, closed-space exposure); perform early intubation before edema progresses
- Estimate ~20 TBSA. Parkland formula: 4 mL x kg x %TBSA over 24 hours; half in first 8 hours from injury time (not presentation). Two large-bore IVs, LR infusion.
- Discuss intubation necessity with patient and family before airway compromise

Difficult Conversations

Wife asks privately if husband will need surgery. Explain severity of burns, high infection risk, prolonged rehabilitation/scarring, and necessity of burn center transfer. Address concern about intubation preventing speech.

Reassessment

90 minutes after arrival (post-intubation, 2L infused): BP 128/76, HR 105, SpO_2 98% on vent. Right upper extremity: radial pulse now absent, cap refill >4 seconds, fingers dusky. Developing compartment syndrome from circumferential eschar and fluid resuscitation requiring emergent surgical consult. Bedside Doppler confirms loss of arterial signal. Perform emergent escharotomy restoring distal pulses in coordination with surgical consult.

Disposition

- Tetanus toxoid IM, fentanyl infusion for analgesia
- Contact regional burn center for emergent transfer
- Discuss hyperbaric oxygen with toxicology for carboxyhemoglobin 8.2 with symptoms

Critical Actions

- Recognize inhalation injury and prioritize early intubation before edema progression
- Calculate fluid resuscitation using Parkland formula from time of injury
- Assess for CO/cyanide poisoning (carboxyhemoglobin, lactate)
- Communicate intubation necessity to patient/family before airway compromise
- Reassess extremity perfusion; recognize compartment syndrome requiring emergent escharotomy
- Ensure analgesia and tetanus prophylaxis
- Coordinate burn center transfer

Nausea and Vomiting

Opening Scenario

A 58-year-old male checks in with abdominal pain, vomiting, inability to pass flatus, and history of gastric bypass surgery. Appears uncomfortable, vomiting in triage.

Initial Assessment

Vitals: BP 142/82, HR 108, RR 18, T 36.8C, SpO_2 98% RA, pain 8/10

History

- HPI: 36 hours of progressive periumbilical cramping now diffuse and constant. Multiple bilious emeses x12 hours, unable to tolerate PO. No BM x3 days, no flatus x24 hours. Denies fever, chest pain, hematemesis, melena.
- PMHx: HTN, diet-controlled type 2 DM (resolved post-bariatric)
- PSHx: Roux-en-Y gastric bypass 5 years ago, remote appendectomy
- Meds: Lisinopril, multivitamin, omeprazole
- Allergies: NKDA
- Social: Retired teacher, no tobacco/alcohol/drugs

Physical Examination

- General: Alert and oriented, moderate distress, diaphoretic, guarding abdomen
- Cardiovascular: Tachycardic but regular rhythm, capillary refill 2 seconds, no peripheral edema
- Abdomen: Distended and tympanitic; hyperactive, high-pitched bowel sounds; diffuse tenderness with voluntary guarding, no rebound tenderness; well-healed midline and laparoscopic scars
- Rectal: Normal tone, hemoccult negative
- GU exam: No appreciable crepitus/bullae, cremasteric reflex present bilaterally, negative prehn sign, no appreciation of inguinal hernias bilaterally
- Remainder of physical examination normal

Diagnostic Studies

- CBC: WBC 14.2, Hgb 14.5, Plt 280
- BMP: Na 138, K 3.8, HCO_3 22, BUN 28, Cr 1.2
- Lactate: 2.8 (elevated)
- Lipase: 45 (normal)
- Coags: Normal
- ECG: NSR, no acute ischemic changes
- KUB Xray: Multiple dilated small bowel loops (>3 cm) with air-fluid levels; no free air
- CT Abd pelvis: dilated small bowel loops up to 4 cm with a transition point related to the Roux-en-Y segment, consistent with a closed loop small bowel obstruction

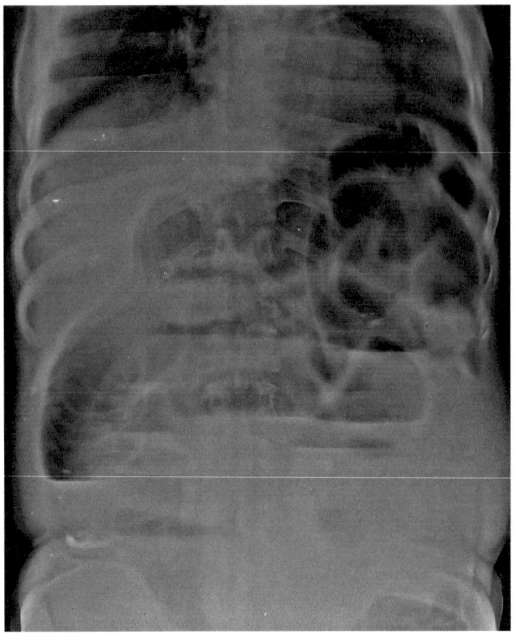

Management

- Two large-bore IVs, 1L LR bolus, NPO, Foley catheter
- Morphine 4mg IV for analgesia
- Labs including lactate, lipase, type and screen
- Urgent surgical consult (Roux-en-Y anatomy increases risk for internal hernia and closed-loop obstruction)
- Elevated lactate is a red flag for potential bowel ischemia

Patient Communication

Patient states: "I don't want another operation. Can't you just give me something to make me have a bowel movement?" Explain mechanical nature of obstruction. Clarify laxatives/enemas are contraindicated (perforation risk). Discuss necessity of NG tube decompression. Address concerns about surgery by explaining risks of non-operative management (necrosis, perforation). Verify understanding with teach-back.

Managing Conflict

Patient requests to leave AMA for a family wedding tomorrow. Explore underlying concerns (fear of surgery, financial worries). Negotiate time-limited observation trial (2 hours) with clear metrics. If patient maintains desire to leave, assess capacity and complete AMA documentation with specific risk discussion including bowel necrosis, perforation, and death.

Reassessment

2 hours later (after 2L crystalloid and NG tube with 800 mL bilious output): BP 98/58 (from 142/82), HR 118, RR 24, T 37.4C, pain 10/10 now localized to RLQ with rebound and rigidity. Patient increasingly toxic and confused.

- Broad-spectrum antibiotics (gram-negative and anaerobe coverage)
- Additional 2L bolus, consider vasopressors
- Urgent surgical re-evaluation for emergent laparotomy (concern for closed-loop obstruction specific to gastric bypass anatomy)

Difficult Conversations

Inform patient and spouse that clinical picture has worsened and emergency surgery is now required. "Warning shot" approach: "I'm afraid I have some serious news about how your condition has changed." Acknowledge prior hesitation about surgery. Explain waiting is no longer safe. Also ask surgery to come to bedside to explain condition to the patient.

Critical Actions

- Recognize high-risk surgical anatomy (Roux-en-Y) predisposing to internal hernia and closed-loop obstruction
- Identify elevated lactate as marker of potential bowel ischemia
- Contraindicate laxatives/promotility agents in mechanical obstruction
- Effectively communicate and negotiate when patient requests AMA
- Recognize clinical deterioration and escalate to antibiotics and emergent surgery
- Deliver urgent news about necessity of emergency surgery empathetically

Seizure and Fever

Opening Scenario

An 18-month-old female arrives by private vehicle with her parents after a "shaking episode" ~10 minutes ago lasting ~5 minutes that stopped spontaneously. She has been difficult to arouse since the event. On monitor with blow-by oxygen.

Initial Assessment

Vitals: HR 162, RR 36, BP 94/62, T 39.6C (rectal), SpO_2 94% RA, weight 12 kg

- Post-ictal, eyes closed, opens briefly to painful stimulus, mildly diaphoretic
- Airway: Patent, handling secretions
- Breathing: Tachypneic, no retractions or flaring, clear bilaterally
- Circulation: Cap refill 2 seconds, 2+ symmetric pulses, warm and well-perfused
- Disability: Opens eyes to voice, withdraws to pain, vocalizes minimally (AVPU: Voice). PERRL. No focal deficits.
- Exposure: Warm to touch, no rashes or petechiae

History

- HPI: Previously healthy, 2-day URI with nasal congestion and low-grade fever. Temperature to 39.6C this afternoon. Witnessed GTC seizure with rhythmic shaking of all extremities, eyes rolling upward, brief lip cyanosis, lasting ~5 minutes. No apnea, no incontinence, no trauma.
- PMHx: Full-term, normal development, immunizations UTD
- Meds: Acetaminophen given at home 45 minutes ago (dose unknown)
- Allergies: None
- Social: Lives with both parents and 4-year-old sibling with similar cold symptoms

Management

- Continuous monitoring, peripheral IV
- Weight-based antipyretic (acetaminophen 15 mg/kg or ibuprofen 10 mg/kg)
- POC glucose: 96

Reassessment

20 minutes post-antipyretic: HR 148, RR 28, T 39.2C, SpO_2 96% RA. Now sleeping but easily arousable, drinking small sips.

45 minutes after arrival: Second generalized tonic-clonic seizure. HR 174, RR 38, BP 102/68, SpO_2 89% RA. Rhythmic bilateral jerking, eyes deviated right, ongoing for 3 minutes. Manage with lateral positioning, suction, supplemental oxygen; prepare rescue benzodiazepine if >5 minutes.

Physical Examination

- General: Post-ictal following second seizure, now sleeping but arousable to voice
- HEENT: Bilaterally erythematous tympanic membranes without bulging or effusion; oropharynx mildly erythematous; anterior fontanelle flat and closed
- Neck: Supple, no nuchal rigidity
- Lungs: Clear to auscultation bilaterally
- Cardiovascular: Regular rhythm, no murmurs, gallops, or rubs

- Abdomen: Soft, non-tender, non-distended
- Skin: No rashes, petechiae, or bruising
- Neurological: Moves all extremities equally when aroused, tracks conjugately, no focal weakness. Remainder of neurological examination normal.

Diagnostic Studies

- CBC: WBC 15.8, Hgb 11.0, Hct 33.2%, Plt 298
- BMP: Na 138, K 4.0, Cl 103, HCO_3 23, BUN 14, Cr 0.3, glucose 102
- UA: SG 1.018, pH 6.5, LE negative, nitrite negative, ketones trace
- LP (if performed): OP normal, WBC 1, RBC 2, protein 22, glucose 65, Gram stain negative

Patient Communication

Parents state: "This is the second time today! Does she have epilepsy? We want a CT scan and we want her admitted." Explain this represents a simple febrile seizure (age-appropriate, generalized, <15 min, normal neuro exam). Discuss benign nature, 30-40 recurrence risk, excellent prognosis with low epilepsy risk. Explain CT/EEG/LP are not routinely indicated.

Disposition

Discharge with return precautions: seizure >15 minutes, focal features, persistent AMS, signs of meningitis. Antipyretic dosing instructions. PCP follow-up within 24-48 hours.

Critical Actions

- Recognize simple febrile seizure based on age, generalized type, duration <15 min, and normal neuro exam
- Manage acute seizure with airway protection, O2, and rescue benzodiazepine if >5 minutes
- Avoid unnecessary testing (routine CT, EEG, LP) when consistent with simple febrile seizure
- Address parental fears about epilepsy with clear education about benign prognosis
- Provide appropriate discharge instructions with return precautions

Early Pregnancy

Opening Scenario

A 28-year-old female arrives via private vehicle with severe lower abdominal pain and heavy vaginal bleeding. Appears pale and requests to lie down immediately.

Initial Assessment

Vitals: BP 92/64, HR 104, RR 14, T 37.1C, SpO_2 99% RA

- Diaphoretic, moderate distress, supine with knees flexed, clutching lower abdomen, conjunctival pallor
- Airway: Patent, speaking in full sentences
- Breathing: Non-labored, clear bilaterally
- Circulation: Cool, clammy extremities, cap refill 3 seconds, weak peripheral pulses

History

- HPI: G3P2 with laparoscopic tubal ligation 18 months ago. Sudden sharp lower abdominal pain and vaginal bleeding starting 6 hours ago, soaking 6 pads. LMP ~6 weeks ago. Dizziness on standing. Home pregnancy test positive 2 weeks ago.
- PMHx: Two prior vaginal deliveries, one first-trimester miscarriage 3 years ago, hypothyroidism
- PSHx: Bilateral tubal ligation, appendectomy
- Meds: Levothyroxine 75 mcg, prenatal vitamins
- Allergies: NKDA
- Social: Lives with partner and two children

Physical Examination

- General: Alert, oriented, anxious, moderate distress
- HEENT: Pale conjunctivae, dry mucous membranes
- Cardiovascular: Regular rhythm, no murmurs, cap refill 3 seconds
- Abdomen: Mild distension, hypoactive bowel sounds, RLQ and suprapubic tenderness, no rebound/ guarding
- Pelvic: Blood in vaginal vault, closed cervical os, cervical motion tenderness, normal uterine size, right adnexal fullness
- Skin: Cool, clammy

Management

- Two large-bore IVs (16g), 1L NS bolus via pressure bag
- POC glucose, continuous cardiac monitoring
- Labs: CBC, CMP, type & screen (crossmatch 2 units PRBC), quantitative hCG, coags
- Urine or serum pregnancy test

Reassessment

After 1L NS: BP 108/72, HR 88, RR 12. Slightly improved dizziness, persistent abdominal pain 7/10. Urine pregnancy test positive.

Diagnostic Studies

- CBC: WBC 11.8, Hgb 9.8, Hct 29.4%, Plt 245

- BMP: Na 138, K 4.0, Cl 105, HCO_3 22, BUN 14, Cr 0.9, glucose 98
- Coags: PT 12.8, PTT 28, INR 1.0
- Type & screen: O-negative, antibody negative
- Quantitative hCG: 8,450 mIU/mL
- TVUS: No IUP identified; heterogeneous right adnexal mass with moderate free pelvic fluid
- FAST: Positive free fluid in hepatorenal space and pelvis

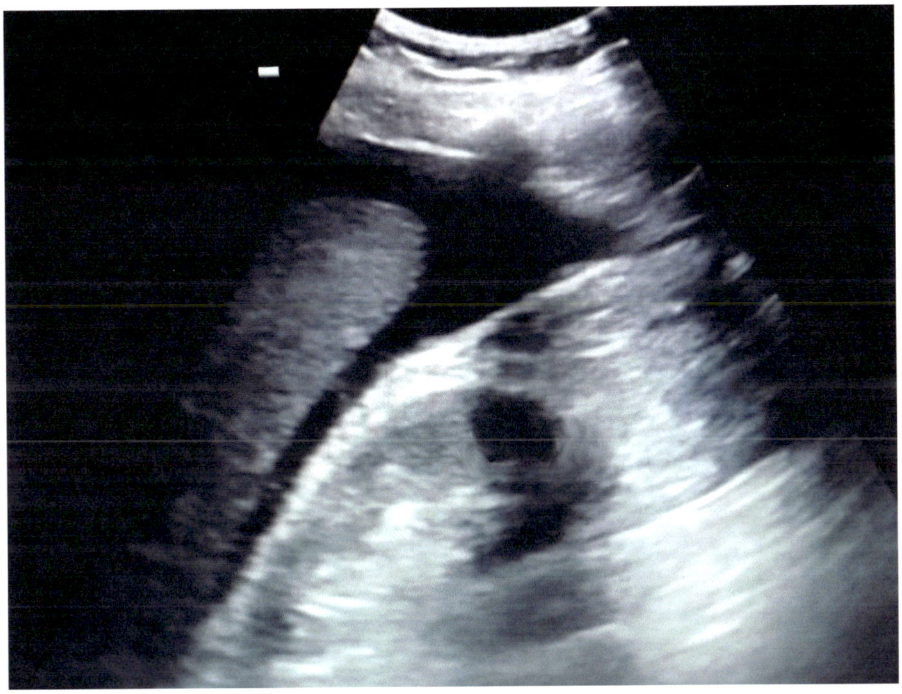

Disposition

- Immediate OB/GYN consult for suspected ruptured ectopic pregnancy
- Rho(D) immune globulin 300 mcg IM (Rh-negative patient)
- Morphine 4-6 mg IV for analgesia
- Continue crystalloid resuscitation
- Prepare for operative intervention (laparoscopy vs laparotomy)
- Update patient and partner regarding diagnosis and need for emergent surgery

Critical Actions

- Obtain pregnancy test in all reproductive-age females with abdominal pain/vaginal bleeding
- Recognize tubal ligation failure as risk factor for ectopic pregnancy
- Perform bedside transabdominal pelvic ultrasound and fast exam in patients with ectopic on differential prior to ordering a formal pelvic ultrasound; recognize no IUP with free fluid and positive hCG as ectopic until proven otherwise
- Initiate aggressive fluid resuscitation; recognize need for blood products
- Administer Rho(D) immune globulin to Rh-negative patient
- Consult OB/GYN emergently for surgical management
- Explain life-threatening nature of ruptured ectopic pregnancy empathetically

Diffuse Abdominal Pain

Opening Scenario

EMS brings a 48-year-old female with severe abdominal pain. Her husband states loudly: "This is ridiculous, we waited three hours. She just needs her insulin fixed and we want to go home." Patient is cachectic, lying in fetal position.

Initial Assessment

Vitals: BP 82/54, HR 138, RR 36, SpO_2 94% RA, T 39.2C, weight 68 kg

- Cachectic, older than stated age, diaphoretic, sunken eyes, speaking in short gasping phrases. Kussmaul respirations.
- Airway: Patent, short phrases
- Breathing: Markedly tachypneic with deep sighing (Kussmaul pattern), clear bilaterally
- Circulation: Cool, clammy, cap refill >4 seconds, weak radial pulses, skin mottling on lower extremities
- Disability: A&O x3, GCS 15
- Exposure: No trauma, skin tenting

History

- HPI: 48 hours of worsening diffuse abdominal pain radiating to back, persistent nausea with 6 bilious emeses, shaking chills. Insulin pump catheter dislodged 3 days ago; no insulin since. Last ate 40 hours ago. No diarrhea. LMP 10 months ago.
- PMHx: Type 1 DM (since age 14), diabetic gastroparesis, hypothyroidism
- PSHx: Cholecystectomy, appendectomy
- Allergies: Penicillin (anaphylaxis), sulfa (rash)
- Meds: Insulin lispro via pump (disconnected), levothyroxine
- Social: Lives with husband, teacher, no tobacco/alcohol/drugs

Physical Examination

- General: Cachectic, dry mucous membranes, poor skin turgor with tenting
- Cardiovascular: Tachycardic, regular, weak distal pulses
- Abdomen: Diffusely tender with voluntary guarding and rebound in epigastrium and RLQ, absent bowel sounds
- Skin: Dry, poor turgor

Diagnostic Studies

- POC glucose: 534
- VBG: pH 6.95, pCO2 16, HCO_3 4
- BMP: Na 126, K 6.2, Cl 94, BUN 58, Cr 2.3, glucose 534
- CBC: WBC 19.2, Hgb 15.1, Plt 298
- UA: SG 1.050, glucose >1000, ketones 4+, LE 3+, nitrites positive, WBC-25/hpf
- Lactate: 4.8
- Beta-hydroxybutyrate: 9.4
- ECG: Sinus tachycardia 134, normal axis, no ST changes, no peaked T waves
- CXR: Clear, no free air

- AXR: Dilated small bowel with air-fluid levels consistent with ileus

Management

- Continuous monitoring, two large-bore IVs, Foley catheter
- Aggressive isotonic fluid resuscitation: 2L NS rapidly (30-50 mL/kg in first hour) BEFORE insulin
- Insulin drip 0.1 units/kg/hr after initial fluid resuscitation
- Withhold potassium initially (K 6.2); replete aggressively as acidosis corrects
- Empiric antibiotics for pyelonephritis
- Ondansetron 4mg IV for nausea

Managing Conflict

Husband insists on leaving AMA, demands oral medications only. Acknowledge frustration and validate prior experience. Explain severe DKA (pH <7.0) is critical illness different from prior episode. Clarify why oral/subcutaneous insulin is impossible in severe dehydration/shock. Explain AMA risks: cardiac arrest from hyperkalemia, cerebral edema, aspiration. Negotiate: "Let's try the insulin drip for one hour and reassess together."

Difficult Conversations

30 minutes into resuscitation: Patient increasingly somnolent. Discuss with husband possible clinical deterioration requiring intubation for airway protection given persistent vomiting and declining alertness.

Reassessment

45 minutes (after 2L NS and insulin drip, K initially hemolyzed): BP 104/72 (improved), HR 112, RR 24. Patient now confused and agitated. Urine output 250 mL (dark amber). Abdomen now rigid with diffuse rebound and guarding. Repeat K: 3.6 (rapid shift), glucose 398.

Actions: - Add dextrose to IVF when glucose approaches 250 - Aggressive potassium repletion (20 mEq/hr peripheral) - CT abdomen/pelvis with IV contrast to differentiate DKA ileus from surgical abdomen - ICU admission

Critical Actions

- Recognize severe DKA (pH <7.0) requiring aggressive isotonic fluid before insulin
- Identify UTI as precipitant; initiate appropriate antibiotics considering allergies
- Manage conflict with resistant family member using non-confrontational approach
- Discuss potential intubation with family given declining mental status
- Reassess and recognize changing abdominal exam may represent surgical abdomen vs DKA ileus
- Manage electrolytes: withhold K if >5.2, then aggressively replete as acidosis corrects
- ICU admission for severe DKA with hemodynamic instability and AMS

Oral Rash

Opening Scenario

A 34-year-old male presents with fever and a painful spreading rash. Visible lip lesions. Recently started allopurinol for joint pain. Condition appears to be evolving.

Initial Assessment

Vitals: BP 98/62, HR 112, RR 22, T 39.1C, SpO_2 97% RA

- Alert, moderate distress due to skin pain and oral discomfort
- Airway: Patent with visible oral ulcerations, speaking in full sentences
- Breathing: Non-labored, clear bilaterally
- Circulation: Tachycardic, weak radial pulses, cap refill 3 seconds

History

- HPI: 4-day history of fever, fatigue, arthralgias. Painful erythematous rash began on face/chest 48 hours ago, spreading to trunk/arms. Painful swallowing and dysuria. No pruritus. Started allopurinol 300mg daily 7 days ago for gout.
- PMHx: Gout, HTN
- Meds: Allopurinol (started 7 days ago), lisinopril
- Allergies: NKDA
- Social: Lives with partner, non-smoker, occasional alcohol

Management

- Two large-bore IVs, isotonic fluid resuscitation
- Labs: CBC with diff, CMP, LFTs, coags, blood cultures, UA with culture
- Acetaminophen for antipyresis
- Continuous cardiac monitoring

Physical Examination

- HEENT: Multiple painful ulcerations on buccal mucosa, palate, and lips with hemorrhagic crusting; injected conjunctivae bilaterally; remainder normal
- Skin: Diffuse erythematous macules with central duskiness involving chest, back, and upper extremities; flaccid bullae covering approximately 10 body surface area; positive Nikolsky sign; targetoid lesions on palms; remainder of examination normal

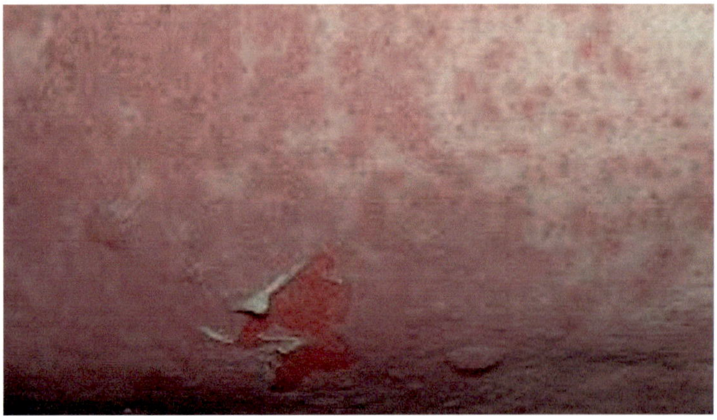

Diagnostic Studies

- CBC: WBC 12.4, Hgb 14.2, Hct 42%, Plt 286
- BMP: Na 138, K 3.8, Cl 102, HCO_3 20, BUN 24, Cr 1.1, glucose 142
- LFTs: AST 45, ALT 38, Alk Phos 88, T.Bili 0.9
- Coags: PT 13.2, PTT 32, INR 1.0
- UA: SG 1.020, pH 6.0, protein neg, blood trace, LE trace, nitrite neg

Reassessment

30 minutes after 2L fluid: BP 88/58, HR 124. Rash extending to lower extremities and genital region with new blisters. Increasing pain and difficulty urinating from mucosal involvement.

- Discontinue allopurinol immediately; document allergy
- Increase fluids to 30 mL/kg; prepare vasopressor support if hypotension persists
- Urgent dermatology and ophthalmology consultations
- Admit to burn unit or ICU for wound care and hemodynamic monitoring
- Communicate diagnosis of Stevens-Johnson Syndrome to patient and family

Critical Actions

- Obtain detailed medication history identifying high-risk drugs (allopurinol) and timing relative to onset
- Perform comprehensive skin exam documenting extent, Nikolsky sign, and target lesions
- Recognize mucosal involvement (oral, ocular, genital) as diagnostic hallmark
- Immediately discontinue offending agent
- Reassess hemodynamic status; recognize third-spacing and hypovolemic shock risk
- Escalate to ICU/burn unit when failing initial fluid resuscitation
- Arrange dermatology and ophthalmology consultations

Procedure Refusal

Opening Scenario

A 58-year-old male with gout and type 2 DM presents with acute left knee pain and fever. Hemodynamically stable initially. Demanding antibiotics and discharge, refusing any physical examination. Patient being disruptive in the waiting room for 45 minutes, nurse calls from triage to ask if you can come speak to the patient in the waiting room..

Initial Assessment

Vitals (initial): BP 144/86, HR 92, RR 14, T 38.9C, SpO_2 97% RA, pain 8/10 Vitals (reassessment): BP 98/52, HR 118

- Uncomfortable, diaphoretic, flushed, holding left knee in slight flexion
- Airway: Patent, speaking full sentences
- Breathing: Non-labored, clear bilaterally
- Circulation: Warm, flushed, cap refill <2 seconds (initially)

History

- HPI: 24 hours of progressive left knee pain, swelling, warmth with fever, rigors, malaise. History of gout in right great toe but "this feels different – more intense and hot." No trauma. Naproxen without relief. Demands antibiotics and states he "doesn't have time for tests."
- PMHx: Type 2 DM (HbA1c 8.2), gout, CKD (baseline Cr 1.8), HTN
- Meds: Allopurinol, metformin, lisinopril, naproxen PRN
- Allergies: NKDA
- Social: Lives with wife who has advanced dementia; construction supervisor; former smoker

Physical Examination

- General: Moderate distress, diaphoretic
- Left Knee: Marked effusion with overlying erythema and warmth; extreme tenderness to palpation; limited active and passive range of motion due to pain (flexed at 30 degrees); unable to bear weight
- Cardiovascular: Tachycardic, regular rhythm, no murmurs
- Skin: Warm, dry (initially); cool and clammy upon reassessment
- Remainder of physical examination: Normal

Diagnostic Studies

- CBC: WBC 14.2, neutrophils 88%, bands 6%, Hgb 13.8, Plt 342
- BMP: Na 138, K 4.2, Cl 102, HCO_3 22, BUN 38, Cr 2.1 (AKI from baseline 1.8), glucose 212
- Blood cultures: Pending

Managing Conflict

Given the physical exam concerning for septic joint, you ask the patient if they would be willing to come back to the main part of the emergency department for arthrocentesis. Patient initially refuses arthrocentesis: "Just give me antibiotics like you do for my gout." Concerned about who will care for wife if admitted. Explain septic arthritis is a joint-threatening emergency requiring drainage; antibiotics alone insufficient. Address caregiver concerns with social work consult. After discussion, patient consents.

Management

- Arthrocentesis under sterile conditions
- Synovial fluid: Turbid yellow-green, WBC 78,000 (92% neutrophils), Gram stain: GP cocci in clusters, no crystals
- Empiric antibiotics
- Orthopedic surgery consult for possible operative I&D

Reassessment

45 minutes later: BP 98/52, HR 118. Increasing pain despite morphine. SpO_2 drops to 92% RA (96% on 2L NC). Progression to sepsis.

- 30 mL/kg crystalloid bolus
- Repeat blood cultures
- Vasopressors if no response to fluids
- Escalate with orthopedics for emergent operative management and admission

Critical Actions

- Recognize monoarticular arthritis with fever as septic arthritis until proven otherwise
- Perform arthrocentesis before antibiotics when feasible
- Elicit patient concerns about caregiving; negotiate consent through shared decision-making
- Recognize deterioration from stable to septic shock; initiate sepsis resuscitation
- Adjust antibiotic coverage based on Gram stain (vancomycin for GP cocci in clusters)
- Admit for IV antibiotics and surgical drainage; ICU if hemodynamically unstable

Cat Bite

Opening Scenario

A 42-year-old male returns to the ED with worsening pain, swelling, and new fever. He initially presented 8 hours after a stray cat bite to his left hand but left AMA refusing antibiotics and tetanus. Now 26 hours post-injury with progressive infection.

Initial Assessment

Vitals (initial, 8 hrs post-injury): BP 142/88, HR 88, RR 16, T 36.9C, SpO_2 97% RA Vitals (reassessment, 26 hrs): BP 138/82, HR 102, RR 18, T 38.2C, SpO_2 98% RA

History

- HPI: Left-hand-dominant male sustained puncture wound to left hand 26 hours ago from a stray cat that could not be located. Initially presented 8 hours post-injury with minimal findings, declined antibiotics/tetanus due to cost concerns and needle anxiety, left AMA. Now with severe throbbing pain, progressive swelling, difficulty making a fist, red streaks up forearm, chills.
- PMHx: HTN
- Meds: Lisinopril (irregular)
- Allergies: NKDA
- Social: Construction laborer; last tetanus unknown

Physical Examination

- Initial examination (8 hours): Small puncture wound (2-3mm) over the dorsal aspect of the left 5th MCP joint with minimal serous drainage; mild surrounding erythema (1cm); intact flexor and extensor tendon function; full sensation to light touch; 2+ radial and ulnar pulses; capillary refill <2 seconds. Remainder of physical examination normal.
- Reassessment (26 hours): Marked fusiform swelling of the 5th digit extending to the dorsal hand; beefy erythema encompassing the entire 5th digit and MCP joint (4×5cm); visible lymphangitic streaking to the mid-forearm; exquisite tenderness with passive extension of the 5th digit; severe pain with axial loading of the 5th digit suggesting possible joint involvement; limited active flexion due to pain but preserved passive ROM. Remainder of physical examination normal.

Diagnostic Studies

- X-ray left hand: No foreign body, fracture, or subcutaneous air; soft tissue swelling over 5th MCP (initial). Interval edema, no new bony changes (reassessment)
- CBC: WBC 16.8 (82% neutrophils, 8% bands)
- CRP 24 mg/L, ESR 45 mm/hr
- Blood and wound cultures: Pending

Management

- IV ampicillin-sulbactam 3g q6h (covers Pasteurella, Staph, Strep; alternatives for penicillin allergy: ceftriaxone + metronidazole, or clindamycin + ciprofloxacin)
- Emergent hand surgery consult for possible operative I&D of 5th MCP joint or flexor tendon sheath
- Rabies PEP: HRIG 20 IU/kg infiltrated around wound (remainder IM) + rabies vaccine 1.0 mL IM deltoid (day 0)
- Tdap given unknown immunization history

- Thorough wound irrigation with NS under pressure; leave open, loose sterile dressing, splint in position of function
- Admit for IV antibiotics and monitoring

Patient Communication

On initial visit: Discuss infection rate for untreated cat bites to hand. Address cost concerns and needle anxiety. Provide detailed return precautions. Document informed refusal.

Critical Actions

- Recognize cat bites to hand as high-risk for rapid infection requiring empiric antibiotics for Pasteurella, Staph, and Strep
- Assess rabies risk: stray/unavailable animal necessitates offering PEP per CDC guidelines
- Obtain radiographs for all hand puncture wounds
- Address barriers to care (cost, anxiety) with patient-centered communication
- Recognize serious infection signs on reassessment (lymphangitis, fever, tachycardia)
- Identify potential septic arthritis/tenosynovitis requiring urgent surgical consult
- Ensure tetanus prophylaxis and never close puncture wounds primarily

Rectal Pain

Opening Scenario

A 32-year-old male with known Crohn disease presents with severe perianal pain worsening over 72 hours. Prior perianal abscess drainage 12 years ago. Unable to sit.

Initial Assessment

Vitals: BP 132/84, HR 96, RR 14, T 37.2C, SpO_2 98% RA

Patient Communication

Patient initially refuses rectal exam due to severe pain and prior traumatic experience. Acknowledge pain, validate concerns. Explain necessity of exam and procedure to prevent deeper space infection. Discuss analgesia plan. Obtain informed consent.

History

- HPI: Constant throbbing perianal pain x3 days, worse with defecation and sitting. Intermittent mucous drainage. No fever, chills, nausea, vomiting, or rectal bleeding. Prior I&D of perianal abscess 12 years ago.
- PMHx: Crohn disease (diagnosed age 16, in remission)
- PSHx: Perianal abscess I&D (12 years ago)
- Meds: Adalimumab, mesalamine
- Allergies: NKDA
- Social: Lives with partner, IT worker, sexually active with men, occasional alcohol

Physical Examination

- General: Alert, moderate distress, diaphoretic, prefers standing or lateral decubitus positioning
- Perianal: 3 cm × 3 cm fluctuant, indurated mass at 5 o'clock position near anal verge with minimal serous drainage; no surrounding erythema, warmth, or crepitus. No rectal fluctuance or evidence of perirectal extension.
- Remainder of physical examination: Normal

Management

- Systemic analgesia (morphine 4mg IV) and local anesthesia followed by I&D
- No labs needed for uncomplicated superficial abscess in stable patient without systemic symptoms

Reassessment

- Pre-procedure: Pain 4/10 (from 10/10) after systemic analgesia; tolerates positioning
- Post-procedure: Adequate drainage, hemostasis, pain 2/10; tolerates sitting

Disposition

- TMP/SMX oral antibiotic for outpatient post drainage
- Surgical follow-up within 24-48 hours given underlying Crohn disease

Critical Actions

- Recognize uncomplicated perianal abscess; differentiate from perirectal abscess
- Provide systemic analgesia before local infiltration and procedure

- Perform I&D with
- Manage anxious patient through empathetic communication and adequate pain control
- If ambiguous during this case, ordering a CT with IV contrast to evaluate for rectal extension is also acceptable.

Reflux Symptoms

Opening Scenario

A 58-year-old woman presents with persistent "indigestion" and upper back discomfort since yesterday evening. Clutching her upper abdomen. Monitored bed.

Initial Assessment

Vitals: BP 118/76, HR 68, RR 16, T 36.4C, SpO_2 92% RA, glucose 156

- Pale, diaphoretic, clutching chest and epigastrium, moderate distress
- Airway: Patent, speaking full sentences
- Breathing: Clear bilaterally, unlabored
- Circulation: Cool, clammy, cap refill 3 seconds, thready radial pulses

History

- HPI: 58-year-old female with type 2 DM and HTN. "Indigestion" and interscapular back discomfort while gardening yesterday. Persisted overnight despite antacids. Nauseous, vomited once this morning. Heavy pressure-like epigastric sensation radiating to back. Lightheaded on standing.
- PMHx: Type 2 DM, HTN, hyperlipidemia
- PSHx: Cholecystectomy
- Meds: Metformin, lisinopril, atorvastatin
- Allergies: NKDA
- Social: Former smoker (quit 3 years ago). Father had MI at 54.

Management

- Continuous monitoring, two large-bore IVs, 500 mL NS bolus
- 12-lead ECG within 10 minutes
- Aspirin 325mg chewed
- O2 via NC 2L to maintain SpO_2 >94%
- CBC, BMP, troponin, coags, type and screen

Diagnostic Studies

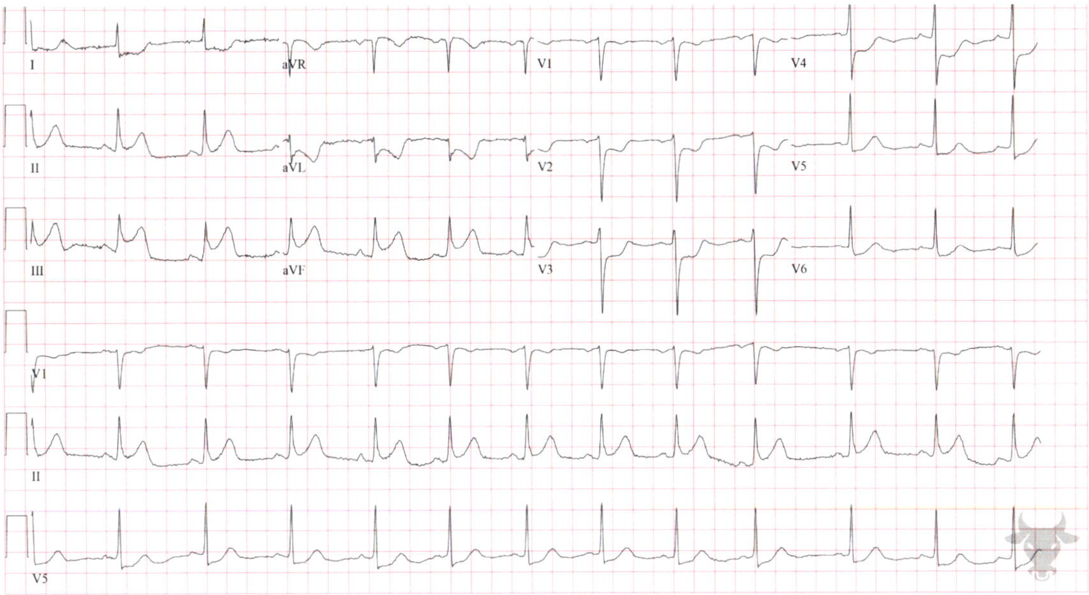

ECG: ST elevation in leads II, III, aVF with reciprocal ST depression in I and aVL. Right-sided V4R shows 2mm ST elevation.

Management

- Obtain right-sided ECG leads (V4R) for RV involvement
- Activate cardiac catheterization lab for inferior STEMI
- Avoid nitroglycerin and preload-reducing agents (RV infarction)
- Additional fluid boluses (250-500 mL) if hypotension persists

Physical Examination

- General: Alert, oriented, pale, diaphoretic
- Cardiovascular: Bradycardic, regular rhythm, no murmurs or rubs
- Respiratory: Clear bilaterally, no wheezes or rales
- Abdomen: Soft, non-tender, no distension, normal bowel sounds
- Skin: Pale, clammy, no peripheral edema or rashes
- Remainder of examination: Normal

Reassessment

Following appropriate fluid resuscitation (1000 mL total):

- BP: 112/70 mmHg
- HR: 64 bpm
- RR: 18 breaths/min
- SpO_2: 97% on 2 L NC
- Patient reports slight improvement in nausea but persistent back discomfort

If nitroglycerin given: BP drops to 78/52, HR 74. Requires Trendelenburg, 500 mL fluid bolus, possible vasopressor.

- CBC: WBC 11.2, Hgb 13.2, Hct 39%, Plt 198
- BMP: Na 140, K 3.9, Cl 104, HCO_3 24, BUN 32, Cr 1.1, glucose 168

- Troponin I: 1.8 (elevated)
- Coags: PT 13.5, PTT 32, INR 1.0

Reassessment

After 1000 mL total fluid: BP 112/70, HR 64, SpO_2 97% on 2L NC. Slight nausea improvement, persistent back discomfort.

Patient Communication

Patient states: "I feel better now. Can't I just go home and see my cardiologist tomorrow?" Explain life-threatening nature of findings and need for immediate cardiac catheterization.

Critical Actions

- Obtain ECG within 10 minutes of arrival
- Recognize atypical ACS presentation (epigastric discomfort, nausea, back pain) in diabetic female
- Identify inferior STEMI (ST elevation in II, III, aVF)
- Obtain right-sided leads; recognize RV infarct
- Administer aspirin; avoid nitroglycerin in suspected RV infarct
- Provide IV fluid to support preload-dependent RV function
- Activate cath lab immediately
- Address patient concerns about admission

Frontal Headache

Opening Scenario

A 48-year-old woman is brought by her husband with worsening headache, fever, and right eye swelling/pain for 12 hours. "Sinus pressure" for one week despite oral antibiotics started 3 days ago. Peripheral IV placed and bloodwork drawn.

Initial Assessment

Vitals: BP 144/82, HR 118, RR 18, T 38.6C, SpO_2 98% RA, glucose 112

- Lying supine with eyes closed (photophobia), moderate distress, cool compress over right periorbital area
- Airway: Patent, speaking full sentences
- Breathing: Normal, clear bilaterally
- Circulation: Warm, cap refill <2 seconds

History

- HPI: One week of nasal congestion, facial pressure, purulent rhinorrhea. Started amoxicillin-clavulanate 3 days ago. Past 24 hours: severe bifrontal headache ("pressure behind eyes"), fever, chills, right periorbital pain/swelling. Now notes double vision looking right.
- PMHx: HTN, seasonal allergies
- PSHx: Cholecystectomy
- Allergies: Penicillin (childhood rash)
- Meds: Lisinopril, amoxicillin-clavulanate (3 days), acetaminophen PRN
- Social: Accountant, lives with husband, no tobacco/alcohol/drugs

Physical Examination

- General: Alert, oriented to person, place, and time, moderate distress
- Eyes:
- Right: Conjunctival injection and chemosis, mild proptosis, complete ptosis of upper eyelid, pupil 4mm, positive afferent pupillary defect, limited abduction (CN VI palsy), decreased visual acuity 20/80,
- Left: Normal examination, pupil 3mm reactive, visual acuity 20/25
- HEENT: Tenderness to palpation over right maxilla and frontal sinus; no nasal discharge currently visible; normal tympanic membranes
- Neck: Supple, full range of motion, no meningismus (negative Brudzinski and Kernig)
- Remainder of physical examination normal including cardiovascular, pulmonary, abdominal, and neurologic (except as noted above)

Management

- O2 2L NC, two large-bore IVs, 1L NS bolus
- Labs: CBC, CMP, coags, blood cultures, lactate, D-dimer
- Antiemetics: ondansetron 4mg IV
- Analgesia: ketorolac 30mg IV
- Dexamethasone 10mg IV
- Empiric antibiotics: vancomycin 15 mg/kg IV, ceftriaxone 2g IV, metronidazole 500mg IV
- Head CT without contrast (must precede LP given focal deficits)

- MRI with MR venography of brain and orbits
- Emergent neurology and ophthalmology consults

Diagnostic Studies

- CBC: WBC 18.2, Hgb 13.2, Plt 285
- BMP: Na 138, K 3.9, Cl 102, HCO_3 24, BUN 24, Cr 1.1, glucose 118
- Coags: PT 13.0, PTT 28, INR 1.0; D-dimer 1.4; lactate 1.9
- ECG: Sinus tachycardia
- CT head: Complete opacification of right sphenoid and posterior ethmoid sinuses; no hemorrhage/ mass effect
- MRI/MRV: Filling defect and expansion of right cavernous sinus consistent with thrombosis; adjacent sphenoid inflammation; no venous infarct
- CSF: Clear, OP 22, WBC 42, RBC 85, protein 48, glucose 58, Gram stain negative

Reassessment

60 minutes: Worsening right eye vision ("colors look dim"), VA declined to 20/200, increased chemosis. Initiate unfractionated heparin drip after discussing risks/benefits with patient and neurology.

Patient Communication

Discuss with patient and husband: diagnosis of cavernous sinus thrombosis (serious complication of sinus infection). Risk of permanent vision loss. Why initial oral antibiotics were insufficient. Need for IV anticoagulation despite infection (bleeding risks vs clot progression). Prolonged IV antibiotics (4-6 weeks) and possible surgical drainage. ICU admission for frequent vision checks.

Disposition

- Medical ICU admission

Critical Actions

- Recognize cavernous sinus thrombosis as complication of sphenoid/ethmoid sinusitis
- Identify focal deficits (CN VI palsy, ptosis, chemosis) as contraindication to immediate LP; obtain CT first
- Initiate broad-spectrum antibiotics covering MRSA, gram-negatives, and anaerobes
- Order MRI/MRV for definitive diagnosis
- Reassess for worsening vision indicating need for anticoagulation
- Consider heparin in consultation with neurology despite active infection
- Communicate serious diagnosis and treatment rationale to patient/family

Pediatric Cardiac Arrest

Opening Scenario

A 5-month-old male arrives via EMS with ongoing CPR. Found unresponsive in car seat ~25 minutes ago; last seen normal 2 hours prior. EMS initiated CPR 15 minutes ago after finding no pulse and apnea. Mother is extremely distressed at bedside.

Initial Assessment

Vitals: BP not obtainable, HR 0, RR 0, SpO_2 not obtainable, T 33.8C (rectal)

- Airway: ETT 3.5mm uncuffed in place, equal breath sounds
- Breathing: Apneic, BVM ventilations with 100 O2
- Circulation: No pulses, ongoing compressions at 100/min
- Disability: Unresponsive, pupils fixed and dilated 6mm
- Exposure: Cyanotic, cool extremities, no external trauma

History

- HPI: Previously healthy 5-month-old male found unresponsive in rear-facing car seat. Mother returned to vehicle after 45-minute shopping trip and noticed infant was blue and limp. No choking episode witnessed. Last fed two hours ago.
- PMHx: Born full-term, uncomplicated pregnancy and delivery, no neonatal intensive care stay
- Medications: None
- Allergies: None
- Social: Lives with single mother and maternal grandmother; no smoking in home; sleeps in crib

Physical Examination

- General: Cyanotic, unresponsive, hypothermic
- HEENT: Endotracheal tube in place at 12cm at lips, dried oral secretions, pupils fixed and dilated
- Cardiovascular: No heart sounds auscultated, no pulses palpable, capillary refill greater than 4 seconds
- Respiratory: No spontaneous respiratory effort, breath sounds equal bilaterally with bagging
- Skin: Cool to touch, mottled appearance, no bruising or abrasions
- Remainder of physical exam: Normal

Diagnostic Studies

- ECG: Asystole
- Glucose: 48
- VBG: pH 6.92, pCO2 82, HCO_3 8, lactate 12
- CBC: WBC 12.5, Hgb 11.2, Plt 245
- BMP: Na 138, K 5.2, Cl 102, HCO_3 9
- Urine tox/blood culture: Pending

Management

- Continue high-quality CPR (15:2 compression-to-ventilation ratio)
- Verify ETT position with waveform capnography
- Bilateral IO access in proximal tibias

- Epinephrine 0.01 mg/kg (1:10,000) IO every 3-5 minutes
- Evaluate H's and T's: hypothermia identified as significant factor
- Active rewarming: warmed NS 20 mL/kg, forced-air warming blanket, warm environment
- Assess for trauma/abuse: none apparent
- Continue resuscitation until normothermia achieved

Reassessment

- 10 minutes: Temperature 34.6°C, rhythm remains asystole, no pulse palpable, end-tidal HCO_3 12 mmHg
- 20 minutes: Temperature 35.8°C, persistent asystole, capnography shows flat line
- 30 minutes: Temperature 36.9°C (normothermic), continued asystole, no cardiac activity on bedside ultrasound, pupils remain fixed and dilated
- Decision: Terminate resuscitation efforts; time of death documented

Patient Communication

Assess mother's understanding: "What have the nurses or paramedics told you about your son's condition?" Provide information about resuscitation efforts. Allow questions and emotional expression.

Difficult Conversations

Request private room. Deliver news directly: "I am so sorry to tell you that despite our best efforts, your son has died." Use "died" and "death," not euphemisms. Address cause: "This appears to be a sudden unexpected infant death." Reassure: "This is not because of anything you did or didn't do." Offer opportunity to hold infant. Discuss medical examiner notification.

Critical Actions

- Initiate appropriate PALS resuscitation for asystole
- Recognize hypothermia as reversible cause; initiate active rewarming
- Systematic reassessment at appropriate intervals
- Terminate resuscitation only after achieving normothermia with persistent asystole
- Deliver death notification using clear, direct language without euphemisms
- Reassure family regarding absence of blame
- Offer family opportunity to hold deceased infant
- Arrange psychosocial support (social work, chaplaincy)

Fever and Confusion

Opening Scenario

A 20-year-old male military recruit presents with sudden onset severe bifrontal headache 8 hours ago, neck stiffness, and photophobia. Bunkmate noted him "staring off" and slow to respond this morning.

Initial Assessment

Vitals: BP 112/78, HR 114, RR 20, T 39.1C, SpO_2 99% RA, glucose 89

- Toxic, lethargic, arousable to voice but confused. Petechial rash on trunk and upper extremities.
- Airway: Patent, short phrases
- Breathing: Clear bilaterally
- Circulation: Tachycardic, cap refill 3 seconds, weak pulses
- Immediately place in droplet isolation

History

- HPI: Sudden severe bifrontal headache 8 hours ago during training. Neck stiffness, photophobia. Acetaminophen without relief. Slow to respond this morning. No nausea/vomiting, no recent travel outside base.
- PMHx: Healthy, vaccinations UTD including meningococcal at age 14
- Meds: None
- Allergies: NKDA
- Social: Lives in crowded barracks with 40 recruits, rare alcohol

Management

- Droplet isolation immediately
- Two large-bore IVs, blood cultures, CBC, BMP, lactate, coags, type and screen
- 1L NS bolus
- Cardiac monitoring

Reassessment

30 minutes later (while awaiting CT): BP 94/64 (from 112/78), HR 132, T 39.6C. Now difficult to arouse, moaning incoherently, opens eyes only to pain.

Physical Examination

- Neck: Severe nuchal rigidity, positive Brudzinski sign (hips and knees flex with neck flexion)
- Skin: Warm and dry, extensive petechial and early purpuric lesions on chest, abdomen, and thighs; remainder of exam normal
- Neurological: GCS 12 (E3, V4, M5), cranial nerves II-XII intact, moves all extremities to pain, no focal deficits; remainder of exam normal

Management

- Recognize septic shock with meningococcemia; do not delay antibiotics for imaging
- Vancomycin 15-20 mg/kg IV + ceftriaxone 2g IV
- Dexamethasone 10mg IV prior to or concurrent with first antibiotic dose
- Additional fluid resuscitation

- LP after hemodynamic stabilization and CT imaging

Diagnostic Studies

- CSF: OP 35, WBC 3800 (96% PMNs), RBC 8, glucose 22, protein 312, Gram stain: gram-negative diplococci
- CBC: WBC 21.4, Hgb 14.2, Plt 82
- BMP: Na 126, K 4.0
- Lactate: 4.8
- CT head: Negative
- CXR: Normal

Patient Communication

Speak with bunkmate: Explain suspected bacterial meningitis with septicemia. Discuss ICU transfer, contagiousness, and need for close contact prophylaxis (ciprofloxacin 500mg PO once or rifampin 600mg PO BID x2 days). Coordinate with military command for contact tracing while maintaining patient confidentiality.

Disposition

- ICU admission for vasopressor support and antibiotics
- Infectious disease consult
- Report to military public health and local health department

Critical Actions

- Immediately implement droplet isolation
- Recognize bacterial meningitis with septicemia (fever, headache, AMS, meningeal signs, petechial rash)
- Do not delay antibiotics for CT in hemodynamically unstable patient
- Select vancomycin + ceftriaxone + adjunctive dexamethasone
- Perform LP with appropriate CSF studies
- Recognize clinical deterioration and escalate care
- Communicate with contacts regarding prophylaxis and coordinate with public health

Altered While Skiing

Opening Scenario

A 38-year-old female attorney is brought by her partner to a community ED at 9,200 feet elevation with worsening confusion, severe headache, and inability to walk straight over the past 12 hours.

Initial Assessment

Vitals: BP 148/92, HR 112, RR 24, T 37.3C, SpO_2 86% RA

- Drowsy but arousable, lying still with eyes closed, clutching head
- Airway: Patent, confused and slurring
- Breathing: Tachypneic, clear bilaterally
- Circulation: Cool extremities, cap refill 3 seconds

History

- HPI: No significant PMH. Flew from sea level to Denver (5,280 ft) yesterday and drove directly to resort elevation (9,600 ft) within 6 hours. Developed headache overnight, became severe this morning with 2 episodes of vomiting. Difficulty with balance, now confused. No fever, cough, chest pain, or visual changes.
- PMHx: None
- Meds: OCPs, occasional ibuprofen
- Allergies: NKDA
- Social: Corporate attorney, non-smoker, social alcohol

Physical Examination

- Neurologic: Alert to person only (not place or time), unable to perform tandem gait, positive Romberg test, intact extraocular movements, pupils equal and reactive to light, no focal motor weakness or sensory deficits
- Remainder of physical examination: Normal

Diagnostic Studies

- ECG: Sinus tachycardia 112, normal intervals
- CT head: Diffuse cerebral edema with sulcal effacement, compressed ventricles, no midline shift, no hemorrhage
- CBC: WBC 9.2, Hgb 15.1, Hct 45%, Plt 310
- BMP: Na 138, K 4.8, Cl 105, HCO_3 21, BUN 20, Cr 1.0, glucose 98
- Coags: PT 12.8, PTT 38, INR 1.1

Management

- 100 NRB at 15 L/min immediately
- Two large-bore IVs, ECG, labs (CBC, BMP, coags)
- Continuous cardiac monitoring
- Ondansetron 4mg IV for nausea
- Dexamethasone 8mg IV immediately
- Acetazolamide 250mg PO if tolerated
- Maintain high-flow O2 via NRB

- Consult hyperbaric medicine or arrange immediate descent/transfer
- NPO for anticipated transfer

Reassessment

Twenty minutes after initial interventions:

- Vital Signs: BP 138/84 mmHg, HR 98 beats/min, RR 20 breaths/min, SpO_2 98% on non-rebreather mask
- Clinical Status: Patient now somnolent but arousable to voice, complaining of severe persistent headache. She becomes agitated when informed she cannot return to her hotel room.
- Neurologic: Remains disoriented to place and time, continues to demonstrate marked truncal ataxia and positive Romberg sign, no new focal deficits

Patient Communication

Patient insists: "I have an important deposition tomorrow. Just give me stronger pain medication and I'll rest at the hotel." Validate professional commitments and disappointment. Explain HACE (brain swelling from altitude). Dexamethasone only "buys time"; definitive treatment requires immediate descent. Without descent: progression to coma, respiratory failure, death. Returning to hotel at 9,600 feet is not an option. Negotiate safe transfer to lower altitude.

Critical Actions

- Recognize HACE based on AMS + ataxia after rapid ascent to >2,500 meters
- Differentiate from benign AMS by presence of neurologic findings
- Administer high-flow O2 immediately
- Administer dexamethasone 8mg IV as soon as HACE suspected
- State that definitive treatment is immediate descent to lower altitude
- Reassess mental status and neuro exam after initial interventions
- Patient-centered communication addressing professional/financial concerns while conveying life-threatening nature
- Appropriate disposition: urgent transfer to lower altitude, not discharge to hotel

Acute Pelvic Pain

Opening Scenario

A 19-year-old female presents with acute left lower quadrant pain. Large-bore peripheral IV placed and labs drawn. Resting uncomfortably on stretcher.

Initial Assessment

Vitals: BP 124/78, HR 108, RR 22, T 37.6C, SpO_2 99% RA

- Obese (BMI 32), diaphoretic, clutching left lower abdomen, unable to find comfortable position
- Airway: Patent, speaking in full sentences
- Breathing: Non-labored, clear bilaterally
- Circulation: Warm, cap refill <2 seconds

History

- HPI: Sudden sharp LLQ pain 8 hours ago while dancing. Constant, non-radiating, 8/10 with nausea and two non-bloody emeses. Similar episode 1 year ago lasting 20 minutes, self-resolved. LMP 2 weeks ago (mid-cycle), irregular menses. Sexually active with one male partner, inconsistent barrier contraception.
- PMHx: PCOS, depression
- Meds: Metformin 500mg BID, sertraline 50mg daily
- Allergies: NKDA
- Social: College student, occasional alcohol

Physical Examination

- General: Alert, oriented, moderate distress due to pain, obese, hirsute (facial hair, abdominal hair)
- Cardiovascular: Tachycardic, regular rhythm, no murmurs, rubs, or gallops
- Respiratory: Clear to auscultation bilaterally, non-labored
- Abdomen: Soft, obese, exquisitely tender to palpation in left lower quadrant without rebound or guarding initially, bowel sounds present, no surgical scars, no hernias appreciated
- Pelvic: External genitalia normal; speculum examination reveals no cervical discharge or blood; bimanual examination reveals enlarged, tender left adnexal mass, no cervical motion tenderness, uterus midline and non-tender
- Remainder of examination: Normal

Diagnostic Studies

- Urine pregnancy: Negative
- CBC: WBC 10.2, Hgb 13.1, Hct 39.2%, Plt 245
- BMP: Na 138, K 4.2, Cl 102, HCO_3 24, BUN 14, Cr 0.8, glucose 98
- Beta-hCG: <5
- UA: Normal
- Pelvic US with Doppler: Left ovary enlarged 8.5 x 6.2 cm with multiple peripheral follicles (polycystic morphology); absent venous flow and diminished arterial flow. Right ovary normal. No free fluid.

Reassessment

After morphine 4mg IV and 1L NS: Pain "a little better" (6/10).

30 minutes later: Sudden worsening pain (10/10), lightheaded, nauseated. BP 98/62 (from 124/78), HR 128. Now with guarding and rebound in LLQ.

Patient Communication

Patient states: "I have PCOS and I'm worried about getting pregnant someday. If you take out my ovary, I'll never have babies. Can't we try antibiotics or wait?" Acknowledge fertility concerns with empathy. Explain time-critical nature of ovarian torsion and relationship between ischemic time and permanent necrosis. Antibiotics are not indicated for mechanical torsion. Prompt detorsion preserves ovarian function better than delay.

Management

- Immediate GYN consult for emergent laparoscopic detorsion
- NPO, repeat type and screen, crossmatch 2 units PRBC
- Additional IV analgesia
- Preoperative cefazolin

Critical Actions

- Recognize ovarian torsion as surgical emergency requiring immediate consult
- Order pelvic ultrasound with Doppler
- Identify PCOS/enlarged ovary (>5cm) as torsion risk factor
- Reassess when condition deteriorates; recognize progressive ischemia
- Communicate urgency while addressing fertility concerns
- Avoid delays for CT when US demonstrates classic torsion findings

Headache and Petechiae

Opening Scenario

A 28-year-old female presents with a severe headache for 2 days and a rash on her legs that she noticed this morning. She also reports easy bruising over the past week and a nosebleed yesterday that took 30 minutes to stop.

Initial Assessment

Vitals: BP 128/78, HR 88, RR 16, T 37.2°C, SpO_2 99% RA

- Alert and oriented, moderate distress from headache
- Airway: Patent
- Breathing: Non-labored, clear bilaterally
- Circulation: Warm, well-perfused, cap refill <2 seconds

History

- HPI: 28-year-old female with no significant medical history presents with a progressively worsening headache over 2 days, now rated 8/10, diffuse, throbbing, with photophobia. She noticed scattered bruises on her arms and legs this week without trauma. This morning she saw a new rash on her lower legs (petechiae). Yesterday she had a spontaneous nosebleed lasting 30 minutes. Denies fever, neck stiffness, vision changes, focal weakness, numbness, vomiting, or recent illness. Last menstrual period 2 weeks ago (heavier than usual). No new medications, supplements, or herbal products.
- PMHx: None
- PSHx: None
- Meds: Oral contraceptive pill only
- Allergies: NKDA
- Social: Graduate student, social alcohol use, no tobacco or drugs
- FHx: No bleeding disorders or autoimmune conditions

Physical Examination

- General: Alert, oriented, moderate distress from headache, holding head in both hands
- HEENT: No papilledema on fundoscopic exam, no retinal hemorrhages, dried blood in left naris, oral mucosa with scattered petechiae on palate and buccal mucosa
- Skin: Diffuse petechiae on bilateral lower extremities and trunk, scattered ecchymoses on arms in various stages, no purpura fulminans
- Neurologic: Alert and oriented x4, cranial nerves II-XII intact, motor strength 5/5 throughout, sensation intact, no pronator drift, no meningismus, no focal deficits
- Remainder of examination: Normal

Diagnostic Studies

- CBC: WBC 8.4, Hgb 11.2, Plt 8 (critically low)
- BMP: Na 140, K 4.0, Cl 104, HCO_3 24, BUN 14, Cr 0.8, Glucose 92
- PT 12.2, PTT 28, INR 1.0, Fibrinogen 310 (normal coagulation studies help distinguish ITP from DIC)
- LDH 180 (normal), Haptoglobin 120 (normal), Reticulocyte 1.2%, Peripheral smear: severely decreased platelets, no schistocytes, no blasts (absence of schistocytes distinguishes ITP from TTP/HUS)
- Urine pregnancy test: Negative

- CT Head non-contrast: Small left convexity acute subdural hematoma, 4 mm maximal thickness, no midline shift, no parenchymal hemorrhage

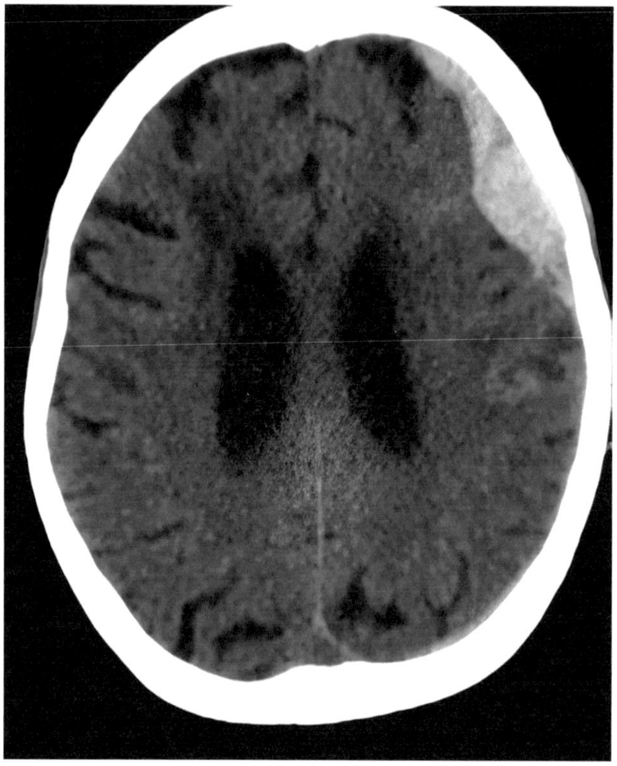

Management

- Recognize immune thrombocytopenic purpura (ITP) with life-threatening complication: intracranial hemorrhage
- This changes management significantly: in ITP without bleeding, platelet transfusion is generally not indicated (antibody-mediated destruction renders transfused platelets short-lived). However, with active intracranial hemorrhage, platelet transfusion IS indicated to temporize while definitive therapy takes effect.
- Platelet transfusion: 1 jumbo pack apheresis platelets IV immediately (will be consumed rapidly but provides temporary hemostasis)
- IVIG 1 g/kg IV (raises platelet count within 24-48 hours by saturating Fc receptors on splenic macrophages and reducing platelet destruction)
- Dexamethasone 40 mg IV daily x4 days (or methylprednisolone 1 g IV; high-dose steroids reduce antibody-mediated platelet destruction)
- Neurosurgery consult for subdural hematoma: given small size without midline shift, likely non-operative with close monitoring, but neurosurgical evaluation is mandatory
- Hematology consult for ITP management and consideration of additional therapies (anti-D immunoglobulin if Rh-positive, romiplostim, rituximab)

Teaching point — When to transfuse platelets in thrombocytopenia: - ITP with life-threatening bleeding (intracranial, GI, mucosal with hemodynamic compromise): YES — transfuse to temporize, even though platelets will be consumed rapidly - TTP: NO — platelet transfusion is contraindicated (may worsen microvascular thrombosis and precipitate organ damage). This is a critical distinction. In TTP, the treatment is plasmapheresis, not platelets. - DIC with bleeding: YES — replace consumed factors and platelets - HIT: NO — heparin-induced antibodies cross-react with transfused platelets

Reassessment

2 hours after IVIG initiation and platelet transfusion:

- Headache slightly improved (6/10 from 8/10)
- Vitals stable: BP 124/76, HR 82, RR 14
- Repeat platelet count: 22 (up from 8; transfused platelets provided transient bump, IVIG effect not yet seen)
- Neurologic exam unchanged: no focal deficits, GCS 15

Neurosurgery recommends: non-operative management with serial CT head in 6 hours, neuro checks q1h, repeat platelet count q6h, goal platelets >50 while intracranial hemorrhage is acute. Continue IVIG (second dose of 1 g/kg tomorrow). Hold anticoagulants and antiplatelet agents.

Patient Communication

The patient is frightened: "I Googled petechiae and it said leukemia. Do I have cancer? And now you're telling me I'm bleeding in my brain?"

- Address the cancer fear directly: explain that her blood smear does not show leukemia cells, and that ITP is an autoimmune condition where her immune system is mistakenly destroying her own platelets
- Explain the subdural hematoma in straightforward terms: a small collection of blood between her brain and skull caused by her extremely low platelet count
- Reassure that the bleeding is small and the neurosurgery team does not think she needs an operation at this time
- Explain the treatment plan: IVIG and steroids will help her body stop destroying platelets, and platelet transfusions are being given as a bridge
- Set expectations: she will need to be in the ICU for close monitoring, and repeat imaging will be done to make sure the bleeding does not worsen

Disposition

- Admit to ICU for neurologic monitoring and serial CT head imaging
- Continue IVIG 1 g/kg IV x2 days total
- Dexamethasone 40 mg IV daily x4 days
- Serial platelet counts q6h with goal >50 during acute intracranial hemorrhage
- Hematology follow-up for outpatient ITP management after discharge
- Neurosurgery follow-up with repeat CT head

Critical Actions

- Recognize isolated severe thrombocytopenia (platelets <10) with normal coagulation studies, no schistocytes, and no blasts as consistent with ITP
- Obtain CT head in the setting of severe thrombocytopenia and headache to evaluate for intracranial hemorrhage
- Initiate IVIG and high-dose corticosteroids as first-line treatment for ITP
- Transfuse platelets for life-threatening bleeding (intracranial hemorrhage) despite ITP — this is an exception to the general rule of avoiding platelet transfusion in immune-mediated thrombocytopenia

- Distinguish ITP from TTP: normal LDH, normal haptoglobin, no schistocytes, normal creatinine, and no fever point away from TTP. This distinction is critical because platelet transfusion is contraindicated in TTP
- Consult neurosurgery for intracranial hemorrhage and hematology for ITP management
- Communicate clearly with a young patient who is frightened about a cancer diagnosis and intracranial bleeding

Facial Swelling

Opening Scenario

A 42-year-old female with insulin-dependent DM presents with 6 days of progressive right lower jaw pain following a broken molar, 4 days of bilateral submandibular swelling, and 24 hours of difficulty swallowing saliva and "wood-like" hardness under the tongue. Could not afford urgent dental care.

Initial Assessment

Vitals: BP 148/84, HR 124, RR 24, T 38.6°C, SpO_2 94% RA

Sitting upright, holding anterior neck, drooling, muffled voice, moderate distress, unwilling to lie supine.

- Airway: Patent but compromised; "hot potato" voice, pooling secretions, trismus, leaning forward
- Breathing: Tachypneic, no stridor at rest, no cyanosis
- Circulation: Warm, flushed, diaphoretic, capillary refill <2 seconds

History

- HPI: 42-year-old female with insulin-dependent diabetes mellitus presents with 6 days of progressive right lower jaw pain following a broken molar, 4 days of swelling under the jaw that has become bilateral, and 24 hours of difficulty swallowing saliva and "wood-like" hardness under the tongue. She reports subjective fever and chills. She attempted to see a dentist but could not afford urgent care.
- PMHx: Type 1 diabetes mellitus (diagnosed age 18), hypertension, hyperlipidemia
- Medications: Insulin glargine, insulin lispro, lisinopril, atorvastatin
- Allergies: Penicillin (anaphylaxis)
- Social History: Unemployed, uninsured, lives with elderly mother whom she cares for full-time, denies tobacco, alcohol, or drug use

Physical Examination

- General: Alert and oriented, moderate distress, sitting upright, unable to tolerate supine position, profuse drooling
- HEENT: Severe trismus (mouth opening <1.5 cm), bilateral submandibular and submental brawny induration with erythema extending to floor of mouth, tongue elevated and displaced posteriorly, palpable crepitus in submandibular region, carious right lower second molar with surrounding gingival edema and purulent drainage
- Neck: Firm, tender anterior cervical lymphadenopathy, no JVD, no meningismus
- Cardiovascular: Tachycardic, regular rhythm, no murmurs
- Respiratory: Clear to auscultation bilaterally, mild accessory muscle use
- Remainder of physical examination normal

Diagnostic Studies

- CBC: WBC 31.2 (H), Hgb 13.8, Plt 285,
- BMP: Na 140, K 3.4 (L), Cl 102, CO_3 22, BUN 28 (H), Cr 1.4 (H), Glucose 428 (H)
- Lactate 3.1 (H)
- CT Neck with contrast: Bilateral submandibular, submental, and sublingual space cellulitis with gas locules; posterior tongue displacement causing oropharyngeal airway narrowing; no drainable abscess

Patient Communication

After initial assessment, you establish IV access, begin fluid resuscitation, administer analgesia, and initiate empiric antibiotics. When you explain the diagnosis of Ludwig's angina and the necessity of immediate admission for airway monitoring and possible operative intervention, the patient becomes tearful and states: "I can't be admitted. My mother has Alzheimer's and I am her only caregiver. If I'm not there tonight, she won't take her medications or eat. I need to go home. Can't you just give me stronger antibiotics and pain medicine? I'll sign whatever says it's not your fault."

Reassessment

Sixty minutes after initial evaluation, despite initial interventions, the patient reports worsening difficulty breathing. New findings include:

- Patient now tripoding on stretcher, unable to speak in full sentences
- Stridor audible at rest
- RR: 32 breaths/min
- SpO_2: 88% on room air, 92% on 15L non-rebreather mask
- Increased agitation and anxiety
- Increased submandibular swelling with extension to floor of mouth

Critical Actions

- Recognize Ludwig's angina based on odontogenic source, bilateral submandibular brawny induration, elevation of tongue, and systemic toxicity
- Identify impending airway obstruction (tripoding, stridor, inability to tolerate supine position, rapidly progressive swelling) requiring immediate definitive airway management
- Select appropriate airway strategy: Awake fiberoptic intubation or surgical airway; avoid RSI with paralysis due to distorted anatomy and risk of complete obstruction
- Initiate broad-spectrum antibiotics covering oral anaerobes and gram-positive organisms (e.g., clindamycin or ampicillin-sulbactam if not penicillin allergic; consider vancomycin plus metronidazole given severe beta-lactam allergy)
- Demonstrate patient-centered communication by acknowledging caregiver concerns, validating anxiety, clearly explaining life-threatening nature of condition using understandable language, and involving social work/case management to arrange care for dependent mother while emphasizing medical necessity
- Perform timely reassessment recognizing clinical deterioration and escalating care before respiratory arrest occurs
- Obtain emergent ENT consultation for operative airway standby and potential surgical drainage

Neonatal Shock

Opening Scenario

An 8-day-old female infant is brought by parents with "not waking up to feed." Increasingly sleepy over 12 hours, won't latch. "Breathes funny" and tires during feeds. Born at term via uncomplicated home delivery, appeared healthy until yesterday.

Initial Assessment

Vitals: BP 105/78 (RUE), BP 50/palp (RLE), HR 182, RR 78, T 36.0°C, SpO_2 94% RA / 97% blow-by, Weight 3.2 kg (down from 3.5 kg)

Lethargic, weak high-pitched cry, subcostal/intercostal retractions, nasal flaring. Mottled, cool skin with differential color (pink UE, dusky LE). Central capillary refill 4 seconds.

- Airway: Patent, weak cry, no stridor
- Breathing: Tachypneic, diffuse crackles bilaterally
- Circulation: Weak brachial pulses, barely palpable femoral pulses, absent pedal pulses
- Disability: Lethargic but arousable, normal tone, fontanelle soft and flat

History

- HPI: Full-term infant born at home 8 days ago. Initially fed well but mother noticed over the past week that the baby "tires out" while breastfeeding and "always breathes fast." Today she refused all feeds, became progressively difficult to arouse, and developed increased work of breathing. No fever, vomiting, or diarrhea. No cough or rhinorrhea.
- PMH: None
- PSH: None
- Medications: None (no vitamin K or erythromycin eye ointment given at birth)
- Allergies: NKDA
- Social: Lives with parents and grandmother; no siblings; no known sick contacts
- Family History: Non-contributory; no congenital heart disease

Physical Examination

- General: Lethargic infant in moderate respiratory distress
- Cardiovascular: S1 and S2 present; grade 2/6 systolic ejection murmur best heard at the left sternal border and between the scapulae; marked discrepancy between strong brachial pulses and weak/absent femoral pulses
- Respiratory: Bilateral fine crackles at bases, subcostal retractions
- Abdomen: Liver edge palpable 3 cm below right costal margin, soft and non-tender
- Extremities: Cool, mottled lower extremities with differential cyanosis (upper extremities pink, lower extremities blue)
- Neurologic: Lethargic, withdraws to pain, symmetric reflexes
- Remainder of examination: Normal

Diagnostic Studies

- WBC 12.5, Hgb 18.5, Hct 55%, Plt 145 (low)
- Na 138, K 5.1, Cl 105, HCO_3 18, BUN 18, Cr 0.9, Glucose 45 (hypoglycemia)
- ABG (RUE): pH 7.28, pCO2 35, pO2 88, HCO_3 16; Lactate 4.8

- CXR: Cardiomegaly with prominent pulmonary vascular markings and mild pulmonary edema
- ECG: RVH, ST depression in lateral leads (strain)

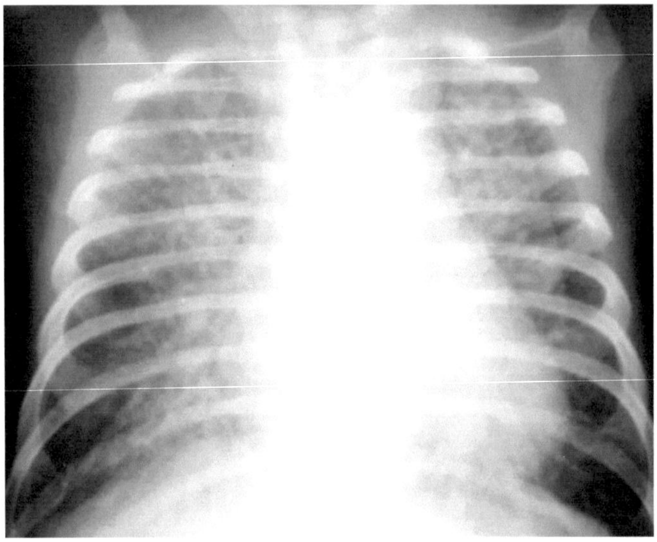

Reassessment

Initial Interventions

- Oxygen via hood (minimal improvement in work of breathing)
- IV access established; D10 bolus 2 mL/kg administered for hypoglycemia
- Coordination with transfer for emergent transfer to pediatric hospital with pediatric cardiology and pediatric surgery.
- Blood culture obtained; Ampicillin and Gentamicin administered after cultures

Reassessment at 15 Minutes

- Vital Signs: BP (RUE) 95/70 mmHg, BP (RLE) 60/40 mmHg (now obtainable), HR 165 bpm, RR 65 breaths/min, SpO_2 98% on oxygen
- Transfer center notifies you of pediatric cardiology on the phone. They ask for a patient summary. After discussion of patient case, they accept and ask that if you can get a second line you start prostaglandin E1 (PGE_1) infusion initiated at 0.05 mcg/kg/min via dedicated IV line for concern of coarctation of the aorta and need to reopen the ductus arteriosus.
- Clinical Status: Improved peripheral perfusion, stronger femoral pulses palpable, decreased retractions, capillary refill 3 seconds
- Monitoring: Continuous cardiorespiratory monitoring shows trending improvement in heart rate variability

Reassessment at 45 Minutes

- Vital Signs: BP (RUE) 90/65 mmHg, BP (RLE) 75/50 mmHg (narrowing gradient), HR 145 bpm, RR 40 breaths/min, SpO_2 99% on room air
- Clinical Status: Awake and crying appropriately with strong cry, capillary refill <2 seconds bilaterally, accepting oral feeding
- Laboratory: Repeat glucose 85; lactate trending down to 2.5

Patient Communication

The candidate must engage with both accepting physician and the family:

- Explanation that the infant has a critical congenital heart defect (coarctation of the aorta) where the aorta is narrowed, preventing blood flow to the lower body
- Clarification that this condition often becomes apparent when a normal fetal blood vessel (ductus arteriosus) begins to close around day 7-10 of life
- Discussion of the temporary nature of the prostaglandin infusion (keeps the ductus open) and the definitive need for surgical repair of the coarctation
- Acknowledgment of parental distress regarding home birth decisions and delayed recognition of illness, providing reassurance without assigning blame
- Clear explanation regarding need for immediate transfer to a tertiary pediatric cardiac center.

Critical Actions

- Recognizes that an 8-day-old infant presenting in shock with differential cyanosis and absent lower extremity pulses likely has duct-dependent congenital heart disease (critical coarctation of the aorta)
- Demonstrates clinical decision-making by obtaining four-extremity blood pressures to document upper-to-lower extremity gradient (>20 mmHg systolic difference) before confirmatory imaging
- Initiates prostaglandin E1 infusion immediately for presumed duct-dependent lesion without awaiting echocardiogram confirmation
- Avoids excessive fluid resuscitation, recognizing the risk of precipitating pulmonary edema in cardiogenic shock while providing cautious correction of hypoglycemia
- Performs complete sepsis evaluation (blood culture, urine culture, lumbar puncture if stable) while acknowledging that the presentation is more consistent with cardiac than infectious etiology
- Demonstrates reassessment skills by monitoring for clinical response to prostaglandin (restoration of femoral pulses, narrowing of BP gradient, resolution of metabolic acidosis) at appropriate intervals
- Communicates empathetically with parents regarding severity of illness, need for emergent transfer, and surgical planning while addressing parental guilt
- Arranges appropriate disposition (urgent transfer to pediatric cardiac ICU) and coordinates with accepting facility and pediatric cardiology for definitive surgical management

Visual Disruption and Bradycardia

Opening Scenario

An 82-year-old female arrives via EMS after syncope while making breakfast. Daughter reports 48 hours of increasing confusion, weakness, nausea, and "strange vision problems." Started clarithromycin 3 days ago for a "chest cold."

Initial Assessment

Vitals: BP 88/46, HR 44, RR 14, T 37.1°C, SpO_2 97% RA, Glucose 118

Physical Examination

- General: Elderly female, alert but oriented only to person and place, mildly diaphoretic, speaking in full sentences
- Cardiovascular: Regular rhythm, marked bradycardia, no murmurs, rubs, or gallops appreciated
- Extremities: 2+ pitting edema bilaterally, warm periphery with normal capillary refill
- Remainder of physical examination normal

History

- HPI: Patient reports progressive dizziness and nausea over two days. She describes her vision as having a "yellow tint" or "looking through yellow sunglasses." She denies chest pain, dyspnea, fevers, or headache. Daughter notes she was started on clarithromycin three days ago by her primary care physician for a "chest cold."
- PMHx: Atrial fibrillation (on rate control), hypertension, chronic kidney disease (baseline creatinine 1.1)
- Medications: Digoxin 0.25 mg daily (dose unchanged for years), lisinopril, clarithromycin (started 3 days ago)
- Allergies: NKDA

Diagnostic Studies

- WBC 11.2, Hgb 12.8, Plt 245
- Na 138, K 5.9 (elevated — severe), Cl 105, HCO_3 24, BUN 32 (elevated), Cr 2.2 (AKI from baseline 1.1), Glucose 110
- Troponin 0.02 (normal); Digoxin level 3.8 (toxic, therapeutic 0.5-2.0)
- ECG: Regular narrow complex rhythm at 34 bpm, no ST elevation and absent p-waves.

- 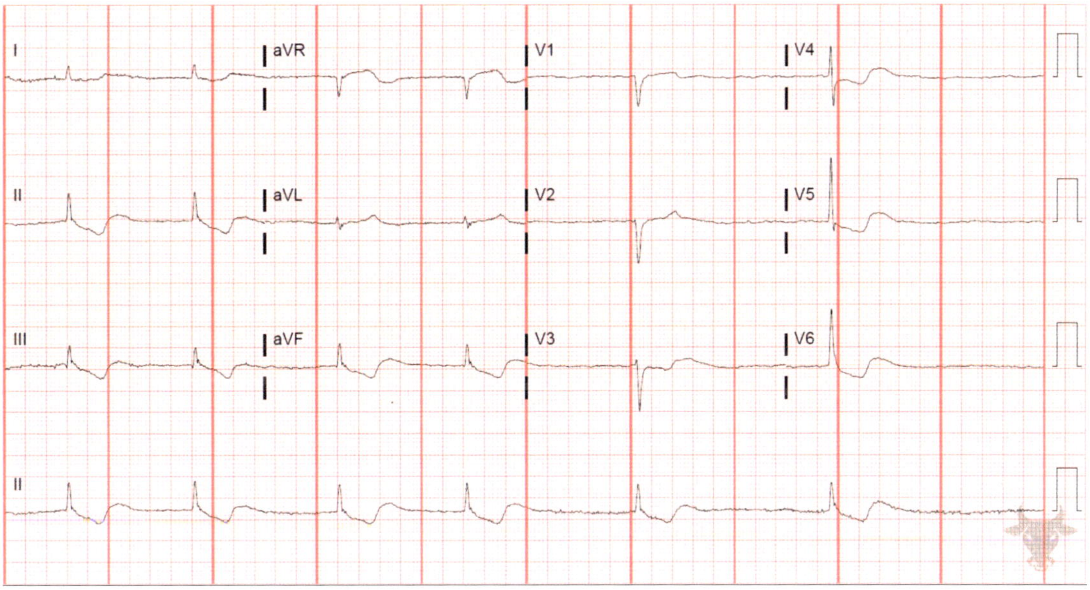

Management

- Two large-bore IVs; continuous cardiac monitoring; Poison Control consultation
- ECG immediately; transcutaneous pacer pads prophylactically for high-degree AV block risk
- Atropine 0.5 mg IV (repeatable to 3 mg total) if hemodynamically unstable
- Digoxin-specific Fab fragments (Digibind) 10 vials IV over 30 minutes
- Treat hyperkalemia: calcium gluconate 1 g IV, insulin 10 units IV with D50, sodium bicarbonate 50 mEq IV

Reassessment

Thirty minutes after Digibind administration:

- Blood Pressure: 105/68 mmHg
- Heart Rate: 68 beats per minute (regular)
- Repeat Potassium: 3.2 (decreased from 5.9)
- Patient reports resolution of nausea and yellow vision, but now complains of mild palpitations

Required Actions:

- Recognize iatrogenic hypokalemia secondary to intracellular shift post-Fab administration
- Administer potassium chloride 10 mEq with cardiac monitoring (trend potassium with schedule continued repletion)
- Recheck potassium in 1 hour

Managing Conflict

The patient's daughter expresses anger and concern: "Her doctor should have known better than to give her that antibiotic with her heart medicine. This is negligence. We want to leave and see her cardiologist tomorrow instead."

Communication Tasks:

- Acknowledge daughter's concerns and validate her vigilance regarding medication safety
- Explain the pharmacokinetic interaction without assigning blame to the outpatient physician
- Clarify that digoxin toxicity can occur even with stable chronic dosing when acute kidney injury develops or new medications are introduced

- Negotiate admission by emphasizing the immediate reversal achieved with Fab fragments but the ongoing risk of rebound arrhythmias and electrolyte shifts requiring telemetry monitoring
- Obtain agreement for admission to monitored setting

Critical Actions

- Recognition of digoxin toxicity classic triad: cardiac bradyarrhythmia, GI symptoms (nausea), and altered color vision (xanthopsia)
- Identification of drug-drug interaction between digoxin and macrolide antibiotics (clarithromycin) as precipitant of toxicity
- Understanding that serum digoxin levels correlate poorly with clinical toxicity in chronic toxicity; clinical presentation guides therapy more than absolute level
- Appropriate prioritization of digoxin-specific Fab fragments as antidote over aggressive hyperkalemia treatment to avoid precipitating profound hypokalemia
- Recognition that hyperkalemia >5.5 in digoxin toxicity indicates severe poisoning and warrants immediate antidote administration
- Placement of transcutaneous pacer pads prior to deterioration for potential high-degree AV block
- Reassessment identifying post-treatment hypokalemia requiring repletion with careful monitoring
- Effective navigation of conflict regarding perceived medical error while maintaining therapeutic alliance and achieving patient-centered outcome (admission)
- Admission to monitored setting (Telemetry/CCU) for ongoing cardiac monitoring and electrolyte management

Agitation and Tachycardia

Opening Scenario

A 42-year-old female police officer arrives via EMS with altered mental status. Husband reports 36 hours of increasing confusion. Known "thyroid issues" never followed up. Recently completed antibiotics for respiratory infection.

Initial Assessment

Vitals: BP 168/56, HR 150, RR 26, T 39.2°C, SpO_2 97% RA, Glucose 118, Weight 68 kg

Physical Examination

- General: Moderately agitated, diaphoretic, speaking in fragmented sentences
- Eyes: Bilateral lid retraction with visible conjunctivae above and below iris (exophthalmos)
- Neck: Firm, non-tender midline mass (goiter), no cervical lymphadenopathy
- Cardiovascular: Tachycardic, regular rhythm, bounding pulses, no murmurs
- Lungs: Tachypneic, crackles at right base, clear elsewhere
- Skin: Warm, moist, flushed; fine tremor noted in outstretched hands
- Neuro: Alert to name only, confused, moving all extremities, no focal deficits
- Remainder of exam: Normal

ECG: Sinus tachycardia at 144, no ST changes. CXR: Right lower lobe infiltrate.

History

- HPI: 42-year-old female with recent "cold" symptoms including productive cough and pleuritic chest pain for 5 days. Husband notes progressive symptoms over 3 months: anxiety, insomnia, 15-pound unintentional weight loss, heat intolerance, and palpitations. She was diagnosed with hypertension at a work screening 4 months ago but declined follow-up. No known drug use.
- PMHx: Hypertension (untreated), presumed hyperthyroidism (undocumented)
- PSHx: None
- Meds: None
- Allergies: NKDA
- Social: Lives with husband and child; police officer; no tobacco/alcohol/drugs per husband

Diagnostic Studies

- WBC 16.8, Hgb 13.2, Plt 385
- Na 140, K 3.2 (low), Cl 106, HCO_3 22, BUN 28, Cr 1.3, Glucose 142
- AST 45, ALT 38, Alk Phos 110; PT 12.8, INR 1.0, PTT 28
- TSH 0.01 (suppressed), Free T4 8.4 (markedly elevated)
- Lactate 3.2; Blood cultures pending; UA normal; Urine tox negative; Pregnancy negative

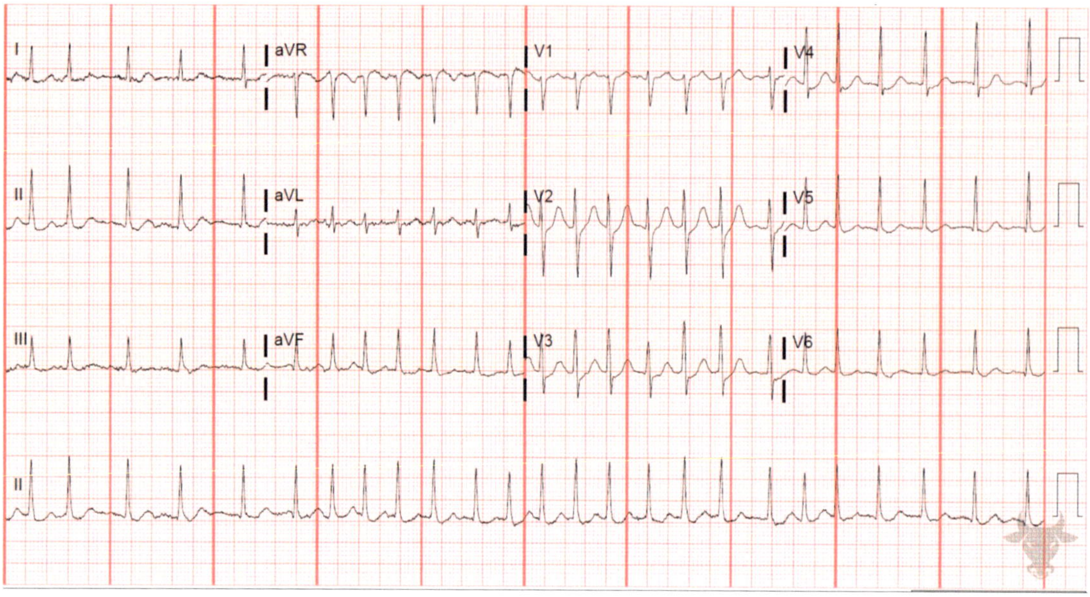

Reassessment (30 minutes)

- Vitals: BP 148/52, HR 128, RR 24, T 38.6°C, SpO_2 99% on 2L NC
- Clinical: Patient remains agitated but less combative; husband at bedside asking "Is she going to be okay?"
- Fluid Status: 1L NS completed, patient making 100mL urine over past hour
- New Finding: Patient has one episode of watery diarrhea

Difficult Conversation

The husband is extremely anxious and asks repeatedly if his wife is "just stressed out like the last doctor said." He mentions they have been arguing about her refusing to see a psychiatrist for her anxiety. Explain th eciritical nature of thyroid storm and the steps you will take to mitigate the severity of the problem.

Management

- O2 via NC 2L; cardiac monitoring; cautious fluid resuscitation; labs: CBC, CMP, LFTs, coags, TSH, free T4, blood cultures, lactate, UA, urine pregnancy, urine tox
- Propranolol 60 mg PO (or 1 mg IV) — blocks adrenergic effects and reduces peripheral T4 to T3 conversion
- PTU 600 mg loading dose (or methimazole), then 200 mg q4h
- Iodine (SSKI or Lugol's) given one hour after antithyroid medication
- Hydrocortisone 100 mg IV (adrenal insufficiency risk and blocks peripheral conversion)
- Acetaminophen for fever; avoid salicylates (increase free hormone levels)
- Antibiotics for precipitating pneumonia: ceftriaxone and azithromycin
- ICU admission

Critical Actions

- Recognizes thyroid storm based on clinical presentation (hyperthermia, tachycardia, altered mental status, gastrointestinal symptoms) in context of hyperthyroidism
- Initiates beta-blockade before or simultaneously with other specific therapies (propranolol preferred for its additional benefit of blocking T_4 to T_3 conversion, but esmolol is an acceptable alternative)
- Administers antithyroid medication (PTU or methimazole) before iodine therapy

- Identifies and treats precipitating infection (pneumonia) with appropriate antibiotics
- Performs focused physical examination noting exophthalmos and goiter
- Orders appropriate labs including TSH and free T_4 to confirm diagnosis
- Provides appropriate fluid resuscitation while monitoring for heart failure
- Communicates effectively with family member about severity of illness, distinguishing thyroid storm from psychiatric illness
- Reassesses patient after initial interventions noting improvement in vitals but ongoing instability
- Consults ICU for definitive management and monitoring
- Avoids contraindicated therapies (aspirin, atropine, excessive fluid administration)
- Considers alternative diagnoses in initial workup (sepsis, sympathomimetic overdose, meningitis, NMS) but prioritizes thyroid storm treatment based on clinical picture

Diarrhea and Discolored Urine

Opening Scenario

A frantic mother brings her 4-year-old daughter with bloody diarrhea for several days and urine that looks "like tea."

Initial Assessment

Vitals: BP 118/78 (elevated for age), HR 112, RR 24, T 37.9°C, SpO_2 98% RA

Pale, irritable preschool-age female in mild distress, clutching her lower abdomen. Airway patent, speaking in short phrases. Mild tachypnea, clear bilateral breath sounds, no retractions. Distal pulses palpable but thready, capillary refill 3 seconds, skin mottled on extremities. Cardiac monitor and pulse oximetry placed, IV access established, isotonic crystalloid bolus initiated. Labs drawn including CBC, BMP, coagulation studies, urinalysis, and stool studies.

History

- HPI: 4-year-old previously healthy female with 5 days of bloody diarrhea (current episode began 8 days after eating undercooked hamburger at a family barbecue). Mother notes urine has been dark and decreased in volume over the past 48 hours. Child complains of crampy pain throughout the abdomen. No vomiting today, but had non-bilious emesis earlier in the illness course. Mother gave acetaminophen for fever.
- PMHx: None
- PSHx: None
- Allergies: NKDA
- Medications: Acetaminophen PRN
- Social: Lives with both parents and older brother; attends preschool
- FHx: Non-contributory

Physical Examination

- General: Pale, irritable, moderate distress due to abdominal pain
- HEENT: Pale conjunctivae and mucous membranes
- Cardiovascular: Tachycardic, regular rhythm, no murmurs
- Abdomen: Soft, mildly distended, diffuse tenderness with voluntary guarding in lower quadrants, no rebound tenderness
- Skin: Pallor noted; scattered petechiae on lower extremities and buttocks
- Remainder of examination normal

Diagnostic Studies

- CBC: WBC 14.2, Hgb 6.2 (low), Hct 18.5% (low), Plt 22 (critically low)
- Peripheral Smear: Schistocytes and helmet cells present
- BMP: Na 138, K 5.2 (high), Cl 102, HCO_3 19 (low), BUN 24 (high), Cr 1.4 (elevated for age), Glucose 94
- Coags: PT 12.8, PTT 28.0, INR 1.0
- Urinalysis: SG 1.025, pH 6.0, protein 2+, blood 3+, RBCs >50/HPF
- Stool Studies: Shiga Toxin EIA positive for Shiga toxin 1 and 2; culture pending, presumptive STEC

Management

- Fluid resuscitation with 40 mL/kg isotonic crystalloid (avoid potassium-containing fluids given hyperkalemia)
- Avoid antibiotics — contraindicated in STEC infection due to risk of increased toxin release and worsening HUS
- Avoid antimotility agents — increased risk of toxic megacolon and systemic complications
- Avoid nephrotoxic agents
- Emergent hematology and nephrology consultation
- Blood pressure management
- Prepare for possible admission to pediatric intensive care unit given multi-organ involvement

Patient Communication

The mother approaches visibly distressed: "I overheard the medical team say something about her kidneys and blood cells. Why didn't you start antibiotics when we first got here? My neighbor said her son got better immediately with antibiotics for his stomach infection. I feel like we wasted precious time waiting."

Address parental concerns empathetically while clearly explaining that antibiotics are harmful in this specific scenario due to the toxin's effect on the microvasculature, not bacterial invasion.

Reassessment

Sixty minutes after initial fluid resuscitation and while awaiting consultant evaluation:

- Patient becomes increasingly lethargic and difficult to arouse
- Sudden onset of generalized tonic-clonic seizure lasting approximately 45 seconds
- Post-ictal state with confusion and irritability
- Repeat vital signs: BP 125/82, HR 120, RR 28
- No witnessed head trauma
- New-onset seizure indicates CNS involvement — consider immediate neuroimaging to rule out alternative causes while managing as HUS-related encephalopathy
- Discuss potential need for plasmapheresis or eculizumab with consultants for severe disease with neurological manifestations

Critical Actions

- Recognize the classic triad of microangiopathic hemolytic anemia (schistocytes on peripheral smear), thrombocytopenia, and acute kidney injury consistent with Hemolytic Uremic Syndrome (HUS)
- Identify the association with Shiga toxin-producing E. coli (STEC) and understand that antibiotic therapy is contraindicated due to risk of toxin release and worsening HUS severity
- Avoid antimotility agents which increase the risk of toxic megacolon and systemic complications
- Demonstrate appropriate fluid resuscitation while avoiding nephrotoxic agents and potassium-containing fluids given emerging hyperkalemia
- Recognize new-onset seizure as an indication of central nervous system involvement requiring emergent hematology and nephrology consultation
- Consider immediate neuroimaging to rule out alternative causes while managing as HUS-related encephalopathy
- Initiate blood pressure management and prepare for possible PICU admission given multi-organ involvement
- Discuss potential need for plasmapheresis or eculizumab with consultants for severe disease with neurological manifestations

Post-Transplant Fever

Opening Scenario

EMS arrives with a 62-year-old female who is 2 weeks post-liver transplant with fever and abdominal pain for 2 days. Uncomfortable, clutching right upper quadrant.

Initial Assessment

Vitals: BP 105/68, HR 118, RR 24, T 102.1°F (38.9°C), SpO_2 97% RA, FS 142

Mildly uncomfortable female with visible scleral icterus and jaundiced skin. Airway patent, speaking in full sentences. Tachypneic but comfortable, no cyanosis or accessory muscle use. Warm to touch, well-perfused peripherally, capillary refill <2 seconds. Cardiac monitor, pulse oximetry, O2 via NC at 2 L/min. Two large-bore peripheral IVs established. Blood cultures (2 sets), urine culture, serum lactate, tacrolimus trough drawn. 1L NS bolus initiated. ECG and chest X-ray ordered.

History

- HPI: 62-year-old female with autoimmune hepatitis cirrhosis, 14 days post-orthotopic liver transplant, presenting with 2 days of fever (max 102.1°F) and constant RUQ pain without radiation. Denies nausea, vomiting, diarrhea, dysuria, hematuria, cough, shortness of breath, or altered mental status. Reports decreased appetite and mild fatigue.
- PMHx: Autoimmune hepatitis with cirrhosis, portal hypertension with esophageal varices (previously banded), orthotopic liver transplantation 14 days ago
- Immunosuppression: Tacrolimus, mycophenolate mofetil, prednisone
- Prophylaxis: TMP-SMX, valganciclovir
- Social: Lives with spouse; retired teacher; denies alcohol, tobacco, or recreational drug use; no recent travel

Physical Examination

- HEENT: Icteric sclera, dry mucous membranes; remainder normal
- Cardiovascular: Tachycardic, regular rhythm, no murmurs/rubs/gallops; remainder normal
- Respiratory: Clear to auscultation bilaterally, no rales/wheezes; remainder normal
- Abdomen: Surgical incision clean/dry/intact, moderate RUQ tenderness to palpation, positive fluid wave, no rebound or guarding; bowel sounds present; remainder normal
- Extremities: Trace pitting edema bilaterally, normal pulses; remainder normal
- Skin: Jaundiced, warm, no rashes or petechiae; remainder normal
- Neuro: Alert and oriented, cranial nerves intact, no asterixis; remainder normal

Diagnostic Studies

- CBC: WBC 2.8 (low), Neutrophils 45%, Bands 12% (high), Lymphocytes 35%, Hgb 9.2 (low), Hct 28%, Plt 180
- BMP: Na 134, K 3.2 (low), Cl 108, HCO_3 22, BUN 28 (high), Cr 1.4 (high), Glucose 156
- LFTs: AST 89 (high), ALT 76 (high), ALP 245 (high), T.Bili 6.8 (high), D.Bili 4.2, Albumin 2.4 (low)
- Coags: PT 16.5, INR 1.5, PTT 38
- Urinalysis: Dark yellow, SG 1.030, pH 5.5, trace protein, LE negative, nitrite negative
- Serum Lactate: 5.4 (elevated)
- Tacrolimus Level: 18.2 (supratherapeutic; target 5-15)

- ECG: Sinus tachycardia at 118 bpm, no ST changes
- RUQ Ultrasound: absent gallbladder extensive ascites and hepatomegaly.

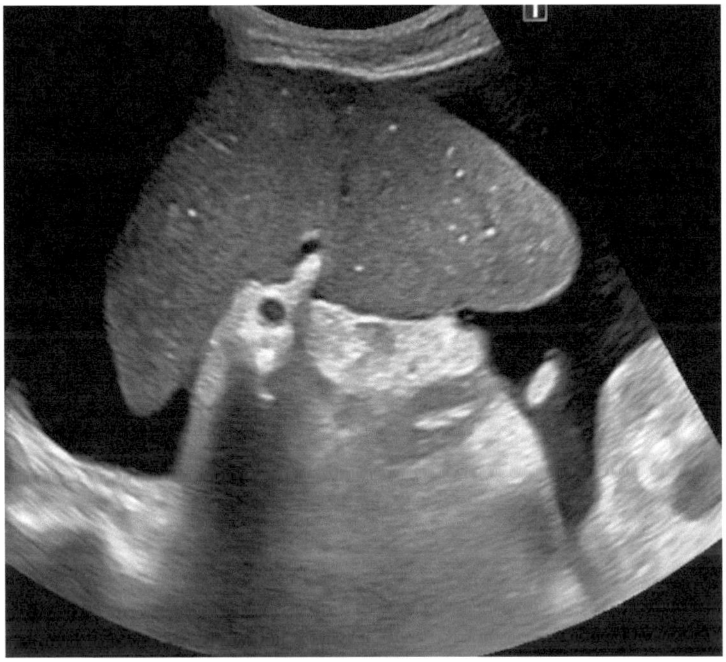

Management

- Obtain blood cultures (2 sets) prior to antibiotic administration
- Perform ultrasound-guided diagnostic paracentesis to evaluate for SBP vs. rejection vs. biliary obstruction
- Initiate broad-spectrum antibiotics: cefepime 2g IV, vancomycin loading dose, metronidazole 500mg IV
- Cautious fluid resuscitation with NS boluses
- Consult transplant surgery/hepatology early for graft dysfunction evaluation
- Consult interventional radiology for possible biliary drainage if obstruction confirmed

Reassessment

- Ascitic Fluid: WBC 850 cells/mm^3 (high), PMN 78%, Gram stain negative, culture pending, protein 1.2, glucose 45

Patient Communication

The patient states: "I've been through so much with the transplant surgery. I don't want any more needles or procedures poking me. Can't you just give me antibiotics through my IV and let me go home to rest? I have my daughter's wedding next week and I need to be there."

Acknowledge anxiety and previous traumatic experiences. Explain rationale for diagnostic paracentesis. Discuss risks of untreated infection in immunosuppressed patients (rapid deterioration, graft loss, sepsis). Negotiate timeline and address concerns about the upcoming wedding. Obtain informed consent for necessary procedures.

Reassessment

After initial 1L NS bolus: BP 92/58, HR 132, RR 26, T 38.6°C, SpO_2 96% on 2L NC. Patient appears more fatigued, capillary refill 3 seconds. Reports worsening abdominal pressure and dizziness upon sitting up.

Recognize septic shock with inadequate response to initial fluid resuscitation. Administer additional 500 mL NS bolus. Place arterial line for continuous hemodynamic monitoring. Prepare for central venous access. Consider norepinephrine if MAP <65 mmHg after additional fluids. Admit to ICU for septic shock management.

Disposition

- ICU admission for septic shock management and ongoing resuscitation
- Continue empiric antibiotics pending culture results
- Discuss with transplant team regarding acute cellular rejection versus cholangitis

Critical Actions

- Obtain blood cultures prior to antibiotic administration in immunosuppressed febrile patient
- Recognize septic shock and initiate early goal-directed therapy with fluids and antibiotics
- Perform ultrasound-guided diagnostic paracentesis to evaluate for SBP in post-transplant patient with ascites and fever
- Identify elevated calcineurin inhibitor level as potential contributor to nephrotoxicity and over-immunosuppression
- Reassess patient after initial interventions and recognize hemodynamic deterioration requiring ICU level care and possible vasopressor support
- Effectively communicate necessity of invasive procedures to anxious patient while addressing goals of care
- Consult transplant team early for admission and possible graft dysfunction evaluation
- Initiate empiric antibiotics covering gram-negative organisms (including Pseudomonas), gram-positives, and anaerobes
- Recognize broad differential including SBP, cholangitis, acute rejection, and opportunistic infections (CMV, fungal, bacterial)

Severe Abdominal Pain

Opening Scenario

A 78-year-old male presents via EMS with acute abdominal pain. Waited 45 minutes in the waiting room; unable to sit still, in obvious distress.

Initial Assessment

Vitals: BP 158/82, HR 98 (irregularly irregular), RR 18, T 37.6°C (99.7°F), SpO_2 96% RA, Pain 10/10

Elderly male, agitated and restless, diaphoretic, continuously shifting position on stretcher. Airway patent, speaking in full sentences. Non-labored breathing, clear bilaterally. Irregular peripheral pulse, capillary refill <2 seconds, no cyanosis. IV access established, cardiac monitor placed, labs drawn including CBC, BMP, coagulation studies, lactate, lipase, type and screen.

History

- HPI: 78-year-old male with sudden onset of severe periumbilical abdominal pain beginning 4 hours prior. Pain is constant, cramping, and out of proportion to physical examination findings. Associated with nausea and two episodes of loose stool with bright red blood. Denies vomiting, chest pain, dyspnea, or urinary symptoms.
- PMHx: Paroxysmal atrial fibrillation, hypertension, CAD s/p CABG (2 years ago), hyperlipidemia
- PSHx: CABG x3, appendectomy
- Medications: Apixaban (held for past 48 hours pending dental extraction), metoprolol, lisinopril, atorvastatin, aspirin 81mg
- Allergies: NKDA
- Social: Lives independently, former smoker (quit 10 years ago), no alcohol or illicit drug use

Physical Examination

- General: Alert and oriented x3, moderate distress, unable to find comfortable position
- Cardiovascular: Irregularly irregular rhythm, no murmurs, rubs, or gallops
- Abdomen: Soft, mildly distended, hypoactive bowel sounds, mild diffuse tenderness without rebound or guarding; periumbilical tenderness to light palpation — pain out of proportion to exam
- Rectal: Brown stool, guaiac positive
- Remainder of physical examination: Normal

Diagnostic Studies

- CBC: WBC 16.2, Hgb 13.8, Hct 41%, Plt 285
- BMP: Na 142, K 3.8, Cl 104, HCO_3 22, BUN 28 (high), Cr 1.1, Glucose 142
- Lactate: 3.8 (elevated)
- INR: 1.1, Lipase: 45 (normal)
- CTA Abdomen/Pelvis: Occlusive thrombus in the SMA approximately 3cm from origin, pneumatosis intestinalis involving the ascending colon, moderate bowel wall thickening of the hepatic flexure and transverse colon, minimal free fluid in the right paracolic gutter

Management

- IV fluid resuscitation
- Broad-spectrum antibiotics covering gut flora

- Therapeutic anticoagulation after CTA results
- Emergent surgical consultation — do not accept delays; request simultaneous surgery and IR involvement
- Recognize anticoagulation interruption as the precipitating factor

Patient Communication

The patient states: "I have a dental procedure scheduled tomorrow morning. Is this serious? I really don't want surgery. Can't you just give me antibiotics and let me go home?"

Acknowledge concerns. Explain this is a life-threatening emergency requiring immediate intervention to prevent bowel death. Discuss the connection between holding anticoagulation and the current event. Clarify that antibiotics alone are insufficient without restoring blood flow.

Managing Conflict

The on-call surgeon states: "This sounds like a medical issue. Start heparin and call interventional radiology. I'm not taking this patient to the OR unless IR declines and he deteriorates further."

Articulate the urgency and CT findings indicating pneumatosis and acute SMA occlusion. Discuss the time-critical nature of mesenteric ischemia and risk of progression to irreversible bowel necrosis. Negotiate simultaneous surgery and IR involvement rather than sequential consultation. Document all communications.

Reassessment

Two hours after initial presentation, despite 2L NS, IV antibiotics, and therapeutic anticoagulation:

- Vitals: BP 142/78, HR 112, T 38.2°C, Pain 8/10 despite analgesia
- Abdomen now demonstrates rebound tenderness and involuntary guarding, rigid on palpation, absent bowel sounds
- Repeat Lactate: 6.4 (rising)
- Clinical deterioration indicates progression to peritonitis and bowel necrosis requiring emergent laparotomy

Critical Actions

- Recognition of acute mesenteric ischemia based on pain out of proportion to examination in a patient with atrial fibrillation and interrupted anticoagulation
- Immediate resuscitation with IV fluids and broad-spectrum antibiotics covering gut flora
- CT angiography as the diagnostic study of choice to confirm arterial occlusion
- Understanding that elevated lactate is a late finding and should not delay definitive imaging or intervention
- Persistence in obtaining surgical consultation despite initial reluctance from consulting services
- Recognition of clinical deterioration on reassessment indicating progression to peritonitis and bowel necrosis requiring emergent laparotomy
- Effective communication with patient regarding life-threatening nature of condition while addressing concerns about elective procedures
- Negotiation between surgical and IR services for definitive management (embolectomy vs. endovascular intervention)

Allergic Reaction

Opening Scenario

A 7-year-old female (22 kg) is brought by parents with acute respiratory distress and facial swelling after eating a cashew-containing snack at a birthday party. Known tree nut allergy. Diphenhydramine given at home; rapidly deteriorated during car ride.

Initial Assessment

Vitals: BP 72/45, HR 185, RR 34, T 36.8°C, SpO_2 91% RA, Weight 22 kg

Airway patent but voice muffled, moderate tongue swelling, pooling secretions. Inspiratory stridor at rest, diffuse wheezing bilaterally, moderate work of breathing with intercostal and subcostal retractions. Tachycardic, thready peripheral pulses, capillary refill 4 seconds, cool mottled skin. Immediate IM epinephrine 0.15 mg (1:1000) into anterolateral thigh. High-flow O2 via NRB at 15 L/min. Two large-bore peripheral IVs. NS 440 mL (20 mL/kg) bolus. Diphenhydramine 25 mg IV, methylprednisolone 40 mg IV, famotidine 15 mg IV. Continuous monitoring. Airway adjuncts prepared.

History

- HPI: Previously healthy 7-year-old with known cashew/pistachio allergy who accidentally ingested a chocolate-covered cashew approximately 25 minutes prior to arrival. Immediate oral pruritus and lip tingling. Parents gave 12.5 mg diphenhydramine orally at home. Within 10 minutes, developed voice changes, cough, and diffuse urticaria. During transport, became increasingly anxious, developed respiratory distress, and appeared pale.
- PMHx: Seasonal allergic rhinitis, atopic dermatitis
- Allergies: Cashews, pistachios (prior reactions limited to urticaria)
- Medications: Cetirizine daily, diphenhydramine PRN
- Social: Lives with parents and younger sibling

Physical Examination

After stabilization:

- HEENT: Moderate upper lip edema, mild oropharyngeal erythema, no tonsillar exudates, trachea midline
- Cardiovascular: Regular rhythm, no murmurs, capillary refill 2 seconds, peripheral pulses full
- Pulmonary: End-expiratory wheezing bilaterally, good air entry throughout, no retractions
- Skin: Diffuse urticarial rash with confluent patches on trunk and proximal extremities, no blistering or target lesions
- Neurological: Alert and appropriate, anxious affect
- Remainder of physical examination normal

Diagnostic Studies

- Serum Tryptase: 18.4 (elevated; ref <11.4)
- CBC: WBC 15.2, Hgb 12.3, Plt 380
- Absolute Eosinophil Count: 720/μL (elevated; ref 0-500)
- BMP: Na 140, K 4.1, Cl 104, HCO_3 22, BUN 14, Cr 0.5, Glucose 124
- High-Sensitivity Troponin I: Negative

Management

- Epinephrine 0.15 mg IM is the first-line treatment — administer immediately without delay
- Correct dosing: 0.15 mg IM for 10-25 kg; 0.3 mg IM for >25 kg; IV epinephrine reserved for cardiac arrest or peri-arrest
- Aggressive isotonic fluid resuscitation (20 mL/kg boluses; multiple boluses may be required due to third spacing and vasodilation)
- Adjunctive therapies (H1/H2 antagonists, corticosteroids, beta-agonists) are secondary to epinephrine
- Prepare airway adjuncts but avoid premature intubation unless complete airway obstruction imminent

Reassessment

Initial response: voice clearer, stridor resolved, speaking in full sentences. Vitals: BP 88/58, HR 128, RR 26, SpO_2 97% on 2L NC.

Then: sudden onset diffuse abdominal cramping, vomiting, recurrence of urticaria spreading to extremities, mild expiratory wheezing returns. Recognize GI manifestations as part of multisystem anaphylaxis (biphasic reaction).

Second dose epinephrine 0.15 mg IM, additional NS 440 mL bolus, nebulized albuterol 2.5 mg, ondansetron 4 mg IV. Extended observation period initiated.

Disposition

- Observation in monitored setting for minimum 6 hours from last epinephrine dose (biphasic reaction risk)
- Allergen avoidance counseling for tree nuts and cross-contamination risks
- Epinephrine autoinjector demonstration with return demonstration by parent (teach-back method)
- Discuss biphasic reactions and return precautions (respiratory symptoms, persistent vomiting, syncope)
- Written anaphylaxis emergency action plan provided
- Prescriptions: Two epinephrine autoinjectors (0.15 mg), cetirizine, prednisolone taper
- Follow-up with pediatric allergy/immunology within 1 week

Critical Actions

- Immediate recognition of anaphylaxis with hemodynamic compromise and airway involvement requiring emergent IM epinephrine without delay
- Correct dosing and route of epinephrine (0.15 mg IM for 10-25 kg; 0.3 mg IM for >25 kg) in anterolateral thigh
- Aggressive isotonic fluid resuscitation (20 mL/kg; multiple boluses may be needed)
- Systematic reassessment identifying biphasic reaction, prompting repeat epinephrine dosing
- Recognition of GI manifestations as part of multisystem anaphylaxis rather than isolated gastroenteritis
- Prescription of epinephrine autoinjectors (two devices minimum) with teach-back demonstration
- Appropriate observation period (minimum 4-6 hours from symptom resolution; longer if biphasic pattern or repeat epinephrine required)
- Adjunctive therapies (H1/H2 antagonists, corticosteroids, beta-agonists) are secondary to epinephrine
- Outpatient follow-up with allergist for testing and long-term management planning

Lower Abdominal Pain with Fever

Opening Scenario

A 22-year-old female presents accompanied by her mother, reporting worsening lower abdominal pain and high fever over the past three days. She appears uncomfortable and flushed upon arrival.

Initial Assessment

Vitals: BP 108/72, HR 118, RR 16, T 102.8°F (39.3°C), SpO_2 99% RA

Lying supine with knees flexed, moderate distress, alert and conversant but diaphoretic. Airway patent, speaking in full sentences. No respiratory distress, lungs clear. Tachycardic, regular rhythm, warm extremities, capillary refill <2 seconds. Two large-bore IVs established, blood cultures drawn prior to antibiotics, urine sent for UA and pregnancy test, 1L NS bolus initiated, analgesia administered. Pelvic examination prepared.

History

Request that the mother step out of the room to conduct a confidential interview regarding sexual history.

- HPI: Three days of constant right lower quadrant pain radiating to suprapubic area, associated with subjective fever to 103°F and rigors. Copious yellow-green vaginal discharge with foul odor for five days. LMP two weeks ago. Sexually active with two current partners; inconsistent condom use. Denies dysuria, hematuria, nausea, vomiting, diarrhea, or constipation.
- PMHx: None
- PSHx: None
- Medications: Oral contraceptive pills
- Allergies: NKDA
- Social: College student, lives with parents during summer break, social alcohol on weekends, denies tobacco and illicit drugs

Physical Examination

- General: Alert, oriented, moderate distress, lying supine with hips flexed
- Abdomen: Soft, tenderness in RLQ and suprapubic region with voluntary guarding; no rebound; negative McBurney's point; no hepatosplenomegaly; positive bowel sounds
- Pelvic: External genitalia normal. Speculum: copious frothy yellow-green discharge from cervical os; cervix friable with contact bleeding. Bimanual: cervical motion tenderness present; positive right adnexal tenderness with fullness; left adnexa non-tender without masses
- Remainder of physical examination: Normal

Diagnostic Studies

- CBC: WBC 16.2, Hgb 12.8, Hct 38.2%, Plt 285
- BMP: Na 140, K 3.8, Cl 104, HCO_3 24, BUN 14, Cr 0.8, Glucose 102
- LFTs: AST 22, ALT 19
- Urinalysis: LE negative, nitrites negative, blood negative
- Urine Pregnancy: Negative
- Blood Cultures: Pending
- Cervical GC/Chlamydia NAAT: Pending

- Pelvic Ultrasound (transabdominal and transvaginal): Right adnexal complex mass 5.2 cm with internal echoes, septations, and irregular walls consistent with abscess. Moderate free fluid in cul-de-sac. Uterus normal. Left ovary normal.

Management

- Obtain cervical cultures for GC/chlamydia
- Initiate empiric broad-spectrum antibiotic therapy covering polymicrobial flora (anaerobes, gram negatives, STI pathogens): cefoxitin and doxycycline
- Order urine pregnancy test early to exclude ectopic pregnancy
- Emergent pelvic ultrasound given persistent symptoms
- Consult gynecology for tubo-ovarian abscess evaluation and possible drainage
- Admit for continued IV antibiotics and possible intervention
- Counseling regarding PID, partner notification, and contraception

Reassessment

Two hours after IV fluids, analgesia, and empiric antibiotics (cefoxitin and doxycycline):

- Vitals: T 102.2°F, HR 112, BP 110/74, RR 14
- Persistent severe pain (8/10) despite analgesia; remains febrile; unable to tolerate oral intake
- Recognize inadequate clinical response — reassess differential and order emergent pelvic ultrasound
- Ultrasound confirms 5.2 cm tubo-ovarian abscess requiring gynecology consultation for drainage

Critical Actions

- Request private interview without family present to obtain sensitive sexual history and ensure patient confidentiality
- Order urine pregnancy test early to exclude ectopic pregnancy
- Perform complete pelvic examination including speculum visualization and bimanual palpation
- Obtain cervical cultures for GC/chlamydia prior to antibiotic administration when possible
- Initiate empiric broad-spectrum antibiotics covering polymicrobial flora
- Reassess after initial interventions; recognize inadequate clinical response and need for advanced imaging
- Recognize indications for admission: TOA on imaging, high fever, inability to tolerate oral medications
- Consult gynecology for complex abscess requiring possible drainage or surgical intervention
- Provide counseling regarding PID, partner notification, and contraception

Sickle Cell and Chest Pain

Opening Scenario

A 19-year-old female with HbSS sickle cell disease arrives with progressive chest pain and worsening shortness of breath over 48 hours. Father reports 3 admissions in the past year for VOC but never ICU.

Initial Assessment

Vitals: BP 94/56, HR 112, RR 28, T 38.2°C, SpO_2 90% RA, Weight 58 kg

Alert female in moderate distress, speaking in short sentences due to breathlessness. Supplemental O2 via NRB to maintain SpO_2 >94%. Two large-bore peripheral IVs established. Isotonic crystalloid bolus (1L) administered with caution to avoid overhydration. IV opioid analgesia (morphine or hydromorphone) initiated. Stat portable CXR ordered. Labs drawn: CBC with differential, CMP, reticulocyte count, LDH, type and screen, blood cultures, ABG.

History

- HPI: 48 hours of progressive substernal chest pain and dyspnea. Pain initially dull, now sharp and pleuritic, worsening with inspiration. Dry cough and subjective fever/chills. States this is "different from my usual pain" which typically involves extremities and back. Home hydrocodone provided minimal relief. No recent travel, sick contacts, or known infections. Three admissions in the past year for VOC, never ICU.
- PMHx: HbSS sickle cell disease
- Allergies: Not reported
- Social: Lives with father

Physical Examination

- General: Alert, moderate distress, speaking in short sentences due to breathlessness
- Cardiovascular: Tachycardic, regular rhythm, no murmurs
- Pulmonary: Decreased breath sounds and dullness to percussion at right lung base; crackles over right lower lung field
- Extremities: No joint swelling or erythema; rest of examination normal

Diagnostic Studies

- CBC: WBC 19.5, Hgb 6.8 (low), Hct 20.5% (low), Plt 82 (low)
- Reticulocyte Count: 11.2 (elevated)
- BMP: Na 135, K 4.8, HCO_3 19 (low), BUN 24 (high), Cr 0.9, LDH 425 (elevated), T.Bili 3.2 (elevated)
- ABG: pH 7.34, pO2 64 (low), pCO2 33, HCO_3 19
- Chest Radiograph: New right lower lobe infiltrate with associated small pleural effusion

- 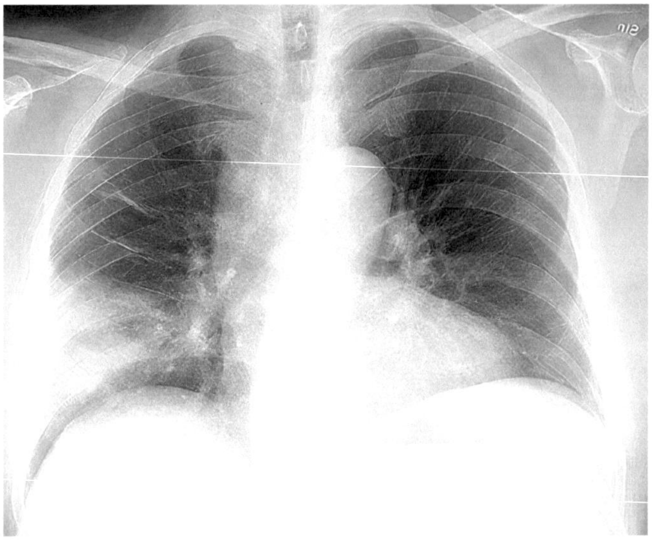

Management

- Supplemental oxygen to maintain SpO_2 >94% — correct hypoxia to prevent further sickling
- IV opioid analgesia accounting for chronic tolerance (typically requiring higher doses than opioid-naïve patients; expect 10-15 mg morphine equivalent or 2-3 mg hydromorphone before adequate relief)
- Empiric antibiotics covering CAP (ceftriaxone and azithromycin) — cannot distinguish infectious from non-infectious etiology clinically
- Cautious fluid resuscitation to maintain euvolemia without volume overload
- Early hematology consultation for consideration of simple vs exchange transfusion
- Incentive spirometry and pulmonary toilet
- ICU admission for hypoxemia and hemodynamic instability
- If hemoglobin drops below 6.0 or cardiopulmonary compromise worsens, initiate exchange transfusion

Managing Conflict

The primary nurse expresses concern: "She's been here several times recently and her pain medications keep escalating. I'm not sure what's going on."

Acknowledge the nurse's concerns while educating that sickle cell patients often require higher opioid doses due to chronic tolerance and that inadequate pain control can precipitate further sickling. Emphasize objective findings (hypoxia, infiltrate, elevated inflammatory markers) supporting acute chest syndrome requiring aggressive analgesia.

Patient Communication

Discuss with the patient and her father: this represents acute chest syndrome, a life-threatening complication distinct from typical pain crises. Explain necessity of ICU admission, potential exchange transfusion, importance of incentive spirometry. Address concerns regarding opioid use by explaining the physiological basis of pain and tolerance. Obtain informed consent for blood transfusion.

Reassessment

- Reassess pain scores 30 minutes after each opioid dose
- Monitor respiratory status every 15-30 minutes; if SpO_2 remains <92% despite supplemental O2 or work of breathing increases, prepare for NIV or intubation
- Re-evaluate vitals after fluid bolus; watch for hypotension or fluid overload

Critical Actions

- Recognize acute chest syndrome based on the triad of chest pain, respiratory symptoms, and new pulmonary infiltrate in a sickle cell patient
- Immediate supplemental oxygen to correct hypoxia and prevent further sickling
- Adequate IV opioid analgesia accounting for chronic tolerance
- Empiric antibiotic therapy covering CAP given inability to distinguish infectious from non-infectious etiology
- Cautious fluid resuscitation to maintain euvolemia while avoiding volume overload
- Early hematology consultation for simple or exchange transfusion
- ICU admission for hypoxemia, multilobar involvement, or hemodynamic instability
- Effective conflict resolution with nursing staff regarding appropriate opioid dosing in sickle cell disease
- Clear communication with patient and family regarding severity and need for escalation
- Serial reassessment of respiratory status, pain control, and hemoglobin trends

Chest Pain After Drug Use

Opening Scenario

A 42-year-old male with chest pain after recreational drug use. Agitated, diaphoretic, demanding to leave for a work meeting. Worried about having a heart attack like his father.

Initial Assessment

Vitals: BP 168/92, HR 118, RR 22, T 36.4°C (97.5°F), SpO_2 97% RA, Pain 8/10 substernal

Agitated male, pacing, diaphoretic, pupils dilated bilaterally (8 mm). Two large-bore peripheral IVs established. Continuous cardiac monitoring and pulse oximetry. 12-lead ECG obtained immediately. Benzodiazepine administered (lorazepam 2 mg IV) for agitation and sympathomimetic symptoms. Aspirin 325 mg PO, sublingual NTG 0.4 mg. Portable CXR ordered. Serial cardiac enzymes and BMP drawn.

History

- HPI: 42-year-old male with hypertension and tobacco use presenting with 90 minutes of crushing substernal chest pain beginning approximately 30 minutes after insufflating a powdered stimulant substance at a social gathering. Pressure-like pain without radiation. Associated dyspnea, diaphoresis, and anxiety. Denies syncope, palpitations, or hemoptysis. Expresses concern about missing work presentation; initially requests to leave AMA, stating he "cannot afford to be here" and fears being labeled as seeking drugs.
- PMHx: Hypertension, tobacco use
- Allergies: Not reported

Physical Examination

- General: Agitated, pacing, diaphoretic
- HEENT: Pupils dilated bilaterally (8 mm), reactive to light
- Cardiovascular: Tachycardic, regular rhythm, no murmurs, radial pulses 2+ bilaterally
- Respiratory: Clear to auscultation bilaterally, no accessory muscle use
- Psychiatric: Anxious, repeatedly checking watch, requesting to leave AMA
- Remainder of physical examination normal

Diagnostic Studies

- CBC: WBC 12.3, Hgb 14.8, Hct 44.2%, Plt 285
- BMP: Na 141, K 3.5, Cl 102, HCO_3 22, BUN 16, Cr 1.0, Glucose 108
- Troponin I: Initial 1ng/dl; 3-hour repeat pending
- ECG (initial): Sinus tachycardia rate 112, no ST elevations or depressions, no T-wave inversions, no pathologic Q waves
- CXR: Normal cardiac silhouette, no pulmonary edema, no pneumothorax, clear lung fields
- Urine Drug Screen: Positive for amphetamines

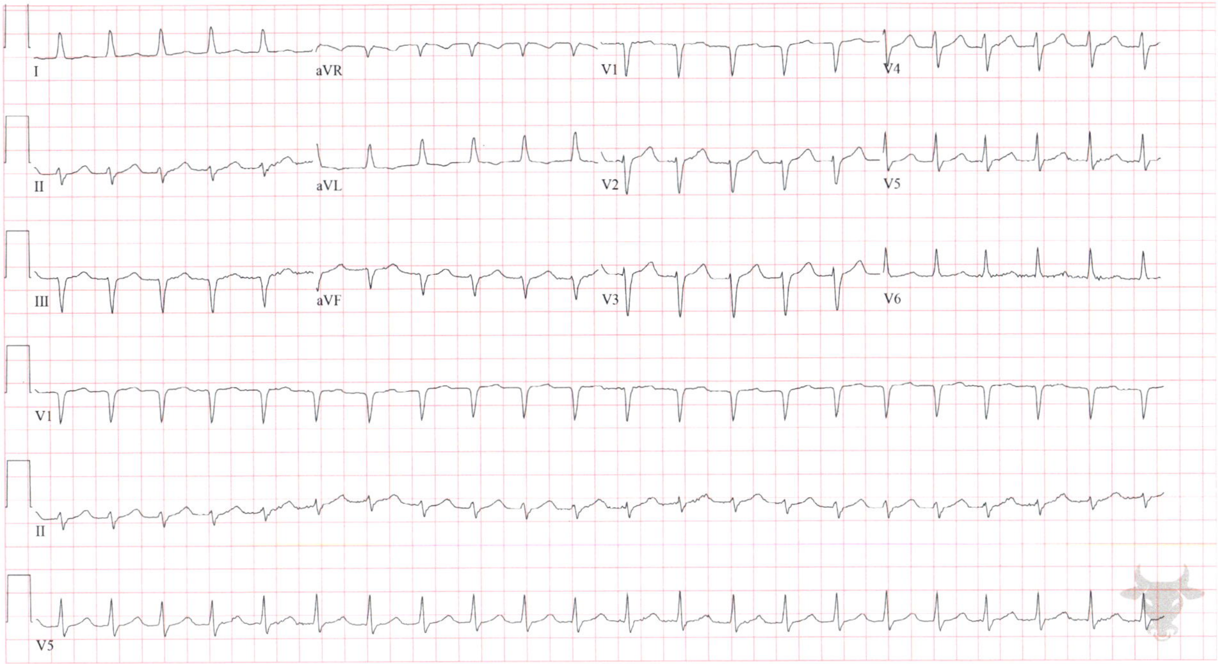

Management

- First-line treatment: benzodiazepines for sympathomimetic toxidrome — reduces myocardial oxygen demand
- Serial troponins and ECGs to monitor for coronary vasospasm vs. ACS
- Therapeutic communication addressing desire to leave AMA: discuss risks, validate concerns, shared decision-making
- Aspirin and nitrate administration
- Consider alternative diagnoses: aortic dissection, pneumothorax, or pneumomediastinum in stimulant users

Reassessment

Initially improves: less agitated, pain 3/10, BP 145/85, HR 95. After 3 hours, recurrent chest pressure develops. Repeat ECG shows persistent sinus tachycardia without Twave changes. Repeat troponin elevated at 115ng/dl (elevated). Cardiology consultation required for possible coronary vasospasm versus evolving NSTEMI. Admit to cardiac monitoring bed.

Critical Actions

- Recognition of sympathomimetic toxidrome with first-line benzodiazepine administration
- Acquisition and interpretation of initial ECG to exclude STEMI
- Therapeutic communication addressing AMA request, including risk discussion and shared decision-making
- Standard ACS protocol (aspirin, nitrates) while avoiding beta-blockers due to unopposed alpha stimulation risk
- Serial troponins and ECGs monitoring for coronary vasospasm versus ACS
- Recognition of dynamic ECG changes on reassessment requiring cardiology consultation and admission
- Consideration of alternative diagnoses including aortic dissection, pneumothorax, or pneumomediastinum in stimulant users

Acute Shortness of Breath

Opening Scenario

At 2 AM, EMS arrives with a 78-year-old male found gasping for air at home. Daughter is in the hallway crying. On NRB at 15 L/min, unable to speak in full sentences.

Initial Assessment

Vitals: BP 210/115, HR 115, RR 32, T 37.0°C, SpO_2 88% on 15L NRB

Elderly male sitting upright in tripod position, markedly diaphoretic, perioral cyanosis, unable to lie flat. Airway patent, speaking in single words only. Severe distress with accessory muscle use, coarse bilateral crackles audible without stethoscope. Pale, cool, clammy skin; capillary refill 3 seconds.

Bedside ultrasound - depressed ejection fraction, no pericardial effusion. B-lines bilateral lung windows.

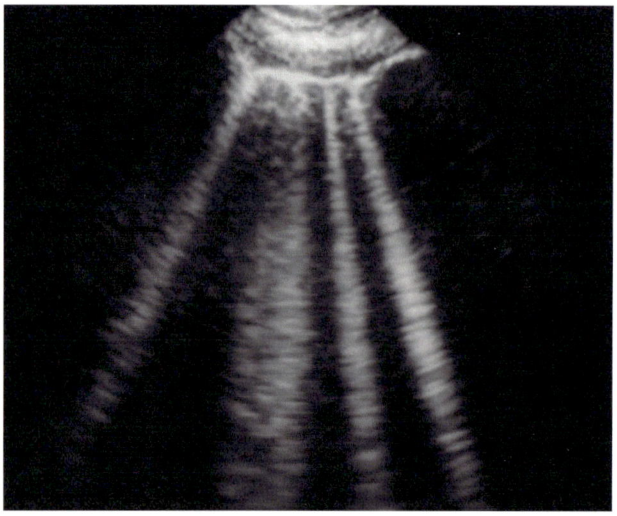

Immediate high-dose nitrates (IV NTG infusion 200 mcg/min or sequential SL NTG 0.4 mg) and BiPAP/CPAP initiated. Labs drawn including BMP, cardiac markers, BNP, ABG.

History

- HPI: Daughter reports history of CAD, hypertension, and type 2 diabetes. Patient ran out of furosemide 3 days ago when pharmacy closed for the holiday. Orthopnea began yesterday, suddenly worsened 1 hour ago with pink frothy sputum. Denies fever, chest pain, recent travel, or unilateral leg swelling.
- Medications: Metoprolol, lisinopril, furosemide (out for 3 days), metformin, atorvastatin, aspirin 81mg
- Allergies: NKDA
- Social: Lives alone in a third-floor walk-up, normally independent with ADLs, daughter checks on him daily

Physical Examination

- General: Severe respiratory distress, anxious, unable to speak in full sentences
- Cardiovascular: Tachycardic, regular rhythm, JVD to angle of jaw at 45 degrees, S3 gallop present, no murmurs or rubs
- Pulmonary: Bilateral diffuse crackles extending to apices, scattered expiratory wheezes, diminished air movement at bases

- Extremities: 2+ pitting edema bilateral lower extremities to knees, warm to touch, no calf tenderness
- Remainder of physical exam normal

Diagnostic Studies

- CBC: WBC 12.5, Hgb 14.2, Plt 280
- BMP: Na 138, K 5.2 (high), Cl 105, HCO_3 18 (low), BUN 48 (high), Cr 2.1 (high), Glucose 142
- Troponin I: 0.08 (elevated), BNP: 3,800 pg/mL (markedly elevated)
- ABG: pH 7.28 (acidotic), pCO2 48 (elevated), pO2 62 (low), HCO_3 22
- Lactate: 2.4 (mildly elevated)
- ECG: LVH normal intervals no peaked T-waves.

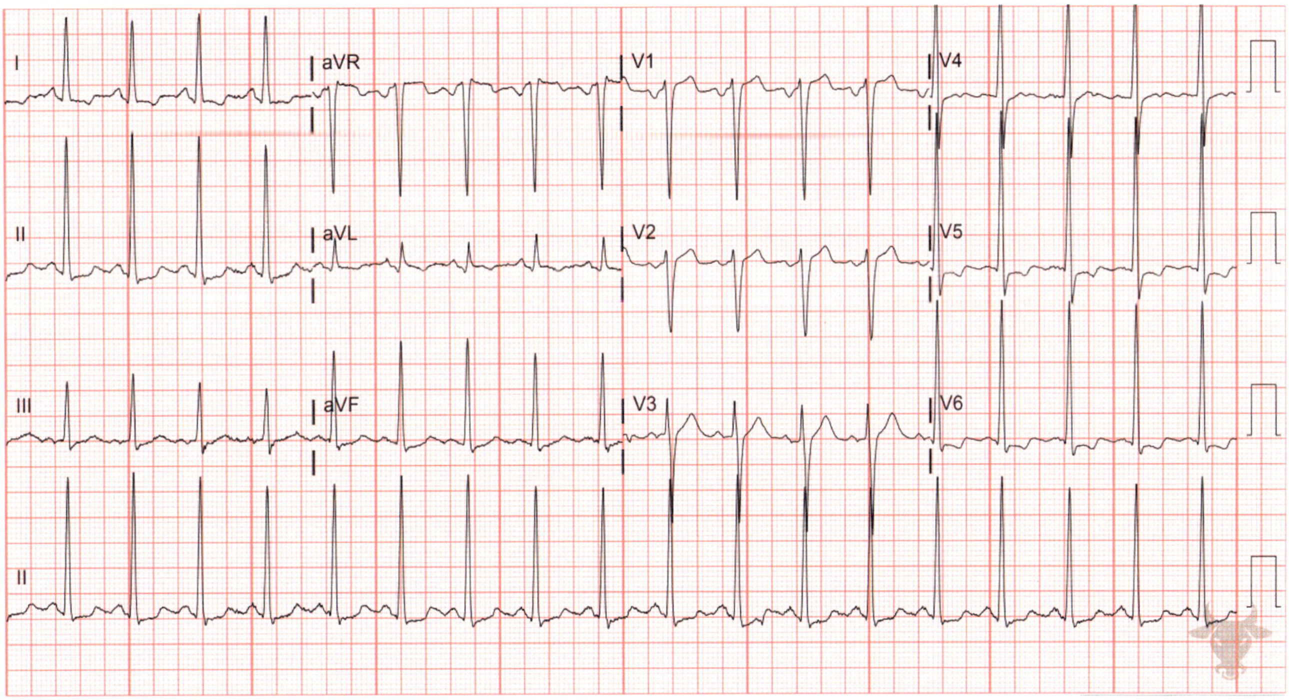

Management

- Prioritize after-load reduction with high-dose nitrates and NIV (BiPAP/CPAP) over immediate diuresis in the acute hypoxic phase — reduces preload and after-load while avoiding intubation
- Identify medication non-compliance (diuretic cessation) as the precipitating factor; address barriers to medication access
- Recognize concomitant AKI and hyperkalemia requiring careful monitoring and adjustment of diuretic therapy
- Consider and exclude alternative diagnoses (ACS, PE, pneumonia) through history, exam, and targeted testing
- CCU/ICU admission with cardiology consultation

Reassessment

Twenty minutes after BiPAP and high-dose nitrates:

- Vitals: BP 165/80, HR 95, RR 24, SpO_2 94% on BiPAP
- Patient now speaking in short phrases, respiratory effort decreased, pink frothy sputum resolved; still tachypneic and cannot tolerate lying flat
- Patient states: "I don't want to be intubated."

Difficult Conversations

Daughter states in the hallway: "He wouldn't want all these machines. He always said he never wanted to be on a breathing machine." No advance directives on file.

Elicit patient's goals of care and code status preferences now that he is temporarily stabilized. Validate daughter's emotional distress. Clarify that BiPAP is non-invasive and helping him improve. Provide clear prognosis information.

Critical Actions

- Recognize acute cardiogenic pulmonary edema secondary to acute decompensated heart failure
- Initiate immediate stabilization: high-dose nitrates and NIV (BiPAP/CPAP) to reduce preload and afterload
- Prioritize afterload reduction with nitrates and NIV over immediate diuresis in the acute hypoxic phase
- Identify medication non-compliance (diuretic cessation) as the precipitating factor and address barriers to medication access
- Timely reassessment after interventions to evaluate response, recognizing improvement while remaining vigilant for deterioration
- Elicit patient's goals of care and code status preferences; address family concerns regarding advance care planning
- Determine appropriate disposition (CCU/ICU) and arrange cardiology consultation
-

Toxic Alcohol Ingestion

Opening Scenario

EMS arrives with a 38-year-old man found unresponsive in his garage. Wife reports he was working on his car radiator earlier. Found 30 minutes ago confused and increasingly somnolent. History of alcohol use disorder. No empty alcohol bottles found; spilled container of green liquid noted near the car.

Initial Assessment

Vitals: BP 118/64, HR 104, RR 30, T 36.4°C, SpO_2 94% RA

Agitated delirium alternating with somnolence. Disheveled, cachectic, dried emesis, sweet odor on clothing and breath. Poor dentition.

- Airway: Patent, gag reflex present
- Breathing: Tachypneic with deep, rapid respirations (Kussmaul pattern), clear bilaterally
- Circulation: Tachycardic, regular rhythm, capillary refill 2 seconds
- Disability: AMS, opens eyes to pain, withdraws to pain, incomprehensible verbalizations
- Exposure: Cool, clammy skin; no track marks; no traumatic injuries; sweet odor on breath

History

- History of Present Illness: Obtained from wife and EMS. Patient was reportedly working on vehicle cooling system. Wife found him 30 minutes ago with confusion. No witnessed seizure activity. No trauma reported.
- Past Medical History: Alcohol use disorder (previous withdrawals), depression, hypertension
- Medications: Lisinopril (non-compliant), thiamine (occasionally)
- Allergies: NKDA
- Social History: Heavy alcohol use (daily), unemployed, lives with wife, 20 pack-year smoking history

Physical Examination

- General: Cachectic male, alternating agitation and somnolence, inappropriate affect
- Head: Normocephalic, no trauma, temporal wasting noted
- Eyes: Pupils equal, sluggishly reactive, horizontal nystagmus present bilaterally, no papilledema
- Cardiovascular: Tachycardic, no murmurs, rubs, or gallops
- Respiratory: Clear to auscultation bilaterally, deep sighing respirations
- Abdomen: Soft, non-distended, normoactive bowel sounds, no masses or tenderness
- Neurological: Cranial nerves intact, tremor noted in upper extremities, ataxia when attempting to sit, asterixis not present due to obtundation
- Skin: Cool, dry, poor turgor; no rashes or needle tracks
- Remainder of physical examination is normal

Diagnostic Studies

- WBC 9.8, Hgb 13.2, Hct 39.8%, Plt 180
- Na 146, K 4.8, Cl 106, HCO_3 8 (critical), BUN 14, Cr 1.0, Glucose 132, Calcium 6.8 (low)
- ABG: pH 7.08, pCO2 24, pO2 95, HCO_3 7; Anion Gap 32
- Lactate 14 (elevated); Measured Osm 345, Calculated Osm 302, Osmolal Gap 43
- Ethanol 8 (negligible), Ethylene Glycol 220 (toxic), Methanol undetectable

- UA: Calcium oxalate monohydrate crystals; positive fluorescence under Wood lamp

Management

- Supplemental O2; two large-bore IVs; cardiac monitoring; 12-lead ECG
- Labs: POC glucose, CMP, CBC, ABG, lactate, serum osmolarity, toxic alcohol levels, UA with microscopy
- Thiamine 100 mg IV; consider naloxone
- Administer fomepizole promptly upon suspicion of toxic alcohol ingestion
- Sodium bicarbonate for severe acidosis (pH <7.1)
- Address hypocalcemia with calcium replacement
- Consult nephrology early for emergent hemodialysis

Reassessment

One hour after fomepizole and bicarbonate: BP 115/60, HR 112, RR 28, SpO_2 98% on 2L NC. Repeat ABG: pH 7.15, pCO2 26, HCO_3 9 (slight improvement but still critical). Patient more obtunded with snoring respirations. Calcium drops to 6.2, QTc prolongs to 520 ms.

- Prepare for definitive airway management if respiratory fatigue develops
- Hemodialysis for toxin clearance and acidosis correction
- Calcium repletion (with caution given precipitation risk)
- ICU admission

Patient Communication

Wife asks, "Is this just his drinking again? Did he try to hurt himself?" Inform her this is life-threatening poisoning, not simple intoxication, requiring immediate treatment. Ask about exact time of last normal behavior, possibility of intentional ingestion, and access to other substances.

Critical Actions

- Recognizes presentation of toxic alcohol poisoning (elevated anion gap metabolic acidosis with elevated osmolal gap) despite low ethanol level
- Orders specific toxic alcohol levels early without waiting for clinical deterioration
- Administers alcohol dehydrogenase inhibitor (fomepizole) promptly upon suspicion
- Initiates sodium bicarbonate therapy for severe acidosis (pH < 7.1)
- Addresses hypocalcemia with appropriate calcium replacement
- Recognizes necessity of hemodialysis for severe acidosis, renal failure risk, and high toxin level
- Communicates effectively with family regarding severity, distinguishes toxic ingestion from ethanol intoxication, and addresses suicide risk
- Performs reassessment recognizing clinical trajectory deterioration and need for airway intervention
- Avoids premature intubation without preparing for hyperventilation maintenance (if intubated, must maintain minute ventilation to compensate for metabolic acidosis)
- Consults nephrology early for emergent dialysis

Drowning

Opening Scenario

A 16-year-old male arrives via EMS after his snowmobile broke through thin ice. Submerged approximately 8 minutes. Bystander CPR for witnessed pulselessness; ROSC after 3 minutes. Arrives intubated with C-collar and backboard.

Initial Assessment

Vitals: BP 76/54, HR 48, RR 12 (ventilated), T 30.8°C (tympanic), SpO_2 97% on 100% FiO2, Glucose 92

Unresponsive adolescent. Pale, cold, wet skin; no shivering. ETT secured at 22 cm.

- Airway: ETT in place, misting observed
- Breathing: Bilateral breath sounds present, coarse, no cyanosis
- Circulation: Bradycardic, weak pulses, capillary refill >4 seconds, mottled extremities
- Disability: GCS 3T, pupils 5 mm bilaterally and sluggish, no spontaneous movement

History

- HPI: 16-year-old male with no past medical history was snowmobiling on frozen lake when ice broke. Submerged for ~8 minutes. Father pulled him out. No pulse initially, CPR started by father (firefighter). ROSC achieved by EMS.
- PMHx: None
- PSHx: None
- Allergies: None
- Meds: None
- Social: Lives with parents, high school student, denies substance use
- FHx: Non-contributory

Physical Examination

- General: No spontaneous movement
- Pulmonary: Bilateral coarse crackles, decreased breath sounds at bases
- Cardiovascular: Regular bradycardic rhythm, no murmurs
- Skin: Pale, cool, mottled extremities with peripheral cyanosis
- Remainder of physical examination: Normal

Diagnostic Studies

- WBC 11.8, Hgb 14.5, Hct 44%, Plt 265
- Na 142, K 5.6 (elevated), Cl 106, HCO_3 19, BUN 16, Cr 1.2, Glucose 110
- PT 12.8, PTT 32, INR 1.0
- VBG: pH 7.26, pCO2 48, HCO_3 21; Lactate 5.8
- ECG: Sinus bradycardia with Osborne waves (J-point notching) in leads II, III, aVF, V4-V6
- CXR: ETT at right mainstem with bilateral patchy opacities (aspiration pneumonitis)

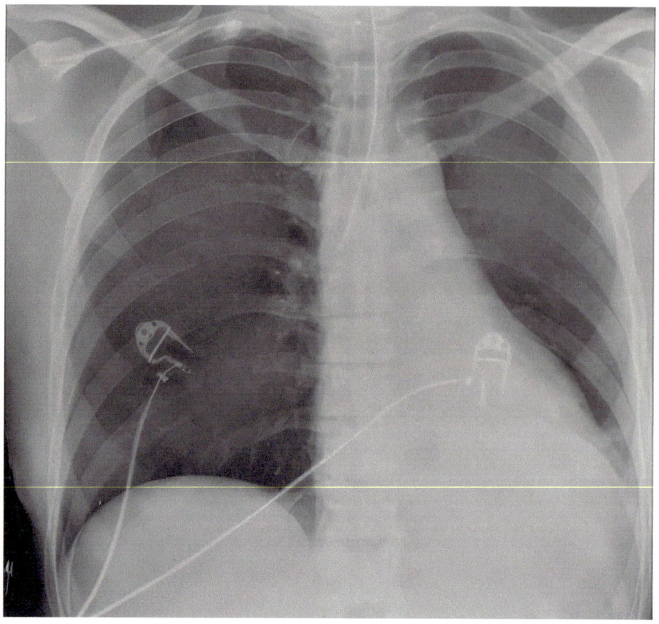

- CT Head: No hemorrhage or mass effect; CT C-Spine: No fracture

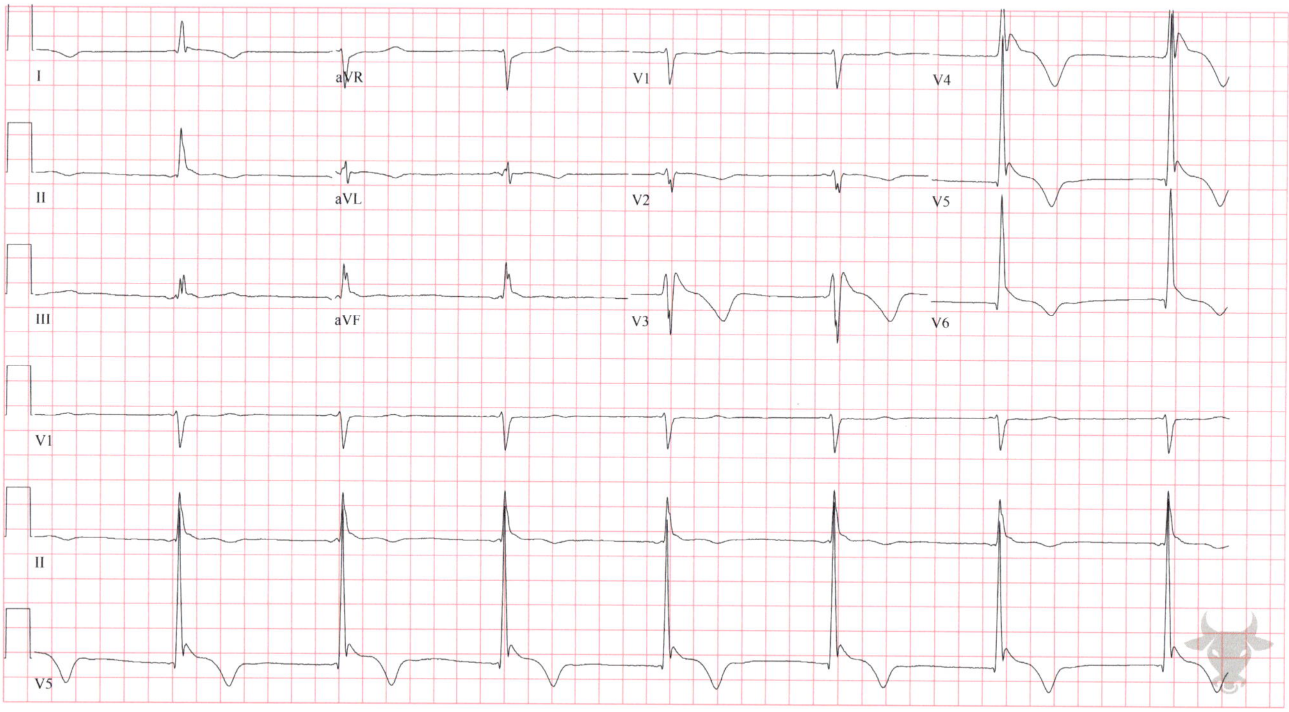

Management

- Confirm ETT with waveform capnography then after xray withdrawl to 2cm above carina. Then repeat xray to verify correct positioning.
- Active rewarming: forced-air warming blanket, warmed IV fluids (40°C), warmed humidified O2 (42°C)
- Temperature-sensing Foley for core monitoring; NG for warmed saline lavage
- 1L warmed NS bolus; cautious handling to avoid precipitating VF

Reassessment

At 45 minutes: BP 102/68, HR 78 (sinus), T 34.8°C (rising), SpO_2 95%. Spontaneous respiratory efforts developing.

- Adjust sedation for ventilator dyssynchrony
- Monitor K+ (5.6); consider insulin/glucose if >6.0 or calcium if ECG changes
- Neurologic: still unresponsive — avoid prognostication until normothermic (>35°C)
- Disposition: Pediatric ICU

Patient Communication

Father is distraught: "Is my son going to die?"

- Acknowledge distress and guilt with empathy
- Explain: critically ill from hypothermia and cardiac arrest, actively warming
- Recovery extent unknown until normothermic
- Offer chaplaincy and social work

Critical Actions

- Recognition that tympanic/axillary temperatures are unreliable in hypothermia; placement of internal temperature monitoring device (esophageal, Foley, or rectal probe) is essential
- Immediate initiation of active rewarming (forced-air warming, warmed IV fluids, warmed humidified oxygen, gastric lavage) for severe hypothermia
- Airway protection with endotracheal intubation followed by adjustment of tube placement.
- Identification of Osborne waves on ECG as pathognomonic for hypothermia (typically <32°C)
- Understanding that defibrillation is unlikely to be successful at core temperatures <30°C; focus on rewarming before repeated shocks if VF occurs
- Recognition that rough handling or unnecessary movement can trigger ventricular fibrillation in severe hypothermia; emphasis on gentle patient manipulation
- Appropriate reassessment of core temperature trends to guide management decisions and detect complications during rewarming (arrhythmias, electrolyte shifts)
- Communication with family using empathetic, clear language regarding prognosis uncertainty and the need to complete rewarming before neurologic assessment
- Knowledge that "nobody is dead until they are warm and dead" — continuation of resuscitation until core temperature >32-35°C before determining futility of resuscitation
- Admission to ICU for continued rewarming and observation

Weakness and Blurred Vision

Opening Scenario

A 28-year-old female graduate student presents with progressive weakness over 5 days. Initially noted difficulty keeping eyelids open, now has difficulty swallowing solids and dyspnea on exertion. Partner reports increasingly nasal voice over 24 hours.

Initial Assessment

Vitals: BP 118/74, HR 92, RR 20, T 37.1°C, SpO_2 94% RA

Physical Examination

- General: Alert, oriented, moderate distress, speaking in full sentences but voice becomes nasal and strained with prolonged conversation
- HEENT: Bilateral ptosis that worsens with sustained upward gaze; diplopia reported with lateral gaze; facial muscle weakness bilaterally affecting eye closure and smile
- Neck: No jugular venous distension, no stridor, weak cough noted
- Pulmonary: Clear breath sounds bilaterally, shallow inspiratory effort with reduced chest expansion, accessory muscle use present
- Neurological: Proximal muscle strength 4/5 bilateral upper and lower extremities; distal strength 5/5 bilaterally. Sensation intact. Deep tendon reflexes normal. No pronator drift. Extraocular movements demonstrate fatigable weakness with sustained lateral gaze.
- Remainder of physical examination normal

Diagnostic Studies

- WBC 5.8, Hgb 13.2, Hct 39.5%, Plt 285
- Na 138, K 3.7, Cl 102, HCO_3 24, BUN 14, Cr 0.8, Glucose 105
- AST 24, ALT 30, Alk Phos 85; PT 11.5, PTT 29, INR 1.0
- TSH 1.8 (normal); Urine pregnancy negative; Urine tox negative
- CXR: Normal; CT Head: No acute pathology

Reassessment

Forty-five minutes after arrival, while awaiting neurology consultation, the patient reports increased difficulty breathing. Repeat vital signs demonstrate:

- Blood Pressure: 122/78 mmHg
- Heart Rate: 105 bpm
- Respiratory Rate: 28 breaths/min
- SpO_2: 89% on room air

The patient is now unable to speak in complete sentences and demonstrates shallow, rapid breathing with paradoxical abdominal movement. Negative Inspiratory Force (NIF) is measured at -15 cm H_2O (normal > -60 cm H_2O). The neurology consultant arrives to perform bedside edrophonium testing to confirm the diagnosis of myasthenia gravis.

Patient Communication

The patient and her partner express significant anxiety about the possibility of intubation and ask about the long-term implications of her diagnosis. They specifically request information about whether she will be able to complete her graduate studies and if this condition is permanent. The patient also expresses fear about the immediate testing and potential need for mechanical ventilation.

Critical Actions

- Identifies pattern of fatigable muscle weakness affecting ocular, bulbar, and proximal extremity muscles consistent with myasthenia gravis
- Performs focused neurological examination demonstrating fatigability of weakness (worsening with sustained effort)
- Monitors respiratory status with objective measures (NIF, vital capacity, or respiratory observations) recognizing risk of respiratory failure
- Recognizes clinical deterioration on reassessment as impending myasthenic crisis with respiratory compromise
- Prepares for immediate airway management prior to diagnostic testing, including selection of appropriate induction agents (avoiding succinylcholine and minimizing non-depolarizing neuromuscular blockers if intubation required)
- Verbalizes need to remain at bedside during edrophonium testing with airway equipment and ventilatory support immediately available
- Initiates appropriate therapy including acetylcholinesterase inhibitors (pyridostigmine or neostigmine) and considers immunomodulatory therapy (IVIG or plasmapheresis) for severe presentations
- Arranges admission to intensive care setting for continuous respiratory monitoring
- Communicates empathetically regarding diagnosis, treatment options, and prognosis while addressing specific concerns about educational and functional outcomes

Hypertension

Opening Scenario

A 62-year-old male found collapsed in his bathroom. Daughter reports "worst headache of my life" and progressive confusion over the past hour. Ran out of BP medications (clonidine and amlodipine) three days ago. Field BP 270/145 mmHg.

Initial Assessment

Vitals: BP 258/138, HR 78, RR 18, T 36.5°C, SpO_2 97% RA, Glucose 89

Lying uncomfortably on stretcher, eyes closed, opens to loud verbal stimuli. Diaphoretic, gripping head.

- Airway: Patent, speaking in short sentences
- Breathing: Non-labored, no cyanosis
- Circulation: Warm and moist skin, capillary refill 2 seconds
- Disability: Alert to person only

History

- HPI: 62-year-old male with hypertension and CKD stage 3. Ran out of clonidine and amlodipine three days ago due to insurance issues. Developed sudden severe occipital headache 3 hours ago associated with nausea and visual blurring. Daughter notes repetitive questioning and confusion.
- PMHx: Hypertension, chronic kidney disease, hyperlipidemia
- PSHx: Appendectomy
- Meds: Clonidine 0.3mg TID (missed x3 days), Amlodipine 10mg daily (missed x3 days), Atorvastatin 40mg
- Allergies: NKDA
- Social: Lives with daughter, retired, no tobacco/alcohol/drugs

History

- HPI: 62-year-old male with hypertension and CKD stage 3. Ran out of clonidine and amlodipine three days ago due to insurance issues. Sudden severe occipital headache 3 hours ago with nausea and visual blurring. Daughter notes repetitive questioning and confusion.
- PMHx: Hypertension, chronic kidney disease, hyperlipidemia
- PSHx: Appendectomy
- Meds: Clonidine 0.3 mg TID (missed x3 days), Amlodipine 10 mg daily (missed x3 days), Atorvastatin 40 mg
- Allergies: NKDA
- Social: Lives with daughter, retired, no tobacco/alcohol/drugs

Physical Examination

- Neurologic: Alert but disoriented to place and time. CN II-XII intact except bilateral papilledema on fundoscopy. No focal motor weakness.
- Cardiovascular: Regular rate and rhythm, S4 gallop appreciated
- Pulmonary: Clear bilaterally
- Abdomen: Soft, non-tender
- Skin: Warm, diaphoretic
- Remainder normal

Diagnostic Studies

- WBC 8.9, Hgb 13.8, Plt 285
- Na 142, K 5.2 (elevated), Cl 100, HCO_3 24, BUN 48 (elevated), Cr 3.1 (elevated), Glucose 95
- PT 13.1, PTT 30, INR 1.1; Troponin 0.06 (elevated)
- UA: Protein 3+, trace blood, RBC 3/HPF
- ECG: Sinus rhythm, LVH with secondary repolarization abnormalities, no acute ST changes
- CT Head: Bilateral posterior parietal/occipital hypodensities consistent with PRES; no hemorrhage or mass effect

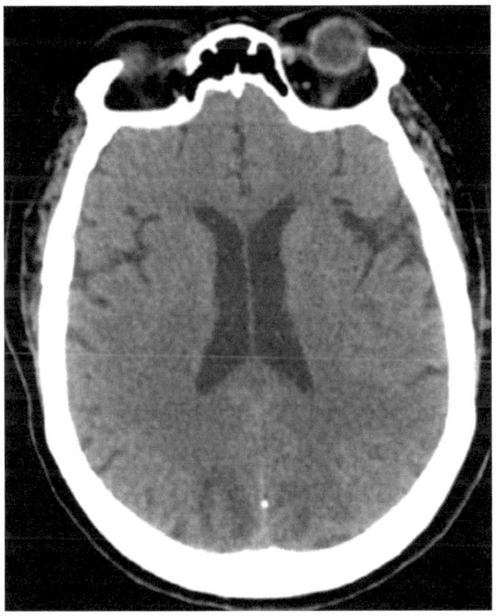

- CXR: Cardiomegaly, cephalization of vessels

Management

- Two large-bore IVs; cardiac monitoring; supplemental O2 2L NC
- Stat labs: CBC, BMP, LFTs, coags, troponin, UA; 12-lead ECG; non-contrast CT head
- IV nicardipine infusion; goal 25% MAP reduction over 1-2 hours
- Avoid precipitous drops that could cause cerebral/coronary hypoperfusion

Reassessment

At 45 minutes: BP 198/110. Patient now oriented x3. Headache improved but present. Papilledema persists.

At 1.5 hours: BP 175/95. Patient requests to leave AMA, feeling "better" and wanting to go to pharmacy. Requires patient-centered discussion about need for monitored admission and risks of early discharge.

Critical Actions

- Recognize hypertensive emergency with end-organ damage (hypertensive encephalopathy, acute kidney injury, PRES on imaging)
- Identify clonidine rebound hypertension as etiology (abrupt cessation of central alpha-2 agonist causing catecholamine surge)
- Order appropriate emergent workup including CT head to exclude hemorrhage and identify PRES
- Initiate controlled IV antihypertensive therapy with goal of 25% MAP reduction in first 1-2 hours, avoiding precipitous drops that could cause cerebral/coronary hypoperfusion
- Interpret imaging findings of bilateral posterior white matter changes consistent with PRES (Posterior Reversible Encephalopathy Syndrome)

- Address barriers to medication adherence through empathetic patient-centered communication regarding insurance/pharmacy access issues
- Counsel patient against leaving AMA by explaining ongoing risks of stroke, renal failure, and recurrent hypertensive crisis
- Admit to monitored setting (telemetry or ICU) for continued IV antihypertensive management and serial neurologic reassessment
- Arrange social work/pharmacy consultation prior to discharge to prevent recurrence

Syncope with Rash

Opening Scenario

A 29-year-old female arrives after syncope while jogging. Increasing fatigue and intermittent dizziness for 3 days. Husband present.

Initial Assessment

Vitals: BP 94/68, HR 38, RR 14, T 37.4°C, SpO_2 98% RA, Glucose 104

Healthy, athletic-appearing female. Alert and oriented, sitting upright, prefers to remain still. Pale and cool skin. Feels "heavy-headed" and weak when attempting to stand.

- Airway: Patent, speaking in full sentences
- Breathing: Clear bilaterally, no tachypnea
- Circulation: Markedly bradycardic, regular rhythm, weak radial pulses, capillary refill 2-3 seconds, no JVD

History

- HPI: 29-year-old physical therapist reports completing a solo backpacking trip along the Appalachian Trail in Pennsylvania two weeks ago. During the final day of hiking, she removed three attached ticks from her lower abdomen and right flank. That evening, she noticed an expanding red lesion on her right flank that developed a clear center with a dark red ring, resembling a "bullseye target." She photographed the lesion with her phone because it was painless but unusual. The rash expanded to approximately 12 cm over three days then faded completely one week ago. She felt well until three days ago when she developed progressive fatigue, myalgias, and episodic lightheadedness culminating in today's syncopal episode while running. She denies chest pain, dyspnea, or palpitations.
- PMHx: None
- PSHx: None
- Medications: Oral contraceptives
- Allergies: No known drug allergies
- Social: Active marathon runner, no tobacco, alcohol, or drug use; lives with husband
- Family Hx: No premature coronary artery disease or conduction abnormalities

Physical Examination

- General: Alert, oriented x3, no acute respiratory distress, reports mild neck stiffness but no headache
- Skin: No visible rash or lesions currently. Patient shows photograph on cellular telephone displaying classic erythema migrans: large annular lesion with bright erythematous border, central clearing, and targetoid appearance with central duskiness on right flank
- Cardiovascular: Bradycardic, regular rhythm, no murmurs, rubs, or gallops, no peripheral edema
- Neurological: Cranial nerves II-XII intact, no facial droop, no meningeal signs, normal strength and sensation
- Remainder of physical examination normal

Diagnostic Studies

- WBC 11.2, Hgb 13.8, Hct 41.5%, Plt 280
- Na 141, K 3.9, Cl 105, HCO_3 24, BUN 12, Cr 0.9, Glucose 98
- Troponin 0.02 (normal), CK-MB 2, Magnesium 1.9
- Lyme serology: Pending
- ECG: Complete heart block (third-degree AV block) with junctional escape rhythm at 32 bpm, no axis deviation, no ST changes

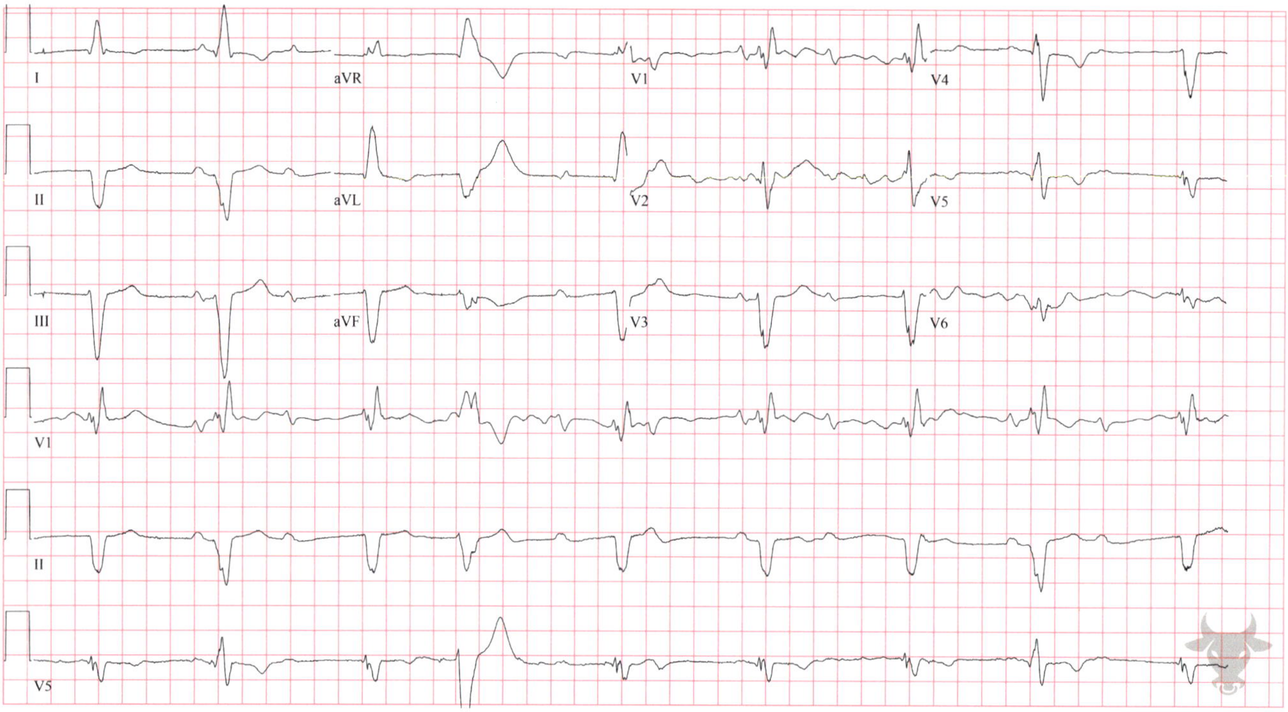

Management

- Continuous cardiac monitoring with defibrillation pads; two large-bore IVs; NS at maintenance
- Begin transcutaneous pacing with adequate sedation and evaluate for both electrical and mechanical capture at 70bpm
- Recognize resolved erythema migrans (documented by patient photograph) with recent tick exposure and new complete heart block as Lyme carditis
- Initiate transcutaneous pacing for symptomatic third-degree block with hypotension
- Doxycycline 100 mg PO BID (or Ceftriaxone 2 g IV daily if unable to tolerate oral)
- Admit to cardiac step-down with continuous telemetry
- Consult cardiology for possible temporary transvenous pacing

Reassessment

HR drops to 32 with worsening dizziness and presyncope. BP 88/58. Rhythm strip shows complete AV dissociation.

Patient Communication

Explain to the patient and her husband that the “bullseye” rash shown in the photograph is pathognomonic for erythema migrans, the hallmark of early Lyme disease, not a spider bite. Clarify that while the skin manifestation has resolved, the bacteria disseminated to the cardiac conduction system, causing inflammation and temporary heart block. Emphasize that this represents early disseminated Lyme disease, not a new infection, and that antibiotic therapy typically leads to complete resolution of the heart block within days to weeks. Discuss that permanent pacemakers are rarely necessary in Lyme carditis unless the block persists despite treatment, and that the prognosis is excellent with appropriate antibiotics. Address that serologic testing may confirm the diagnosis but treatment should not be delayed while awaiting results when the clinical picture is classic.

Diagnosis

Early Disseminated Lyme Disease with Lyme Carditis (Complete Heart Block)

Critical Actions

- Recognized history of erythema migrans (target/bullseye rash) documented by patient photograph as diagnostic of Lyme disease despite resolution of visible skin findings
- Identified appropriate temporal relationship between tick exposure (2 weeks prior), initial rash, and current cardiac manifestations consistent with early disseminated Lyme disease
- Interpreted third-degree AV block in young healthy female with recent endemic exposure as Lyme carditis rather than acute coronary syndrome or intrinsic conduction system disease
- Distinguished between early localized disease (resolved rash) and early disseminated disease (cardiac manifestation) based on timeline
- Selected appropriate empiric antibiotic therapy (Doxycycline or Ceftriaxone) without awaiting serologic confirmation
- Demonstrated clinical decision-making by initiating transcutaneous pacing for symptomatic complete heart block with hemodynamic compromise
- Performed timely reassessment identifying progression to complete AV dissociation with hypotension requiring immediate intervention
- Communicated effectively regarding delayed presentation of disseminated disease, distinction from spider bite, and reversible nature of conduction abnormality
- Arrange CCU admission due to need for potential transvenous pacing if needed

Hypercyanotic Spell in an Infant

Opening Scenario

A 4-month-old male infant with known tetralogy of Fallot (diagnosed at 2 weeks of age, surgical repair scheduled for next month) is brought by his parents after turning "dark blue" during a feeding. The episode began 20 minutes ago and has not resolved. The infant is inconsolably crying and appears deeply cyanotic.

Initial Assessment

Vitals: HR 178, RR 62, T 37.1°C (axillary), SpO_2 58% RA, Weight 5.8 kg

Deeply cyanotic infant, irritable, inconsolable crying. No respiratory distress at rest but tachypneic. Crying worsens the cyanosis.

- Airway: Patent, vigorous cry
- Breathing: Tachypneic, clear bilaterally, no retractions or wheezes
- Circulation: Capillary refill 3 seconds centrally, pulses equal in all extremities

Immediate actions: Place on 100% NRB (SpO_2 improves minimally to 62%), cardiac monitor, IV access, knee-to-chest positioning.

History

- HPI: 4-month-old male with known tetralogy of Fallot diagnosed after a murmur was detected at a 2-week well-child visit. Echocardiogram confirmed large VSD, overriding aorta, RVH, and moderate right ventricular outflow tract obstruction. Surgical repair planned for age 5 months (next month). Parents report the infant was feeding normally when he suddenly became deeply blue, began crying inconsolably, and became diaphoretic. He has had brief episodes of perioral cyanosis with crying before (lasting <1 minute) but nothing this severe or prolonged. No fever, vomiting, diarrhea, or recent illness.
- PMHx: Tetralogy of Fallot; otherwise healthy
- Meds: None (no beta-blocker prescribed)
- Allergies: None known
- Social: Lives with both parents and a 3-year-old sibling
- FHx: No additional congenital heart disease

Physical Examination

- General: Deeply cyanotic infant, inconsolable, diaphoretic
- HEENT: Anterior fontanelle soft and flat, no dysmorphic features
- Cardiovascular: Tachycardic, regular rhythm, previously documented loud systolic murmur is now ABSENT (the absence of murmur during a tet spell indicates severely reduced flow across the RVOT — this is an ominous sign, not an improvement)
- Pulmonary: Clear bilaterally, tachypneic without accessory muscle use
- Abdomen: Soft, nondistended
- Extremities: Diffuse cyanosis, cool peripherally, pulses equal
- Neurologic: Irritable but interactive, strong cry, normal tone

Management

Recognize this as a hypercyanotic ("tet") spell: acute dynamic increase in right-to-left shunting across the VSD due to infundibular spasm of the RVOT, causing severely reduced pulmonary blood flow and profound cyanosis.

Step 1 — Immediate interventions: - Knee-to-chest positioning (increases systemic vascular resistance, reduces right-to-left shunt, and increases pulmonary blood flow) - Calm the infant; minimize stimulation (crying increases oxygen consumption and worsens the spell) - 100% oxygen via blow-by or NRB - IV fluid bolus: 10-20 mL/kg NS to increase preload

Step 2 — If no improvement in 5 minutes: - Morphine 0.1 mg/kg IV/IM (reduces infundibular spasm, decreases systemic venous return, and sedates the infant to reduce oxygen demand) - Continue knee-to-chest positioning

Step 3 — If refractory: - Phenylephrine 5-20 mcg/kg IV bolus (increases SVR, forces blood across the RVOT into the pulmonary circulation) - Ketamine 1-2 mg/kg IV (increases SVR and provides sedation; useful if intubation is needed) - Esmolol 0.5 mg/kg IV over 1 minute, then infusion (relaxes infundibular spasm)

Reassessment

After knee-to-chest positioning and morphine 0.1 mg/kg IV:

- HR 156, RR 48, SpO_2 78% on NRB (improved from 58%)
- Infant calms, cyanosis improving, murmur becomes audible again (indicates improved pulmonary blood flow)
- Lactate 2.8 (was not obtained initially)

Pediatric cardiology consulted. They recommend admission to pediatric ICU and acceleration of surgical timeline given the severity of this spell. Propranolol 0.5 mg/kg PO q6h started as bridge to surgery.

Patient Communication

The parents are panicking: "His surgery is next month! The cardiologist said he was stable enough to wait. What happened? Is he going to die before they can fix it?"

- Acknowledge their fear and validate their distress; they have been living with the anxiety of knowing their child has a heart defect
- Explain in simple terms: the blood vessels in his heart sometimes allow blood to bypass the lungs, and today that happened more severely than before
- Reassure that the treatment is working (the baby is pinking up) and that the cardiology team has been called
- Explain that this episode means surgery will likely need to happen sooner rather than later, and that is actually good because it means the team will prioritize his repair
- Describe what will happen next: admission, monitoring, medication to prevent another spell, and surgical planning

Disposition

- Admit to pediatric cardiac ICU
- Continuous cardiorespiratory monitoring and pulse oximetry
- Propranolol for spell prophylaxis
- Pediatric cardiothoracic surgery consult for expedited repair
- NPO status pending surgical planning

Critical Actions

- Recognize a hypercyanotic (tet) spell in a known ToF patient: acute cyanosis, absent murmur (reduced RVOT flow), and failure to improve with supplemental oxygen
- Initiate knee-to-chest positioning immediately as the first-line intervention
- Minimize stimulation and calm the infant (crying worsens the dynamic obstruction)
- Administer morphine for sedation and reduction of infundibular spasm
- Escalate to phenylephrine or ketamine if refractory (increase SVR to overcome right-to-left shunting)

- Recognize that the disappearance of the murmur during a spell is an ominous sign indicating near-complete RVOT obstruction
- Differentiate a tet spell from other causes of infant cyanosis (sepsis, pneumonia, foreign body, congenital heart disease with fixed shunt)
- Consult pediatric cardiology emergently and discuss acceleration of surgical repair
- Communicate effectively with terrified parents, providing reassurance while being honest about the seriousness of the event

Industrial Burn

Opening Scenario

You are working in a busy urban emergency department when a 42-year-old male industrial technician presents with hand pain. The charge nurse alerts you that the patient appears diaphoretic and uncomfortable in the triage area, holding his left hand elevated.

Initial Assessment

Vitals: BP 148/92, HR 118, RR 18, T 37.2°C, SpO_2 98% RA

Moderate distress, diaphoretic, guarding left hand.

- Airway: Patent, speaking in full sentences
- Breathing: No respiratory distress
- Circulation: Peripheral pulses equal, capillary refill <2 seconds

History

- HPI: Patient reports sudden onset of deep, burning pain to left thumb that began approximately 3 hours ago while at work. Pain is throbbing, unrelenting, and seems disproportionate to the visible skin changes. He denies direct trauma or impact. Upon specific questioning, he reveals employment as a semiconductor manufacturing technician where he handles hydrofluoric acid (HF) for silicon wafer etching. He notes that while he wears protective gloves, he discovered a small tear in his left glove upon completing his shift.
- PMHx: Hypertension (well-controlled)
- PSHx: None
- Allergies: NKDA
- Social: Lives with partner, denies tobacco use, occasional alcohol consumption
- FHx: Non-contributory

Physical Examination

- General: Moderate distress, focused on guarding left hand
- Extremities: Left thumb with edematous, grayish-white discoloration and vesicle formation extending from the interphalangeal joint to the fingertip, including involvement of the nail bed and surrounding cuticle. Severe pain with passive movement and palpation out of proportion to visual findings. Full active range of motion present but limited by pain. Distal capillary refill intact. Remainder of physical examination normal.

Diagnostic Studies

- BMP: Na 140, K 4.2, Cl 98, CO_3 24, BUN 14, Cr 1.0, Ca 7.8 (low)
- Ionized Ca: 4.1 (low)
- Mg: 1.8

ECG: Normal sinus rhythm, QTc 440 ms

Management

- Immediate copious irrigation with tepid water; IV access; ECG monitoring

- Topical calcium gluconate gel to affected digit
- Intradermal 5 calcium gluconate (0.5-1 mL/cm2) into burn margins
- IV calcium gluconate 2 g slowly
- At 30-minute reassessment: persistent severe pain 9/10, no relief from topical/intradermal/IV calcium
- Consult toxicology or burn surgery for intra-arterial calcium gluconate infusion

Critical Actions

- Recognize hydrofluoric acid exposure based on occupational history (semiconductor manufacturing, glass etching, or metal processing) and characteristic presentation of severe pain out of proportion to visible tissue injury
- Understand the pathophysiology of fluoride ion penetration causing calcium and magnesium chelation, leading to hypocalcemia, hypomagnesemia, and potential hyperkalemia with subsequent cardiotoxicity
- Order appropriate diagnostic monitoring including ECG and serial calcium assessments (total and ionized)
- Initiate immediate decontamination with copious irrigation and escalate calcium therapy through multiple modalities (topical, intradermal, IV)
- Perform timely reassessment after initial interventions to evaluate treatment efficacy and recognize therapeutic failure
- Identify when initial calcium measures fail and escalate to intra-arterial calcium gluconate for severe digital exposures
- Communicate effectively with the patient regarding the serious nature of HF burns, rationale for invasive treatment options, and necessity of admission when outpatient therapy is insufficient
- Consult appropriate specialist (toxicology or burn service) for refractory cases requiring intra-arterial therapy
- Admit patient for ongoing intra-arterial calcium infusion, pain control, and cardiac monitoring when ED-based interventions fail to achieve adequate pain control and fluoride neutralization

Progressive Weakness

Opening Scenario

A 41-year-old female presents with her spouse for progressive fatigue and proximal muscle weakness over 10 weeks. PCP referral after noting new-onset hypertension and borderline hypokalemia on outpatient labs. Patient appears anxious, rubbing her thighs, noting they "feel weak."

Initial Assessment

Vitals: BP 152/96, HR 96, RR 18, T 37.2°C, SpO_2 97% RA, Fasting glucose 312, Weight 95 kg (13 kg gain over 10 weeks)

History

- HPI: 41-year-old female with 10-week history of progressive proximal muscle weakness (difficulty rising from seated position and climbing stairs), facial rounding, dorsocervical fat pad prominence, and easy bruising without trauma. She reports amenorrhea for 3 months, increased irritability, and new acne. She denies headache, visual field deficits, chest pain, or dyspnea. She was started on spironolactone 2 weeks ago by PCP for hypertension but stopped after 5 days due to dizziness.
- Past Medical History: Previously healthy; no chronic conditions
- Medications: None currently (specifically denies exogenous steroid use)
- Allergies: No known drug allergies
- Social History: Nonsmoker, rare alcohol use, marketing executive, lives with spouse and two children
- Family History: Maternal grandmother with type 2 diabetes mellitus

Physical Examination

- General: Pleasant, alert, oriented; rounded facial appearance with facial plethora; supraclavicular fullness evident
- HEENT: PERRLA, mild periorbital edema, posterior cervical fat pad (buffalo hump) present
- Cardiovascular: Regular rate and rhythm, no murmurs
- Pulmonary: Clear to auscultation bilaterally
- Abdomen: Obese, soft, non-tender, no organomegaly; purple striae (>1 cm width) noted on abdomen and flanks
- Skin: Thin, fragile skin with visible vessels on dorsal hands; multiple ecchymoses (2—5 cm) on forearms and thighs; acne on face and upper back
- Musculoskeletal: Proximal muscle weakness (4/5 strength hip flexors and shoulder abductors), distal strength 5/5
- Neuro: Sensation intact; gait normal though patient declines deep squat due to weakness
- Remainder of physical examination normal

Diagnostic Studies

- Na 142, K 2.4 (critically low), Cl 106, HCO_3 30 (elevated), BUN 20, Cr 0.8, Glucose 342
- WBC 11.5, Hgb 14.1, Hct 42.8%, Plt 260
- PT 12.0, aPTT 31, INR 1.0
- UA: Glucose 4+, Ketones trace

Reassessment

Upon review of the laboratory results, you identify severe hypokalemia (K 2.4) and significant hyperglycemia. While awaiting further studies, the patient reports increasing muscle cramps and palpitations.

- Repeat vital signs: BP 158/100, HR 108, patient appears anxious
- 12-lead ECG: Sinus tachycardia at 108 bpm, flattened T waves in precordial leads, prominent U waves in V2—V4, QTc 540 ms
- The patient asks, "Is this serious? My mother had diabetes and I'm scared this is something worse."
- Random serum cortisol: 48 mcg/dL (elevated, normal 5-20)

Patient Communication

- Acknowledge patient's anxiety regarding physical appearance changes and potential serious underlying diagnosis
- Explain likely endocrine etiology (Cushing syndrome) requiring hospital admission without causing undue alarm
- Address concerns regarding family obligations and work responsibilities during proposed admission
- Discuss need for further confirmatory testing and specialist involvement

Management

- Immediate placement on cardiac monitor for hypokalemia-related arrhythmia risk
- IV potassium chloride repletion with cardiac monitoring (goal K >3.0 before any imaging)
- Endocrinology consultation for suspected Cushing syndrome/hypercortisolism
- Additional endocrine studies: 24-hour urine free cortisol, serum ACTH level, dexamethasone suppression test (when hemodynamically stable)
- CT abdomen/pelvis with contrast (after potassium stabilized and QTc normalized) to evaluate for adrenal mass
- Insulin sliding scale for hyperglycemia management
- Admission to monitored bed for electrolyte correction and comprehensive endocrine workup

Critical Actions

- Recognize clinical constellation of Cushing syndrome (central obesity, purple striae >1 cm, dorsocervical fat pad, proximal myopathy, easy bruising, amenorrhea)
- Identify severe hypokalemia (K 2.4) as immediate life threat requiring urgent intervention and continuous cardiac monitoring
- Interpret ECG manifestations of hypokalemia (flattened T waves, prominent U waves, prolonged QT interval)
- Order appropriate endocrine diagnostic studies (random cortisol, ACTH, 24-hour urine free cortisol, dexamethasone suppression test)
- Consult endocrinology for suspected hypercortisolism prior to disposition
- Perform timely reassessment when critical lab values return, specifically monitoring for cardiac manifestations of electrolyte abnormalities
- Communicate empathetically with patient regarding concerning findings, addressing fears while maintaining appropriate urgency for metabolic derangements
- Prioritize stabilization of potassium and QT interval before sending patient to radiology for CT imaging
- Recognize necessity for admission given severe metabolic derangements (hypokalemia, hyperglycemia) and need for further diagnostic workup

- Differentiate from polycystic ovary syndrome and simple metabolic syndrome based on specific stigmata of hypercortisolism (thin skin, purple striae, proximal weakness)

Exertional Collapse

Opening Scenario

A 32-year-old male construction worker presents via private vehicle with "legs giving out" and feeling like he is dying. Ambient temperature 98°F with high humidity. Diaphoretic, flushed, clutching bilateral thighs.

Initial Assessment

Vitals: BP 88/62, HR 132, RR 20, T 103.4°F (oral), SpO_2 97% RA

- Airway: Patent, speaking in full sentences
- Breathing: Clear bilaterally, no cyanosis
- Circulation: Warm, flushed, diaphoretic; weak radial pulses; capillary refill 3-4 seconds; no JVD

History

- HPI: 32-year-old male was performing heavy roofing work in extreme heat for approximately 8 hours with limited fluid breaks. Yesterday evening he participated in an intense CrossFit workout after several months of inactivity. He reports severe aching pain in bilateral thighs that began 4 hours ago and has progressed to involve his lower back and arms. He noticed dark urine this morning with decreased urine output. Associated symptoms include nausea, vomiting, and generalized weakness. He admits to using methamphetamine 24 hours prior "to stay awake for the double shift." He took naproxen 440mg this morning for back stiffness.
- PMHx: Occasional mechanical back pain, denies known kidney disease
- PSHx: None
- Allergies: No known drug allergies
- Medications: Naproxen sodium OTC PRN for back pain
- Social: Methamphetamine use (last use 24 hours ago), tobacco 1 pack per day for 12 years, denies alcohol use. Employed as commercial roofer.
- FHx: Father with end-stage renal disease (dialysis dependent), mother with hypertension

Physical Examination

- General: Alert and oriented ×3, diaphoretic, uncomfortable, moderate distress
- Extremities: Diffuse tenderness to palpation of bilateral thighs and calves, compartments soft and compressible, full range of motion present, 2+ pitting edema to knees bilaterally, diminished but palpable dorsalis pedis pulses
- Skin: Warm and moist, flushed, no rashes or ecchymoses
- Neurological: Cranial nerves II—XII intact, strength 5/5 upper extremities, 4/5 lower extremities secondary to pain, sensation intact to light touch, gait not tested due to pain
- Remainder of physical examination normal

Diagnostic Studies

- WBC 11.8, Hgb 16.2, Hct 48%, Plt 165
- Na 134, K 5.3 (elevated), Cl 101, HCO_3 17 (low), BUN 82 (elevated), Cr 5.2 (elevated), Glucose 108
- AST 680, ALT 145, Alk Phos 110; CK 24,500 (markedly elevated)
- UA: SG 1.030, blood large (no RBCs — myoglobinuria), pigmented granular casts, dark amber
- VBG: pH 7.28, pCO2 30, HCO_3 14; Lactate 3.2
- ECG - normal intervals, no ST changes or peaked Twaves.

Reassessment

Interval Assessment (60 minutes after initial presentation):

- Patient has received 3 liters of normal saline total
- Reports pain improved from 9/10 to 5/10
- New development: Patient requests to leave against medical advice stating, "I can't lose this job, they're already short-staffed and warned me about missing days"
- Repeat Vital Signs: BP 108/74 mmHg, HR 98 bpm, T 101.2°F, RR 16, SpO_2 98%
- Physical Exam: Still warm but less diaphoretic, stronger radial pulses. Urine output 180mL over last hour (dark amber color).
- New Data: CK 28,500 (trending up), repeat creatinine 5.4 (worsening from 5.2).

Critical Actions

- Recognizes exertional rhabdomyolysis with acute kidney injury secondary to the triad of hyperthermia, dehydration, and NSAID use in the setting of stimulant use
- Prioritizes aggressive isotonic fluid resuscitation targeting urine output of 200—300 mL/hour while avoiding further nephrotoxic agents
- Initiates active cooling measures for hyperthermia rather than antipyretics, addressing heat stroke/ exhaustion component
- Obtains ECG to evaluate for life-threatening dysrhythmias from hyperkalemia or QT prolongation secondary to methamphetamine use
- Performs timely reassessment after initial intervention, noting hemodynamic improvement but laboratory deterioration (rising CK and creatinine)
- Engages in patient-centered communication when patient requests to leave AMA by exploring underlying concerns (employment security), explaining risks of permanent renal failure/dialysis need, and negotiating temporary observation period
- Consults nephrology early for progressive renal failure and potential need for renal replacement therapy

Postpartum Seizure

Opening Scenario

A 38-year-old female, 5 days postpartum from uncomplicated vaginal delivery, arrives via EMS in a post-ictal state after a witnessed 3-minute generalized seizure at home with tongue biting and incontinence. Field BP 190/110. Husband present, agitated.

Initial Assessment

Vitals: BP 188/112, HR 102, RR 18, T 36.4°C, SpO_2 97% RA, Glucose 98

History

- HPI: 38-year-old G1P1, delivered healthy infant 5 days ago via uncomplicated SVD, discharged postpartum day 2. Developed severe frontal headache and "dark spots" in vision yesterday evening. Epigastric pain and nausea this morning. Collapsed at kitchen counter with generalized tonic-clonic seizure lasting 2-3 minutes. Remained confused since. Husband reports she stopped labetalol 2 weeks before delivery because she "felt fine" and has not restarted any antihypertensives.
- PMHx: Chronic hypertension (diagnosed 2 years ago), generalized anxiety disorder
- Medications: Prenatal vitamins only (noncompliant with antihypertensives)
- Allergies: NKDA
- Social: Lives with husband and newborn. Former smoker (quit during pregnancy). Currently breastfeeding.
- Family: Mother with preeclampsia

Physical Examination

- General: Post-ictal, confused, drowsy but arousable to voice, oriented only to self and place
- Neurological: Confused, follows commands intermittently. Pupils 4 mm, equal, reactive. No focal motor deficits appreciated. Deep tendon reflexes 3+ bilaterally with sustained clonus at ankles.
- Cardiovascular: Tachycardic, regular rhythm. No murmurs, rubs, or gallops.
- Respiratory: Clear to auscultation bilaterally. No respiratory distress, accessory muscle use, or cyanosis.
- Abdomen: Soft, non-tender, non-distended. Uterine fundus at umbilicus, appropriate for postpartum day 5. No guarding or rebound.
- Skin: Warm, dry. No rashes or petechiae. 2+ pitting edema bilateral lower extremities to knees.
- Remainder of physical examination: Normal

Diagnostic Studies

- CBC: WBC 11.2, Hgb 11.8, Hct 35.2%, Plt 198
- BMP: Na 140, K 3.8, Cl 102, HCO_3 24, BUN 18, Cr 1.3 (elevated), Glucose 104
- LFT:AST 68 (elevated), ALT 42, Alk Phos 145, T Bili 1.3, LDH 320 (elevated)
- UA: Protein 2+, otherwise negative
- Lactate 3.2 (elevated), Uric acid 7.8 (elevated), Magnesium 1.8

Managment

- Two large-bore IVs placed in antecubital fossa
- Magnesium sulfate 4 g IV bolus over 15 minutes, followed by continuous infusion at 2 g/hour
- Labetalol 20 mg IV bolus administered

- Cardiac monitor, pulse oximetry, and continuous fetal monitoring (if applicable) discontinued given postpartum status
- Foley catheter placed for strict urine output monitoring
- Emergency Obstetrics consultation requested

Reassessment at 30 Minutes:

The patient becomes more alert and oriented ×3. However, she begins rubbing her temples and states, "The spots are back and my head is pounding."

Updated Vital Signs: SBP:172/98 mmHg (improved but severely elevated; HR: 96 beats/min; RR: 14 breaths/min; SpO_2 97% RA

Nurse Update

The nurse reports the patient is complaining of worsening headache and photophobia. Suddenly, the patient develops rhythmic eye deviation to the right and begins generalized tonic-clonic activity lasting approximately 90 seconds.

Managing Conflict Event

During the second seizure, the husband enters the resuscitation bay despite staff attempts to stop him, shouting: "This is because you gave her that magnesium! She was fine until you started that drip. I read online it causes respiratory problems. Stop it immediately---we're leaving against medical advice. Our baby needs her mother at home."

Patient Communication

The physician must de-escalate the situation, acknowledge the husband's anxiety, explain the pathophysiology of eclampsia versus medication side effects, discuss the life-threatening risks of recurrent seizures (intracranial hemorrhage, aspiration, status epilepticus), and negotiate a care plan that addresses his concerns while ensuring the patient receives definitive therapy.

Final Reassessment (60 Minutes Post-Arrival):

Following the second magnesium bolus and antihypertensive therapy, the patient remains seizure-free for 30 minutes. Blood pressure stabilizes at 158/92 mmHg. Patient is now alert and oriented, though amnestic to the events. She endorses continued headache but denies visual changes. Urine output is 40 mL/hour via Foley. Brisk reflexes.

Critical Actions

- Recognize eclampsia in the postpartum period (can occur up to 10 days post-delivery, occasionally later) in a patient with risk factors including chronic hypertension and medication noncompliance
- Immediate seizure management: Prioritize airway protection, administer magnesium sulfate 4—6 g IV loading dose followed by 1—2 g/hour continuous infusion, and utilize benzodiazepines (lorazepam or diazepam) for breakthrough seizures

- Blood pressure control: Administer antihypertensive therapy (labetalol, hydralazine, or nifedipine) with target systolic <160 mmHg and diastolic <110 mmHg; strictly avoid ACE inhibitors in breastfeeding patients
- Reassessment: Recognize warning signs of recurrent seizure (worsening headache, visual changes, hyperreflexia, rising blood pressure) and respond with additional magnesium bolus and airway preparation
- Patient Communication: Address family concerns regarding treatment necessity, explain the difference between post-ictal somnolence and magnesium toxicity, discuss breastfeeding safety with magnesium therapy, and provide frequent updates on clinical status
- Managing Conflict: De-escalate family anxiety using empathy and clear explanations; clarify that seizures are caused by eclampsia, not the treatment; explain the legal and ethical implications of leaving AMA in an actively seizing patient; offer to involve chaplaincy or social work support
- Disposition: Admit to ICU or high-obstetric surveillance unit for continued magnesium therapy (typically 24 hours after the last seizure), strict blood pressure management, and seizure monitoring; obtain CT head to rule out intracranial hemorrhage given severe range hypertension
- Safety monitoring: Monitor for magnesium toxicity (loss of deep tendon reflexes, respiratory depression <12 breaths/min, bradycardia); maintain urine output >25—30 mL/hour; keep calcium gluconate 1 g IV immediately available as antidote for magnesium toxicity

Multiple Trauma Patients

Opening Scenario

You are the trauma team leader in a Level II trauma center at 14:30 on a weekday. The trauma surgeon is scrubbed in an elective case for the next hour. You have one emergency medicine resident, one trauma nurse, and one ED technician available. Three ambulances arrive simultaneously: one with a construction site amputation injury with active hemorrhage, and two separate low-speed motor vehicle collisions from the same parking lot incident. You must prioritize evaluations, allocate limited personnel, and anticipate deteriorations while managing competing patient and family demands.

Patient A: Critical Hemorrhage

History of Present Illness 34-year-old male construction worker with left arm caught in industrial table saw. Witnessed arterial bleeding with prehospital tourniquet placed 45 minutes ago. Patient reports numbness in hand and inability to move fingers.

Vital Signs BP 88/56, HR 132, RR 24, T 35.8°C (96.4°F), SpO_2 95% on RA

Patient A Physical Examination

12cm gaping laceration proximal forearm with exposed muscle, tendon, and pulsatile arterial bleeding around tourniquet margin. Radial and ulnar pulses absent distal to injury. Median nerve distribution anesthesia and inability to flex thumb/index finger. Capillary refill >4 seconds in fingertips. Remainder of examination normal.

Patient A Diagnostic Studies

- CBC/Coags: Hgb 8.4 , Hct 25 , INR 1.1
- Type & Crossmatch: O negative, antibody screen negative
- BMP: K 5.4 , Lactate 4.8
- X-ray (Forearm): Comminuted fracture of proximal radius with bony fragments

Patient B: Low-Speed MVC with Anticoagulation

History of Present Illness 79-year-old female driver backed into concrete barrier at approximately 5 mph in grocery store parking lot. Airbag did not deploy. Developed midsternal chest pain 10 minutes post-impact while still in vehicle.

Vital Signs BP 148/82, HR 96, RR 18, T 36.6°C (97.9°F), SpO_2 97% on RA

Patient B Physical Examination

Sternal tenderness to palpation without step-off or crepitus. Horizontal seat belt sign across anterior chest at level of sternum. Remainder of examination normal.

Diagnostic Studies

- CBC: Hgb 11.2
- Coags/Renal: INR 3.4, Cr 1.3
- Cardiac: Troponin I 0.02 (normal)
- ECG: Normal sinus rhythm, rate 96, no ST changes
- CXR: Sternal fracture, mediastinum unremarkable
- CT chest/abd/pelvis with IV contrast. 4cmx2cm peri-sternal hematoma with no evidence of extravasation

Patient C: Low-Speed Rear Impact with Pregnancy

History of Present Illness 27-year-old female, 28 weeks gestation, rear-ended at stop sign by vehicle traveling 10 mph. Immediate neck pain and lower abdominal tightening. Felt fetal movement initially but decreased over 15 minutes.

Vital Signs BP 108/68, HR 102, RR 20, T 36.9°C (98.4°F), SpO_2 98% on RA

Patient C Physical Examination

Horizontal seat belt sign across lower abdomen suprapubic region. Uterine tenderness on palpation, fundal height 28cm. Fetal heart rate 140 bpm (initial auscultation). Remainder of examination normal.

Patient C Diagnostic Studies

- CBC: Hgb 10.8
- Coags: Fibrinogen 380 (normal)
- Type & Screen: A positive, antibody negative
- CT Abdomen/Pelvis: Declined by patient due to pregnancy concerns
- Ultrasound: Intrauterine pregnancy with FHR 155, no obvious free fluid seen

Initial Prioritization and Resource Allocation

Immediate activation of massive transfusion protocol for Patient A with blood bank notification. Assignment of available trauma nurse to Patient A for continuous monitoring and tourniquet time documentation. Delegation of Patient B and Patient C evaluations to emergency medicine resident with explicit instructions for immediate notification of any vital sign changes. Direct communication with trauma surgeon regarding Patient A requiring emergent operative intervention. Placement of Patient B on continuous cardiac monitoring given mechanism and anticoagulation status. Initiation of fetal monitoring for Patient C with OB consultation requested.

Clinical Decision-Making: The Tourniquet Dilemma

Recognition that tourniquet time approaching 60 minutes mandates a decision on definitive managment. Decision to forego CT angiography in Patient A given hemodynamic instability and obvious vascular injury requiring operative exploration regardless of imaging. Balancing need for immediate limb-salvage attempt against potential systemic effects of prolonged ischemia and reperfusion injury. Determination that Patient B requires admission for observation despite low mechanism due to age, anticoagulation, and sternal fracture with anticoagulation. Decision to proceed with limited CT imaging of abdomen/pelvis with fetal shielding for Patient C given concerning physical examination findings despite patient hesitation.

Patient Communication

Patient A: Capacity and Consent Patient becomes increasingly agitated and hypotensive, questioning tourniquet tightness and demanding removal to "save the arm." Discussion of risks: irreversible muscle necrosis if tourniquet removed without surgical control, potential need for primary amputation versus revascularization attempt with unknown functional outcome. Recognition of diminishing decisional capacity due to hypoperfusion and hypothermia. Attempt to obtain informed consent for possible amputation versus limb-salvage surgery while explaining time-critical nature of decision.

Patient C: Pregnancy Counseling Patient refuses CT imaging citing internet-based concerns about fetal radiation exposure. Shared decision-making discussion regarding fetal radiation exposure versus undetected intraabdominal trauma. Negotiation to proceed with serial ultrasounds with continuous monitoring and obstetrics reexamination.

Patient B: Anticoagulation Reversal Discussion with patient regarding reversal of warfarin given sternal fracture and risk of delayed mediastinal hematoma expansion. Patient initially refusing reversal agents citing recent mechanical valve replacement.

Managing Conflict: Resource Competition

Family Confrontation Family members of Patient B arrive and demand immediate physician attention, questioning why "a broken arm" (Patient A) takes priority over their elderly mother's chest pain. De-escalation technique utilizing privacy area for family discussion regarding hemodynamic instability and immediate surgical needs of Patient A. Setting clear expectations regarding evaluation timeline for Patient B while ensuring continuous cardiac monitoring is visible to family.

Consultant Disagreement Orthopedic surgery consulting on Patient A recommends immediate transfer to tertiary center for limb replantation versus salvage, estimating 3-hour transfer time. Trauma surgery recommending immediate operative exploration given tourniquet time constraints and hemodynamic instability. Conflict resolution regarding appropriateness of transfer versus local damage control surgery with possible completion amputation.

OB-ED Interface Obstetrics resident suggesting immediate delivery for Patient C based on seat belt sign and uterine tenderness despite reassuring initial fetal heart rate. Disagreement regarding necessity of emergent C-section versus expectant management with tocolysis. Negotiation for trial of monitoring with clear triggers for operative intervention.

Reassessment: Clinical Deterioration

Patient A BP 72/44 despite 2 units PRBCs. Tourniquet time 90 minutes. Patient increasingly confused and combative (reperfusion syndrome developing). New finding: dark, tea-colored urine output via catheter suggesting rhabdomyolysis and acute kidney injury.

Patient B BP 126/50, HR 140 irregularly irregular (new atrial fibrillation with RVR). ECG: remains unchanged from initial presentation.

Patient C BP 92/58. FHR 90 bpm (bradycardia). Vaginal examination: Patient starting to have >150mL bright red blood per vagina increasing concern revealed placental abruption. Patient now reporting severe continuous abdominal pain with contractions.

Final Dispositions

Patient A: Emergent operative exploration.

Patient B: Surgery agrees to inpatient observation and repeat imaging to asses expansion of hematoma.

Patient C: Discussion with OB for patient to go immediately to the OR given development of fetal bradycardia and concern for abruption; neonatology team present; massive transfusion protocol activated for mother.

Critical Actions

Recognized hemodynamic instability in Patient A as immediate priority requiring massive transfusion and surgical intervention over diagnostic imaging.

Demonstrate understanding of tourniquet time limitations and the pathophysiology of reperfusion injury with crush syndrome.

Identified Patient B as high-risk trauma despite low mechanism due to advanced age, anticoagulation, and anatomical location of injury (sternum).

Recognized placental abruption in Patient C based on reassessment findings of vaginal bleeding, uterine tetany, and fetal bradycardia despite initially reassuring vital signs.

Managed conflict between surgical specialties regarding Patient A's disposition while maintaining patient safety and timeline awareness.

Navigated patient-centered communication challenges including informed consent with diminishing capacity, refusal of imaging in pregnancy, and family demands during concurrent critical events.

Prioritized limited resources effectively by delegating stable evaluations while maintaining personal oversight of unstable patients.

Demonstrated appropriate reassessment frequency leading to recognition of delayed manifestations of injury: cardiac tamponade in Patient B and abruption in Patient C.

Balanced maternal and fetal interests in Patient C while recognizing that maternal stability ultimately determines fetal outcomes. Applied clinical decision-making regarding anticoagulation reversal in the setting of traumatic injury with competing thrombotic and hemorrhagic risks.

Multiple Medical Emergencies

Opening Scenario

You are the sole attending physician in a community emergency department. Three ambulances arrive simultaneously with critically ill patients. You must evaluate, prioritize, and manage all three patients concurrently while anticipating deterioration, communicating with families, and navigating limited ICU bed availability.

Patient A: Cardiac Concern

History of Present Illness 68-year-old male with crushing substernal chest pain radiating to jaw and left arm, onset 45 minutes ago. Associated diaphoresis and nausea. History of hypertension and hyperlipidemia.

Vital Signs BP 88/52, HR 110, RR 22, T 36.8°C (98.2°F), SpO_2 94% on RA

Physical Examination Cool, clammy skin. Bilateral crackles at lung bases. Remainder of examination normal.

Patient A Diagnostic Studies

- Cardiac Markers: Troponin I 2.8 (elevated), BNP 650 (elevated
- Renal/Lytes: Cr 1.4 (elevated), K 4.8
- CBC: Hgb 13.2
- ECG: ST depressions, T-wave inversions

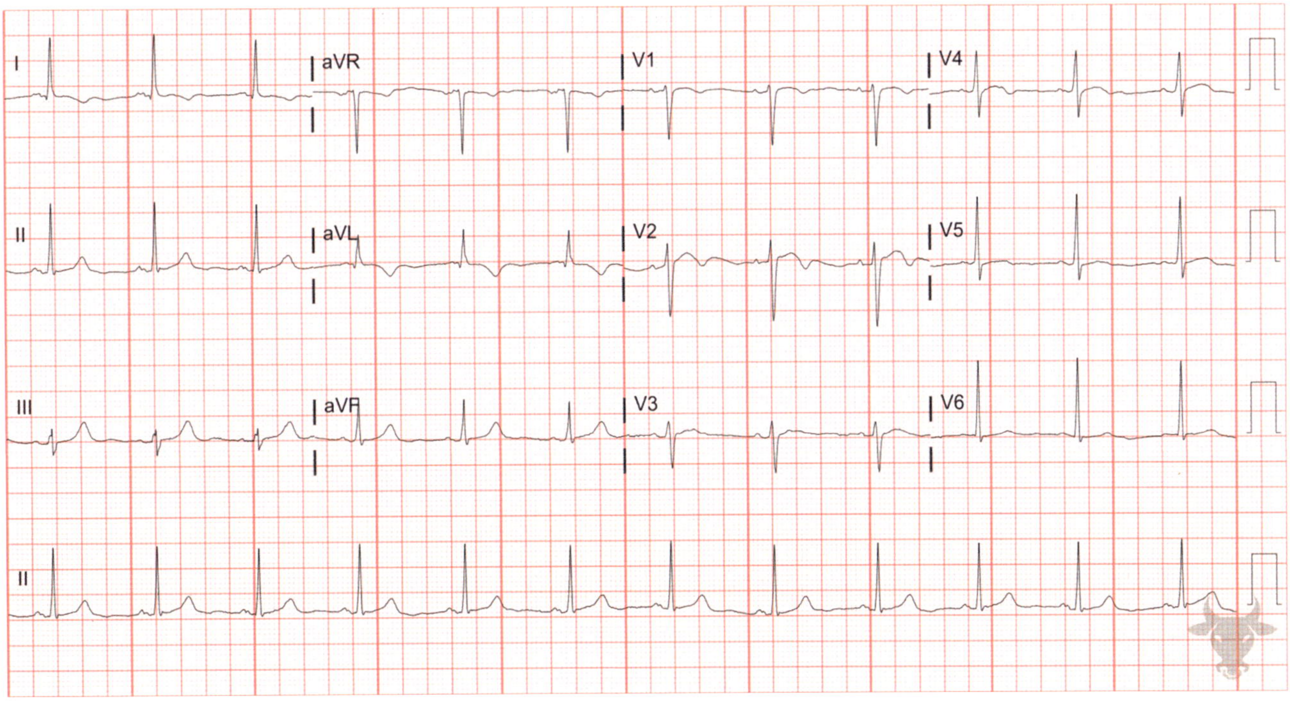

Patient B: Septic Shock

History of Present Illness 54-year-old female with fever, confusion, and flank pain. History of diabetes mellitus and recurrent urinary tract infections. Found by family confused at home.

Vital Signs BP 76/40, HR 128, RR 28, T 39.2°C (102.6°F), SpO_2 91% on RA

Physical Examination Altered mental status (GCS 13). Right costovertebral angle tenderness. Remainder of examination normal.

Patient B Diagnostic Studies

- CBC: WBC 18.5
- BMP: Cr 2.8 , Glucose 342
- Lactate: 6.2
- UA: Positive nitrites, >100 WBC/hpf, many bacteria

Patient C: Gastrointestinal Hemorrhage

History of Present Illness: 72-year-old male with hematemesis (approximately 500mL coffee-ground emesis). History of cirrhosis and prior variceal bleeding. Witnessed by spouse at home.

Vital Signs: BP 92/58, HR 118, RR 20, T 36.4°C (97.5°F), SpO_2 96% on RA

Physical Examination Patient C

Jaundiced sclerae. Mild hepatic encephalopathy (asterixis present). Remainder of examination normal.

Diagnostic Studies Patient C

- CBC: Hgb 7.8 , Plt 85
- Coags/Liver: INR 2.4 , T Bili 4.2 , Albumin 2.4
- Ammonia: 68 µmol/L
- Type & Screen: Type O+, antibodies negative

Initial Prioritization and Interventions

Identify Patient B (septic shock) as highest priority due to profound hypotension and altered mental status requiring immediate source control. Initiate simultaneous resuscitation for all three patients with appropriate nursing assignments. Assign physician assistant to Patient A (cardiac monitoring, IV access, aspirin administration). Personally attend to Patient B (central line placement, blood cultures, aggressive fluid resuscitation). Activate massive transfusion protocol for Patient C and initiate octreotide infusion.

Clinical Course: First Reassessment

Patient A BP 82/48 (worsening), HR 115. Now with worsening dyspnea and new jugular venous distension.

Patient B BP 78/44 (no improvement after 2L crystalloid). Urine output 5mL in 30 minutes. Remains febrile and confused.

Patient C BP 88/56 (stable). Second emesis: 200mL fresh red blood. Now agitated and combative.

Patient Communication

Family Discussion for Patient C Wife expresses desire for "everything done" but patient previously stated he would not want prolonged intubation or heroic measures. Discuss goals of care considering high-risk variceal bleeding and hepatic decompensation. Explore code status and potential need for emergent intubation for airway protection. Address alcohol use history sensitively while obtaining additional history from spouse.

Patient B Communication Patient now briefly alert after initial fluid resuscitation. Discuss need for ICU admission, central line placement, and possible vasopressors. Address concerns about diabetes management during critical illness and need for insulin protocol.

Clinical Decision-Making: Tertiary Triage

Decision to intubate Patient C for airway protection prior to endoscopy given ongoing hematemesis and altered mental status. Decision to start vasopressors on Patient B (norepinephrine) given persistent hypotension despite adequate fluid resuscitation. Decision to activate cardiac catheterization lab for Patient A despite hypotension (non-STEMI with cardiogenic shock requiring invasive hemodynamic support). Coordinate timing of interventions to allow for adequate staffing.

Reassessments

Patient A BP 74/40, HR 45 (new bradycardia responsive to 1mg atropine). Mentation remains normal

Patient B BP 82/54 on norepinephrine at 15 mcg/min. Developing diffuse macular rash (possible antibiotic reaction). Lactate 5.8 (minimal improvement).

Patient C Post-intubation, sedated. Hemoglobin 6.4 (further drop from 7.8). BP 76/42 despite blood product administration

Managing Conflict and Resource Allocation

ICU Bed Allocation Crisis Only one ICU bed available; two patients require ICU-level care immediately. ICU attending suggests Patient A needs immediate catheterization lab rather than ICU admission first. Medical floor refuses admission of Patient B due to vasopressor requirement. Gastroenterology available for urgent endoscopy on Patient C but concerned about blood pressure.

Resolution Approach Negotiate with cardiology to accept Patient A directly to cath lab, bypassing ICU temporarily. Advocate with hospitalist for step-down unit with continuous monitoring for Patient B until ICU bed available. Request emergent transfer of Patient C to tertiary center with interventional gastroenterology capabilities if local resources insufficient.

Final Dispositions and Critical Actions

Patient A: Emergent cardiac catheterization] for cardiogenic shock, subsequent cardiac ICU admission.

Patient B: Continued resuscitation, antibiotic change to ceftriaxone if penicillin allergy suspected, ICU admission for septic shock management.

Patient C: Emergent upper endoscopy with variceal banding, massive transfusion completion, transfer to tertiary center for continued care.

Critical Actions

Recognized need for immediate triage of three simultaneous critical patients with appropriate assignment of clinical resources. Correctly identified septic shock (Patient B) as highest mortality risk requiring immediate source control, blood cultures prior to antibiotics, and early vasopressor initiation. Demonstrated appropriate reassessment frequency with recognition of clinical deterioration in all three patients (cardiogenic shock progression, allergic reaction, continued hemorrhage). Managed conflict regarding limited ICU resources while advocating for patient-centered outcomes and appropriate level of care. Utilized patient-centered communication techniques including shared decision-making when discussing goals of care with Patient C's family. Prioritized interventions based on acuity: airway protection for Patient C, vasopressors for Patient B, invasive hemodynamic support for Patient A. Recognized changing clinical scenarios (bradycardia in Patient A suggesting conduction system involvement, allergic reaction in Patient B requiring antibiotic adjustment, continued bleeding in Patient C requiring transfer). Coordinated multidisciplinary care including cardiology, gastroenterology, critical care, nursing, and transfer services while maintaining situational awareness of all three patients simultaneously.

Multiple Patients and Boarding Issues

Opening Scenario

You are the sole attending physician in a 30-bed community emergency department at 02:00. The department is at capacity with 15 boarding patients awaiting inpatient beds. You have one emergency medicine resident and two nurses available. The trauma bay is occupied by an overdose patient who cannot yet be cleared or moved. EMS arrives with a 24-year-old male status post high-speed motorcycle collision. Simultaneously, charge nurse reports that your two sickest boarding patients are deteriorating: a six-year-old with presumed appendicitis who has been awaiting surgical admission for six hours, and a 68-year-old with COPD exacerbation who has been boarding for four hours. The CT scanner has one slot available in the next hour. You must stabilize the trauma patient while preventing harm to your deteriorating boarders and navigate limited resources.

Patient A: New Trauma

History of Present Illness:

- 24-year-old male unrestrained motorcyclist collided with vehicle at approximately 50 mph, thrown approximately 20 feet. Complains of severe chest pain and abdominal pain. Denies loss of consciousness per witnesses

Vital Signs: BP: 92/58 mmHg; HR: 132 beats/min; RR: 28 breaths/min; Temp: 35.8°C (96.4°F); SpO_2: 94% RA

Patient A Physical Examination

Paradoxical chest wall movement right lower ribs; Distended neck veins; Absent breath sounds right hemithorax with tracheal deviation to the lef; Abdominal guarding with distension and seat belt sign across upper abdomen; Pelvic instability on compression; Remainder of examination normal

Patient A: Diagnostic Studies

- Hbg: 9.2; Base Deficit -8; Lactate 5.4; INR 1.1;
- FAST US: Positive right upper quadrant (free fluid), positive pericardial (effusion) Negative
- Pelvis X-ray Open book pelvic fracture with 8cm pubic symphysis diastasis

Patient B: Pediatric Boarder

History of Present Illness Six-year-old female with 36-hour history of right lower quadrant pain initially diagnosed with appendicitis six hours ago. Awaiting surgical bed assignment and operating room availability. Parents report worsening pain and new fever since arrival.

Vital Signs (Current vs Previous) BP 88/52 (previously 105/68); HR 142 (previously 118); RR 26, T 39.2°C (previously 37.8°C); SpO_2 97% on RA

Patient B Physical Examination

Rigid abdomen with rebound and guarding in right lower quadrant. Pain now generalized with positive psoas sign. Capillary refill 3.5 seconds. Remainder of examination normal.

Patient B Diagnostic Studies

- CBC: WBC 22, Bands 18%
- BMP: K 3.2 low, Lactate 3.8
- Ultrasound (Previous): Non-compressible appendix 11mm, periappendiceal fluid
- Repeat Ultrasound: New fluid collection suggesting perforation

Patient C: Adult Boarder

History of Present Illness 68-year-old male with known severe COPD (FEV1 40% predicted) admitted four hours ago for exacerbation. Awaiting medical floor bed. Now requesting to leave against medical advice due to length of wait.

Vital Signs (Current vs Previous) BP 158/92 (previously 138/82), HR 118 (previously 96), RR 32 (previously 22), T 37.4°C (99.3°F), SpO_2 86% on 2L NC (previously 94% on same)

Patient C Physical Examination

Tripod positioning with accessory muscle use. Paradoxical breathing pattern. Prolonged expiratory phase with diffuse wheezing. Altered mental status with somnolence. Remainder of examination normal.

Diagnostic Studies

- ABG: pH 7.26, pCO_2 78, pO_2 52 HCO_3 32
- CBC: WBC 11
- CXR: Hyperinflation without infiltrate

Initial Prioritization and Resource Allocation

- Immediate recognition of tension pneumothorax in Patient A requiring decompression followed by chest tube prior to full trauma survey completion
- Assignment of one nurse to Patient A for massive transfusion protocol activation and blood product preparation
- Directing second nurse to page respiratory therapy to place Patient C on BiPAP given hypercapnic respiratory failure
- Requesting charge nurse to page surgery urgently for Patient B regarding deterioration suggesting perforation

Clinical Decision-Making: Parallel Resuscitation

- Decision to perform immediate tube thoracostomy for Patient A prior to CT imaging given hemodynamic instability and positive FAST
- Recognition that Patient B now meets criteria for sepsis with source control emergency requiring operative intervention within one hour
- Determination that Patient C requires immediate ICU-level care for COPD exacerbation with acute-on-chronic hypercapnic respiratory failure, not medical floor admission
- Triage of CT scanner: Patient A requires CT trauma series but must be stabilized first; decision to defer CT for Patient B given clear surgical abdomen; Patient C does not require CT

Patient Communication

Patient A: Capacity and Family Notification

- Patient becomes obtunded during chest tube insertion due to hypotension and hypothermia
- Attempt to obtain informed consent for blood products and possible exploratory laparotomy while patient still has marginal capacity
- Phone discussion with parents regarding critical condition, need for emergent surgery, and uncertainty regarding outcomes

Patient B: Parental Anger and Expectation Management

- Parents confront you in trauma bay demanding immediate surgery for daughter, expressing frustration that "she has been ignored for six hours"

- De-escalation technique acknowledging their concerns while explaining new findings suggest perforation requiring more urgent intervention than originally anticipated
- Discussion regarding risks of perforation including peritonitis and sepsis
- Negotiation to allow parents to accompany child to operating room threshold while maintaining sterile field

Patient C: Against Medical Advice Discussion

- Patient removing BiPAP mask stating he will leave because "you clearly don't have room for me"
- Discussion of acute respiratory failure and risk of intubation if departs
- Exploration of barriers to admission including specific request for single room due to claustrophobia
- Shared decision-making regarding trial of high-flow nasal cannula as compromise to avoid intubation while awaiting bed

Managing Conflict: Resource Competition

Operating Room Allocation

- Trauma surgeon demanding immediate OR for Patient A for exploratory laparotomy and external pelvic fixation
- Pediatric surgeon simultaneously requesting OR for Patient B for appendectomy
- Conflict resolution regarding parallel trauma laparotomy versus pediatric case; decision to transfer Patient B to neighboring pediatric hospital for surgery while stabilizing Patient A.

ICU Bed Dispute

- ICU charge nurse refusing admission of Patient C stating "if patient was wheened from BiPAP they could go to the floor". Explain calmly that the hypercapnia warrants continued BiPAP that exceeds floor abilities.

Reassessment

Patient A

- Chest tube placed with 800mL immediate blood return and air leak
- Blood pressure: 78/42 mmHg despite 2 units O negative blood
- Pelvic binder applied with transient improvement then renewed instability
- FAST now positive in left upper quadrant (new bleeding)
- Decision for emergent exploratory laparotomy without CT imaging

Patient B

- Now hypotensive to 76/40 mmHg with altered mental status
- Parents consenting to transfer to pediatric facility for emergent surgery
- Paramedic crew expressing concern regarding transporting unstable septic child
- Decision to intubate for airway protection prior to transfer given altered mental status and risk of aspiration

Patient C

- Initially improved on BiPAP with pCO_2 dropping to 58 mmHg
- Sudden somnolence with BiPAP non-compliance
- Repeat blood gas: pH 7.18, pCO_2 78 mmHg
- Decision for emergent intubation and mechanical ventilation

Initial Actions

- Patient A: Emergent exploratory laparotomy revealing splenic laceration and mesenteric hematoma; damage control surgery with temporary abdominal closure; ICU admission
- Patient B: Intubated for airway protection; emergent transfer to pediatric facility with critical care paramedic crew; successful appendectomy with peritoneal washout
- Patient C: Intubated using rapid sequence intubation with ketamine and rocuronium; admitted to medical ICU for ventilator management and weaning

Critical Actions

- Recognized immediate life-threat in Patient A (tension pneumothorax) requiring intervention before complete primary survey
- Demonstrated appropriate delegation to resident while maintaining oversight of deteriorating boarders
- Identified sepsis progression in Patient B (previously stable boarder) requiring escalation from urgent to emergent surgical intervention
- Recognized acute-on-chronic hypercapnic respiratory failure with altered mental status in Patient C requiring ICU-level care rather than medical floor admission
- Managed conflict between surgical services regarding operating room allocation while prioritizing based on immediate survival needs (hemorrhage control versus source control)
- Navigated patient-centered communication challenges including informed consent with diminishing capacity, angry family members, and patients threatening to leave against medical advice
- Balanced resource limitations by triaging imaging studies and making disposition decisions based on clinical deterioration rather than original admission plan
- Demonstrated reassessment of "stable" boarding patients leading to recognition of clinical decompensation requiring immediate intervention
- Applied clinical decision-making regarding transfer versus local management for pediatric patient weighing risks of transport against risks of surgical delay
- Coordinated multidisciplinary care involving trauma surgery, pediatric surgery, critical care, anesthesia, nursing, and transport teams while managing three concurrent critical events with limited staff

Multiple Triages and Limited Beds

Opening Scenario

You are the attending physician assigned to triage in a busy urban emergency department on a Monday evening. The department has three distinct patient care areas:

- Fast Track: Low acuity (ESI 4-5)
- General Purpose Pod: Medium to high acuity (ESI 2-3)
- Critical Care Pod: Life-threatening conditions (ESI 1)

Your role is to evaluate incoming patients, order initial diagnostic studies, assign them to the appropriate care area, and provide brief handoffs for critically ill patients. You will not follow patients once they are placed in a pod. However, patients who remain in the waiting room will require reassessment when results return. Five new patients have just arrived simultaneously.

Patient 1: Janice. Washington- Chest Pain in the Waiting Room

Chief Complaint: Chest pain

Vital Signs: BP 145/92, HR 118, RR 22, SpO_2 96% RA, Temp 98.6°F, Pain 8/10

Brief History: 58-year-old male with hypertension and diabetes presents with 2 hours of substernal chest pressure radiating to left arm. Associated diaphoresis and shortness of breath. No prior cardiac history.

Physical Exam:

- Diaphoretic, moderate distress
- Remainder of exam normal

Initial Orders:

- ECG (STAT)
- Troponin I
- CBC, BMP, magnesium
- Chest X-ray
- Aspirin 325 mg chewable
- Nitroglycerin 0.4 mg SL q5min x3 if SBP > 90

Location Decision: Critical Care Pod

Handoff to Critical Care Pod Physician: "58-year-old male with 2 hours of substernal chest pressure, diaphoretic, hypertensive, diabetic. ECG pending. I've given aspirin and ordered troponin, labs, and chest X-ray. Pain is 8/10. May need nitro. Over to you."

Patient 2: Maria Hernandez- Abdominal Pain

Chief Complaint: Right lower quadrant pain

Vital Signs: BP 128/76, HR 92, RR 18, SpO_2 99% RA, Temp 100.8°F, Pain 6/10

Brief History: 24-year-old female with 12 hours of progressive RLQ pain, nausea, no vomiting. Last menstrual period 3 weeks ago. Denies vaginal bleeding or discharge.

Physical Exam:

- Tender RLQ with guarding, no rebound
- Remainder of exam normal

Initial Orders:

- Urine hCG
- CBC with differential

- BMP
- Transvaginal pelvic ultrasound

Location Decision: General Purpose Pod

Patient 3: Ronald White - Work-Related Laceration

Chief Complaint: Finger laceration

Vital Signs: BP 122/68, HR 74, RR 14, SpO_2 100% RA, Temp 98.2°F, Pain 3/10

Brief History: 35-year-old construction worker with 2 cm clean laceration to left index finger from utility knife. Bleeding controlled with direct pressure. No neurovascular compromise. Tetanus up to date.

Physical Exam:

- 2 cm linear laceration, superficial, distal phalanx
- Cap refill <2 sec, sensation intact
- Remainder of exam normal

Initial Orders:

- Wound care supplies
- No imaging or labs required

Location Decision: Fast Track

Patient 4: Alice Rodriguez - Elderly Fall with Head Injury

Chief Complaint: Head injury after fall

Vital Signs: BP 158/88, HR 88, RR 16, SpO_2 95% RA, Temp 97.8°F, Pain 4/10

Brief Complaint: 78-year-old female on warfarin for atrial fibrillation. Tripped on rug, struck forehead on table. No loss of consciousness. GCS 15. Minor frontal headache. Family reports she seems "a little off."

Physical Exam:

- 3 cm frontal hematoma
- Minor confusion with orientation to person and place only
- Remainder of exam normal

Initial Orders:

- Head CT non-contrast (STAT)
- INR/PTT
- CBC, BMP
- Type and screen

Location Decision: Patient remains in waiting room for initial CT results

Patient 5: Terrance O'Malley - Demanding Patient with Chronic Pain

Chief Complaint: Back pain

Vital Signs: BP 145/95, HR 102, RR 20, SpO_2 98% RA, Temp 99.1°F, Pain 10/10

Brief History: 42-year-old male with history of chronic low back pain, multiple prior ED visits. States he "needs Dilaudid" and is "allergic to everything else." Previous records show multiple negative workups. Today reports acute exacerbation after lifting boxes.

Physical Exam:

- Diffusely tender lumbar spine, no focal deficits
- Remainder of exam normal

Initial Orders:

- Urine drug screen
- Lumbar X-ray
- No opioids at triage

Location Decision: General Purpose Pod

Patient Communication & Managing Conflict:

- Acknowledge pain and frustration
- Set clear boundaries: "I understand you're in significant pain. I'm going to evaluate you appropriately, but I cannot provide opioids at triage. We'll get you seen and develop a safe treatment plan."
- Offer alternatives: NSAIDs, muscle relaxants
- Explain need for objective evaluation

Reassessment: Patient 4 (Alice Rodriguez)

Time Elapsed: 45 minutes

New Data: Head CT results available - 5mm right front subdural

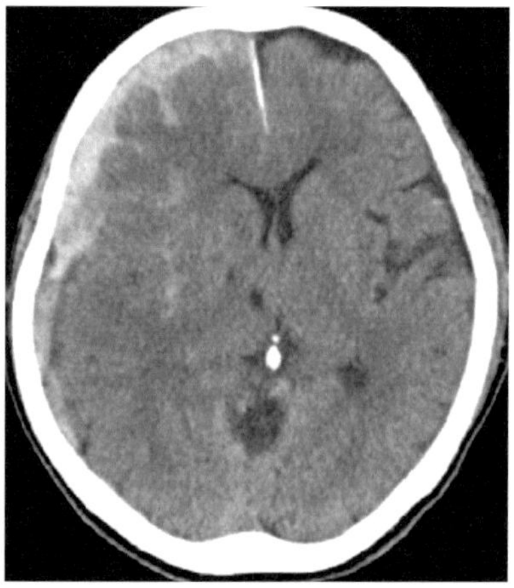

Repeat Vital Signs: BP 165/92, HR 95, RR 18, SpO_2 94% RA, Temp 98.0°F

Patient Status: Increased confusion, now only oriented to self. Headache worsened to 7/10. Vomited once.

Reassessment Decision: Escalate to Critical Care Pod immediately

Handoff to Critical Care Pod Physician: "78-year-old female on warfarin with subdural hematoma, INR 3.8. Initially stable but now deteriorating: worsening confusion, headache, vomiting. CT shows 5mm bleed. I've ordered reversal agents. She needs neurosurgery consult and ICU-level care now."

Critical Actions

Clinical Decision-Making:

- Recognized Patient 1 as potential ACS and ordered appropriate initial workup (ECG, troponin, aspirin)
- Identified Patient 2 as possible appendicitis with appropriate rule-out of ectopic pregnancy
- Appropriately triaged Patient 3 to Fast Track based on low acuity and stable exam
- Recognized Patient 4 as high-risk for intracranial hemorrhage due to anticoagulation and age
- Ordered appropriate initial evaluation for Patient 5 while maintaining safety boundaries

Prioritization:

- Correctly identified Patient 1 and Patient 4 as highest acuity requiring critical care resources
- Appropriately assigned Patient 2 to general pod for further workup

- Correctly assigned Patient 3 to Fast Track
- Recognized Patient 5 required evaluation but not immediate critical resources

Reassessment:

- Monitored Patient 4 in waiting room appropriately
- Recognized clinical deterioration based on new imaging and vital sign changes
- Escalated care promptly based on objective findings (subdural hematoma, elevated INR)
- Provided clear handoff with critical information for ongoing management

Patient Communication:

- Demonstrated empathy while maintaining professional boundaries with Patient 5
- Used clear, non-judgmental language with the challenging patient
- Explained rationale for decision-making without being confrontational
- Acknowledged patient's reported pain while prioritizing safe medical practice

Managing Conflict:

- Successfully de-escalated potential conflict with opioid-seeking behavior
- Set firm but respectful boundaries with Patient 5
- Offered alternative treatment options rather than simply refusing care
- Maintained therapeutic relationship despite patient's demands

Handoff Communication:

- Provided concise, structured handoffs for critical patients (Patient 1 and reassessed Patient 4)
- Included key clinical data, pending tests, and interventions performed
- Clearly communicated level of urgency and patient stability

Safety:

- Administered aspirin appropriately for potential ACS
- Recognized need for anticoagulation reversal in Patient 4
- Avoided opioid administration in ambiguous clinical scenario at triage
- Ordered pregnancy testing in fertile female with abdominal pain

Multiple Pediatric Patients

Opening Scenario

You are the attending physician in the pediatric emergency department at 19:00 during peak respiratory season. Three patients present simultaneously with moderate respiratory distress: a three-month-old with apneic episodes, a four-year-old with moderate asthma exacerbation, and an eighteen-month-old with suspected pneumonia and dehydration. Only two monitored beds remain, and the pediatric ward has one available inpatient bed. You must determine admission criteria, manage parental expectations, and monitor for deterioration while balancing limited resources.

Patient A: Infant with Bronchiolitis

History of Present Illness Three-month-old former 36-week gestation infant presenting with three days of nasal congestion and cough. Mother witnessed two apneic episodes at home lasting five seconds each with color change to pale. Decreased oral intake to 50% of baseline over past 24 hours. Two wet diapers in past 24 hours.

Vital Signs BP 85/55, HR 165, RR 58, T 38.2°C (100.8°F), SpO_2 92% on RA

Patient A Physical Examination

Moderate intercostal and subcostal retractions. Nasal flaring present. Occasional grunting with expiration. Scattered wheezes and fine crackles bilaterally. Capillary refill 3 seconds. Remainder of examination normal.

Patient A Diagnostic Studies

- Viral Panel: RSV PCR positive , Influenza A/B negative
- CBC: WBC 12.5, Hgb 10.8
- BMP: Na 138
- CXR: Hyperinflation with perihilar markings, no infiltrate

Patient B: Preschool Asthma Exacerbation

History of Present Illness Four-year-old with history of two prior hospitalizations for asthma, one requiring PICU admission. Developed wheezing and cough after playing at indoor playground six hours ago. Three albuterol treatments at home with minimal relief. Parents requesting "natural remedies only" and refusing steroids.

Vital Signs BP 95/60, HR 142, RR 36, T 37.6°C (99.7°F), SpO_2 91% on RA

Patient B Physical Examination

Moderate respiratory distress with tripod positioning. Diffuse expiratory wheezing with prolonged expiratory phase. Intercostal retractions present. Peak expiratory flow 60% predicted. Remainder of examination normal.

Patient B Diagnostic Studies

- CBC: WBC 14.200, Absolute Eosinophil Count 850 (high), Hgb 11.5
- BMP: K 3.4
- Capillary Blood Gas: pH 7.38, pCO_2 42
- CXR: Hyperinflation without infiltrate

Patient C: Toddler with Pneumonia and Dehydration

History of Present Illness Eighteen-month-old with four days of fever to 39.5°C and rhinorrhea. Refusing oral intake for 36 hours, vomiting twice. Parents report rapid breathing and lethargy. No urine output in past 12 hours.

Vital Signs BP 88/52, HR 158, RR 48, T 39.1°C (102.4°F), SpO_2 93% on RA

Patient C Physical Examination

Tachypnea with mild nasal flaring. Decreased breath sounds and crackles at right base. Dry mucous membranes. Sunken fontanelle (still open). Skin tenting noted. Capillary refill 4 seconds. Remainder of examination normal.

Diagnostic Studies

- CBC: WBC 18.8 , Bands 15% , Hgb 11.2
- BMP: Na 152 hypernatremic, BUN 28 , Cr 0.6
- CXR: Right lower lobe consolidation
- Viral Panel: Influenza B positive

Initial Clinical Decision-Making and Prioritization

Recognition that Patient A meets criteria for apnea-related admission and requires continuous cardiorespiratory monitoring given age and prematurity history. Decision to place Patient A in remaining monitored bed with pulse oximetry and apnea monitor. Assignment of Patient B to observation area with frequent reassessment given moderate distress but stable appearance. Initiation of oral rehydration trial for Patient C with rapid reassessment of hydration status. Delegation of resident to obtain detailed asthma history from Patient B parents while initiating bronchodilator therapy. Calculation of fluid deficit for Patient C using 10mL/kg for mild dehydration plus 4-1-1 rule for maintenance fluids.

Patient Communication

Patient B: Treatment Refusal Discussion Parents express strong preference for herbal remedies and honey over "chemicals" and steroids. Exploration of parental concerns regarding side effects and previous steroid experiences. Shared decision-making discussion explaining pathophysiology of airway inflammation and evidence for corticosteroids in preventing progression to respiratory failure. Negotiation to accept single dose of dexamethasone versus three-day prednisolone course. Documentation of informed refusal risks including possible intubation if asthma progresses.

Patient C: Fluid Management Preferences Parents requesting IV fluids be avoided due to fear of needles and preference for oral rehydration. Explanation of hypernatremic dehydration risks and need for controlled rehydration. Offer oral rehydration solution with strict parameters for failure requiring IV access. Discussion regarding antibiotic selection given influenza-positive status and concern for secondary bacterial pneumonia.

Reassessment

Patient A Oxygen saturation dropped to 89% while feeding attempt. Apneic episode witnessed lasting eight seconds with desaturation to 78%. Respiratory rate increased to 68 with severe retractions. Capillary refill now 4 seconds with mottled extremities.

Patient B Remains in moderate distress despite three back-to-back albuterol treatments. Peak flow unchanged at 60% predicted. Parents still refusing steroids but requesting admission to avoid "hospital at home" responsibility. Blood gas now showing pCO_2 46 with dropping bicarbonate.

Patient C Vomited twice after 50mL oral rehydration solution. Decreased responsiveness with weak cry. Urine output still zero. Sunken eyes and doughy skin texture noted on reassessment.

Clinical Decision-Making: Resource Allocation Crisis

Recognition that only one monitored bed remains and two patients now require continuous observation. Decision to move Patient B to the ward bed with q15min vitals versus keeping Patient A in ED with higher observation capabilities. Calculation that Patient C now meets criteria for moderate dehydration requiring IV fluids and possible admission. Conflict arising between pediatric ward charge nurse refusing second admission (Patient C) until Patient B is discharged or transferred.

Managing Conflict: Disposition Negotiations

Bed Availability Dispute Ward nurse stating hospital policy prohibits two respiratory patients on same unit due to isolation requirements. Suggestion to transfer Patient A to NICU step-down for apnea monitoring met with resistance from neonatal team regarding bronchiolitis infection risk. Negotiation for admission of Patient C to general pediatrics while Patient A remains in ED observation unit overnight.

Parental Demands for Patient B Parents now demanding admission after witnessing Patient A's apnea episode and becoming frightened. Explanation that admission criteria not yet met for moderate asthma if steroids accepted and adequate follow-up arranged. Discussion of observation unit alternative versus home with strict return precautions.

Reassessment: Hour Two with Interventions

Patient A High-flow nasal cannula initiated at 2 L/kg/min. Apneic episodes decreased to isolated brief pauses <5 seconds. Feeding improved with smaller, frequent volumes. Capillary refill improved to 2.5 seconds.

Patient B Accepted single dose dexamethasone after social work consultation. Peak flow improved to 75% predicted. Oxygen saturation 95% on room air. Discharged home with asthma action plan and follow-up in 24 hours.

Patient C IV placed after topical anesthetic application. Normal saline bolus 20mL/kg given with improvement in mentation. Ceftriaxone administered for presumed bacterial superinfection. Urine output 2mL/kg in following hour.

Final Dispositions

Patient A: Admission to pediatric ward with continuous pulse oximetry and apnea monitoring given persistent apnea episodes and prematurity history.

Patient B: Discharge home with oral steroid taper, albuterol inhaler, and strict return precautions for respiratory distress; follow-up with primary pediatrician in 24 hours.

Patient C: Admission for IV antibiotics and hydration given persistent vomiting and documented bacterial pneumonia with influenza co-infection.

Critical Actions

- Recognized high-risk criteria for bronchiolitis admission including apnea episodes, prematurity history, and age under three months in Patient A.
- Demonstrated appropriate reassessment frequency leading to escalation of care when Patient A desaturated and Patient C failed oral rehydration.

- Managed conflict regarding parental refusal of evidence-based treatment in Patient B through motivational interviewing and shared decision-making.
- Prioritized resource allocation effectively by matching patient acuity to appropriate monitoring levels while negotiating ward bed availability.
- Identified hypernatremic dehydration in Patient C requiring controlled fluid resuscitation rather than aggressive free water replacement.
- Applied clinical decision-making regarding admission criteria balancing over-admission risks versus safety for moderate respiratory conditions.
- Demonstrated patient-centered communication techniques including developmentally appropriate explanations and parental anxiety acknowledgment.
- Recognized changing clinical status requiring intervention escalation: high-flow oxygen for Patient A, IV fluids for Patient C, and steroid acceptance for Patient B.
- Balanced infectious disease considerations including RSV isolation for Patient A and droplet precautions for Patient C's influenza.
- Coordinated multidisciplinary care involving nursing, respiratory therapy, social work, and admitting teams while managing three concurrent moderate-acuity patients.

Triage with Pediatric Patient in Waiting Room

Opening Scenario

You are the attending physician in triage on a chaotic Monday evening. The waiting room is at capacity with 28 patients, and the department is operating at 120 capacity. The charge nurse informs you that wait times are approaching 3 hours for non-urgent complaints. Your role is to evaluate five newly arrived patients, order initial diagnostics, assign them to the appropriate care area (Fast Track, General Purpose Pod, or Critical Care Pod), and manage any conflicts that arise. Patients who remain in the waiting room will require reassessment when results return. Once patients are placed in a pod or handed off, you will not follow them further.

Patient 1: Mr. Henderson - Chest Pressure

Chief Complaint: Chest pressure

Vital Signs: BP 178/105, HR 112, RR 24, SpO_2 94% RA, Temp 99.0°F, Pain 9/10

Brief History: 45-year-old male with uncontrolled hypertension and 40-pack-year smoking history. One hour of crushing substernal chest pressure with radiation to jaw. Diaphoretic, nauseated, no vomiting. No prior cardiac history but strong family history of early MI.

Physical Exam:

- Diaphoretic, moderate respiratory distress
- Remainder of exam normal

Initial Orders:

- ECG (STAT)
- Troponin I (STAT)
- CBC, BMP, magnesium, phosphate
- Chest X-ray
- Aspirin 325 mg chewable
- Nitroglycerin 0.4 mg SL q5min x3 if SBP > 90

Location Decision: Critical Care Pod

Handoff to Critical Care Pod Physician: "Mr. Henderson is a 45-year-old male, heavy smoker, one hour of crushing chest pressure radiating to jaw, diaphoretic, hypertensive emergency. ECG and troponin pending. I've given aspirin, nitro in the waiting room."

Patient 2: Emily Chen - Febrile Child with Anxious Parent

Chief Complaint: Fever and rash

Vital Signs: BP 92/58, HR 145, RR 36, SpO_2 97% RA, Temp 103.8°F (rectal)

Brief History: 3-year-old female (15 kg) with 2 days of fever, today developed diffuse erythematous rash that blanches. Tylenol provides temporary relief. Decreased oral intake, no vomiting, one episode of diarrhea. Immunizations up to date. Parent is visibly anxious and states: "We've been waiting 20 minutes already and she's getting worse!"

Physical Exam:

- Febrile and tired but not lethargic
- Diffuse blanching erythematous maculopapular rash
- Cap refill 2 seconds
- Remainder of exam normal

Initial Orders:

- Blood culture

- CBC with differential
- BMP
- CRP
- Urinalysis (catheterized)
- Acetaminophen 15 mg/kg PO now
- Ibuprofen 10 mg/kg PO now

Location Decision: Patient remains in waiting room for initial labs and fever control

Patient Communication: "I can see how worried you are, and you're right to be concerned. We're going to get some tests started right away and control her fever. The wait is frustrating, but we're prioritizing based on how sick patients are. Your daughter is stable right now, and we're going to keep a close eye on her while these tests are running."

Patient 3: Sarah Mitchell - Right Lower Quadrant Pain

Chief Complaint: Abdominal pain

Vital Signs: BP 118/72, HR 98, RR 20, SpO_2 99% RA, Temp 100.4°F, Pain 7/10

Brief History: 28-year-old female with 18 hours of progressive RLQ pain, anorexia, nausea. Last menstrual period 2 weeks ago. Denies vaginal bleeding or discharge. No prior abdominal surgeries.

Physical Exam:

- RLQ tenderness with voluntary guarding
- Negative Rovsing's sign
- Remainder of exam normal

Initial Orders:

- Urine hCG
- CBC with differential
- BMP
- Transvaginal pelvic ultrasound

Location Decision: General Purpose Pod

Patient 4: Marcus Johnson - Agitated Patient with Migraine

Chief Complaint: Severe headache

Vital Signs: BP 165/95, HR 105, RR 18, SpO_2 99% RA, Temp 98.9°F, Pain 10/10

Brief History: 38-year-old male with history of migraines, frequent ED visits. States he has been waiting for 2.5 hours, pacing the waiting room, and loudly complaining to staff and other patients: "This is ridiculous! I'm in agony and nobody cares! I can see people going back before me!" He demands "the shot that works" (referring to hydromorphone). Previous records show multiple negative neuro workups.

Physical Exam:

- Photophobia present
- Normal neuro exam, no focal deficits
- Remainder of exam normal

Initial Orders:

- Urine drug screen
- CBC, BMP (to assess for other causes)
- Non-contrast head CT
- Acetaminophen 1000 mg PO
- Metoclopramide 10 mg IV

- Normal saline 500 mL IV bolus

Location Decision: Patient remains in waiting room pending CT results

Managing Conflict & Patient Communication: "Mr. Johnson, I understand you've been waiting a long time, and I can see you're suffering. The wait is truly unacceptable, and I apologize. We're dealing with life-threatening emergencies like heart attacks and strokes that have to go first. I'm going to evaluate you right now, but I need to be honest—I cannot give you hydromorphone at triage without a full evaluation. Let's get a CT scan to make sure this is your typical migraine, and I'll start some treatment while we wait. I know this isn't what you wanted to hear, but my job is to keep you safe."

Patient 5: Robert Torres - Occupational Laceration

Chief Complaint: Hand laceration

Vital Signs: BP 132/78, HR 82, RR 16, SpO_2 99% RA, Temp 98.6°F, Pain 4/10

Brief History: 50-year-old chef with 3 cm clean laceration to right thumb from kitchen knife while preparing food. Bleeding controlled with pressure. No tendon or neurovascular compromise. Last tetanus booster 8 years ago.

Physical Exam:

- 3 cm linear laceration, superficial, good cap refill
- Sensation intact, full range of motion
- Remainder of exam normal

Initial Orders:

- Wound care supplies
- Tetanus toxoid 0.5 mL IM

Location Decision: Fast Track

Reassessment: Patient 2 (Emily Chen)

Time Elapsed: 60 minutes

New Data: Initial labs resulted

- CBC/Inflammatory: WBC 18.5, Neutrophils 82% , CRP 145
- BMP: Na 141, Glucose 110
- UA: Negative for nitrites/leukocytes
- Blood Culture: Pending, no growth

Repeat Vital Signs: BP 88/55, HR 152, RR 38, SpO_2 96% RA, Temp 102.4°F (rectal)

Patient Status: Child appears more ill, less interactive. Parent is now standing at triage desk demanding to speak to a supervisor: "Her fever isn't coming down and these results are bad! Why isn't she in a room yet?"

Reassessment Decision: Escalate to General Purpose Pod immediately

Managing Conflict & Handoff: To parent: "Ms. Chen, you're absolutely right to be concerned. These results show a significant infection, and I'm moving her to a bed right now. I know the wait has been stressful, but we needed these results to get her the right care. Your daughter is stable, but she needs more monitoring. Let's go." To receiving physician: "Emily Chen, 3-year-old female, 15 kg, with high fever, rash, and labs showing leukocytosis with left shift, CRP 145. Appears more ill now. Blood cultures pending. Given acetaminophen and ibuprofen. Needs sepsis workup and empiric antibiotics."

Reassessment: Patient 4 (Marcus Johnson)

Time Elapsed: 90 minutes

New Data: CT resulted - no acute intracranial pathology; Labs within normal limits

Repeat Vital Signs: BP 148/92, HR 95, RR 16, SpO_2 99% RA, Temp 98.7°F

Patient Status: Patient is sleeping in waiting room chair after receiving medications. Headache improved to 4/10. Staff reports he has been quiet for past 30 minutes.

Reassessment Decision: Discharge from waiting room with outpatient follow-up

Patient Communication: "Mr. Johnson, good news—your CT scan is completely normal, and your labs look great. I know the wait was frustrating, but we had to make sure this wasn't something serious. The medications we gave are helping. I'm going to send you home with a prescription for your migraine and a referral to a headache clinic to help prevent these ER visits. Here's a work note for tomorrow."

Critical Actions

Clinical Decision-Making:

- Recognized Mr. Henderson as potential ACS and ordered appropriate STAT workup (ECG, troponin, aspirin)
- Identified Emily Chen as potentially septic with appropriate pediatric workup including cultures and weight-based dosing
- Correctly triaged Sarah Mitchell to General Purpose Pod for appendicitis workup with appropriate pregnancy testing
- Appropriately ordered comprehensive evaluation for Marcus Johnson despite history of frequent visits
- Correctly assigned Robert Torres to Fast Track based on low-acuity, stable wound

Prioritization:

- Immediately identified Mr. Henderson as ESI 1 requiring critical care resources
- Appropriately kept Emily Chen in waiting room initially while ordering essential labs, recognizing need for data before escalation
- Correctly prioritized Sarah Mitchell as ESI 3 for General Purpose Pod
- Recognized Marcus Johnson required evaluation but not immediate critical resources
- Appropriately assigned Robert Torres to Fast Track

Reassessment:

- Monitored Emily Chen appropriately while in waiting room, recognized clinical deterioration and critical lab values
- Escalated pediatric patient promptly based on objective findings (WBC 18.5, CRP 145, persistent tachycardia)
- Reassessed Marcus Johnson after CT results, recognized improvement and appropriate for discharge
- Did not inappropriately follow patients after handoff or pod placement

Patient Communication:

- Demonstrated empathy with anxious parent of pediatric patient while setting realistic expectations
- Acknowledged Ms. Chen's frustration and provided clear rationale for wait times
- Used age-appropriate language and included parent in decision-making process
- Maintained therapeutic relationship despite time pressures

Managing Conflict:

- Successfully de-escalated angry Mr. Johnson using acknowledgment, apology, and boundary-setting
- Did not capitulate to inappropriate opioid demands but offered alternative treatment plan
- Explained triage rationale without being defensive or dismissive
- Managed second conflict with pediatric parent by validating concerns and taking immediate action when warranted
- Maintained professionalism despite being challenged publicly in waiting room

Pediatric-Specific Care:

- Used weight-based dosing (15 kg child) for antipyretics
- Recognized tachycardia and fever as concerning in pediatric patient
- Ordered appropriate pediatric workup including catheterized urine sample
- Communicated effectively with anxious parent while maintaining safety standards

Handoff Communication:

- Provided concise, structured handoff for life-threatening Mr. Henderson including key risk factors and interventions
- Delivered clear handoff for deteriorating pediatric patient including weight, vital sign trends, and treatment given
- Included critical lab values and clinical changes in handoff communication

Safety:

- Administered aspirin appropriately for potential ACS
- Avoided opioid administration in ambiguous chronic pain scenario at triage
- Ordered pregnancy testing in fertile female with abdominal pain
- Recognized need for tetanus update in laceration patient
- Maintained sepsis precautions for pediatric patient with concerning presentation

Hypotension After a Fall

Opening Scenario

EMS arrives with a 78-year-old male who fell at home while getting up from a chair 45 minutes ago. He hit a coffee table and landed on his left side. He takes warfarin for atrial fibrillation. His wife reports he has been increasingly confused since the fall and "looks pale."

EMS Report:

- GCS 14 (E4, V4, M6); confused but following commands
- BP 88/52, HR 112, RR 22, SpO_2 94% on 2L NC
- IV established with NS running wide open
- Fingerstick glucose 118

Initial Assessment

Vitals: BP 86/50, HR 114, RR 24, SpO_2 94% on 2L NC, T 36.0°C

- Airway: Patent, speaking in short sentences
- Breathing: Tachypneic, clear bilaterally
- Circulation: Pale, diaphoretic, weak radial pulses, cap refill 4 seconds
- Disability: GCS 14, confused to time and place
- Exposure: Left flank ecchymosis, no open wounds

Immediate actions: Two large-bore IVs, type and crossmatch for 4 units PRBCs, activate massive transfusion protocol standby, place on monitor with continuous vitals, obtain FAST exam, send labs including INR.

History

- HPI: Ground-level fall onto left side striking a coffee table. No head strike or LOC per wife. Progressive confusion and pallor since the fall. No chest pain, no antiplatelet agents.
- PMHx: Atrial fibrillation, hypertension, hyperlipidemia, mechanical aortic valve (2019)
- Medications: Warfarin 5 mg daily, metoprolol 50 mg BID, atorvastatin 40 mg
- Allergies: Penicillin (rash)
- Social: Lives with wife, independent ADLs, no alcohol

Physical Examination

- General: Elderly male, pale, diaphoretic, anxious
- HEENT: No scalp lacerations or hematoma, pupils equal and reactive
- Neck: No JVD, no cervical tenderness
- Cardiovascular: Tachycardic, irregularly irregular, mechanical click at aortic position, no rub
- Pulmonary: Tachypneic, clear bilaterally
- Abdomen: Soft, diffusely tender with involuntary guarding in left upper quadrant, no rebound, no distension
- Pelvis: Stable to compression
- Extremities: No deformity, no long bone tenderness
- Neurological: Confused, follows commands, moves all extremities symmetrically

Diagnostic Studies

Bedside FAST Exam:

Using a curvilinear (3-5 MHz) probe, perform a 4-view FAST examination:

- Right upper quadrant (Morrison's pouch): Anechoic free fluid in the hepatorenal recess
- Left upper quadrant (splenorenal recess): Anechoic free fluid surrounding the spleen with perisplenic clot
- Suprapubic: Free fluid in pelvis
- Subxiphoid cardiac: Small pericardial effusion; however, the right ventricle fills normally in diastole, there is no RV diastolic collapse, and no respiratory variation in mitral inflow — findings consistent with a small incidental or reactive effusion, not tamponade. The IVC is collapsed (<1 cm), consistent with hypovolemia.

The candidate must differentiate the pericardial effusion from tamponade by assessing RV diastolic collapse, IVC plethora, and clinical context. This patient's shock is hemorrhagic (collapsed IVC, positive abdominal FAST), not obstructive.

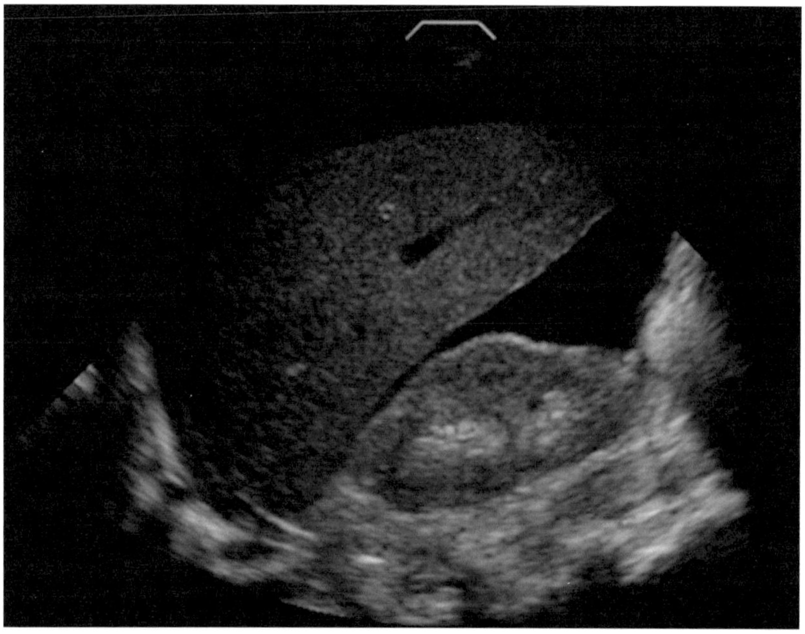

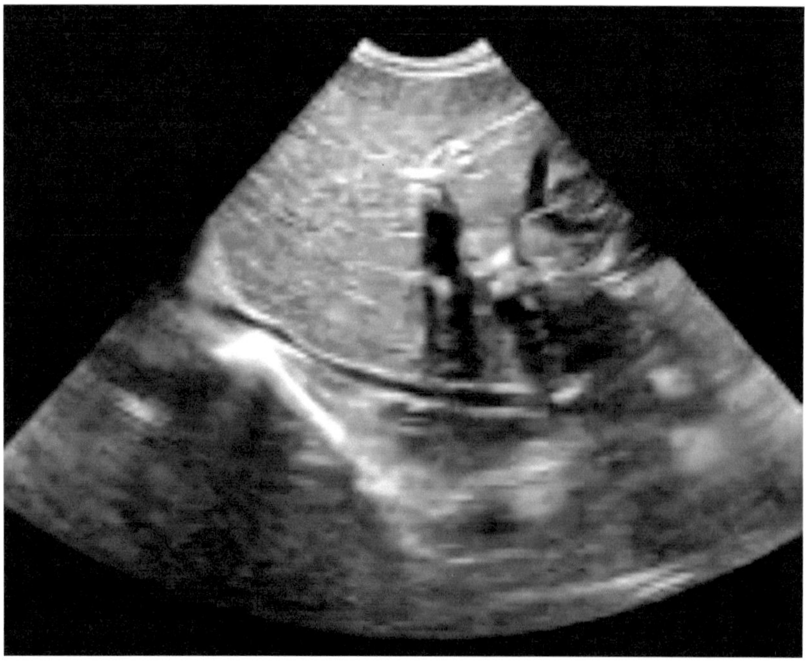

- CBC: WBC 9.8, Hgb 9.2, Hct 27%, Plt 198

- BMP: Na 141, K 4.8, Cl 106, HCO_3 18, BUN 34, Cr 1.4, Glucose 118
- INR 3.8, PT 42 seconds
- Lactate 4.6
- Type and screen: Sent

Management

- Hemorrhagic shock from intra-abdominal injury in an anticoagulated patient. Most likely splenic injury given mechanism, left flank ecchymosis, and perisplenic fluid/clot on FAST.
- Activate massive transfusion protocol: 1:1:1 ratio PRBCs, FFP, platelets
- Anticoagulation reversal: 4-factor PCC (Kcentra) 25-50 units/kg IV for immediate INR reversal (preferred over FFP alone for speed); administer vitamin K 10 mg IV concurrently for sustained reversal
- Hold warfarin; discuss anticoagulation risks with cardiology given mechanical valve (bridge with heparin once hemostasis achieved)
- Consult Trauma Surgery immediately for operative management
- Foley catheter, arterial line for continuous BP monitoring

Reassessment

Thirty minutes later: Despite 2 units PRBCs and PCC, BP remains 82/48, HR 118. Repeat FAST shows significantly increased free fluid in all abdominal windows with new clot formation around the spleen. Repeat Hgb 7.4 (from 9.2). INR now 1.4 (improved from 3.8 with PCC).

- Continue MTP; transfuse additional PRBCs, FFP, and platelets
- Patient requires emergent operative intervention — surgery prepping the OR for exploratory laparotomy
- If patient stabilizes with transfusion, CT abdomen/pelvis with IV contrast to fine grade splenic injury with active extravasation
- If hemodynamically unstable despite resuscitation, proceed directly to OR without CT

Critical Actions

- Recognize hemorrhagic shock in anticoagulated elderly patient after ground-level fall
- Correctly perform and interpret bedside FAST exam using curvilinear probe
- Differentiate pericardial effusion from tamponade physiology (assess RV diastolic collapse, IVC diameter, clinical context)
- Integrate FAST findings with clinical picture — collapsed IVC and positive abdominal FAST confirm hemorrhagic rather than obstructive shock
- Reverse anticoagulation emergently with 4-factor PCC and IV vitamin K
- Activate MTP with 1:1:1 transfusion strategy
- Repeat FAST to assess for interval change and guide surgical decision-making
- Consult Trauma Surgery for operative management; avoid delays for CT if hemodynamically unstable

Shortness of Breath with Leg Swelling

Opening Scenario

A 45-year-old female presents via ambulance with acute-onset shortness of breath that started 2 hours ago while walking up stairs. She had a right knee arthroscopy 2 weeks ago and has been mostly sedentary during recovery. She is anxious and tachypneic on arrival.

Initial Assessment

Vitals: BP 102/68, HR 118, RR 28, SpO_2 88% on RA (94% on 15L NRB), T 37.1°C

- Airway: Patent, speaking in 3-4 word sentences
- Breathing: Tachypneic, clear to auscultation bilaterally, no wheezes or crackles
- Circulation: Tachycardic, regular rhythm, JVD present, right calf swollen and tense
- Disability: Alert, anxious, GCS 15
- Exposure: Right lower extremity wrapped in ACE bandage from recent surgery, calf visibly larger than left

Immediate actions: Continuous monitoring, two large-bore IVs, high-flow oxygen, obtain ECG, bedside echocardiography, lower extremity venous compression ultrasound.

History

- HPI: Sudden-onset dyspnea 2 hours ago while climbing stairs. Associated with pleuritic chest pain, right-sided, worse with inspiration. Progressive right calf swelling and pain over past 4 days — attributed to postoperative swelling. No hemoptysis. Immobilized with knee brace for 2 weeks; minimal ambulation.
- PMHx: Obesity (BMI 34), combined oral contraceptive use, right knee meniscal tear
- PSHx: Right knee arthroscopy 14 days ago
- Medications: Norgestimate-ethinyl estradiol, acetaminophen, oxycodone PRN (postoperative)
- Allergies: NKDA
- FHx: Mother with DVT during pregnancy
- Social: Non-smoker, no alcohol, works as an accountant (desk job)

Physical Examination

- General: Anxious, dyspneic, diaphoretic
- HEENT: Normal
- Neck: JVD to 10 cm at 45 degrees
- Cardiovascular: Tachycardic, regular, loud P2, right-sided S3, no murmurs
- Pulmonary: Clear bilaterally, no crackles, no wheezes — absence of crackles is notable and inconsistent with heart failure or pneumonia
- Abdomen: Soft, nontender, no hepatomegaly
- Extremities: Right calf circumference 4 cm greater than left, pitting edema to mid-calf, tender along posterior calf, positive Homan's sign; surgical incisions well-healed without erythema
- Neurological: Alert, oriented, no focal deficits

Diagnostic Studies

Bedside Echocardiography (Cardiac POCUS):

- Parasternal long axis: RV visibly dilated, RV:LV ratio >1:1

- Parasternal short axis: Interventricular septum bowing into the LV during systole and diastole (D-sign), consistent with RV pressure and volume overload
- Apical 4-chamber: RV dilation with hypokinesis of the RV free wall and preserved apical contractility (McConnell's sign — highly specific for acute PE)
- Subcostal IVC: IVC dilated (>2.1 cm) with <50% respiratory variation, consistent with elevated right atrial pressure
- 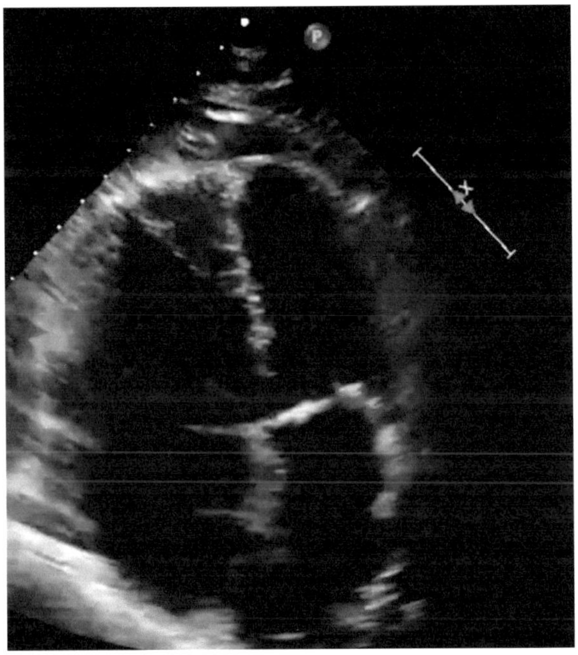

Lung Ultrasound:

- Normal lung sliding present bilaterally (rules out pneumothorax)
- A-line pattern throughout — no B-lines (rules out pulmonary edema and alveolar pathology)
- No consolidation or pleural effusion

The absence of B-lines in a dyspneic patient with RV strain strongly supports PE over cardiogenic pulmonary edema.

Lower Extremity Compression Ultrasound:

- Common femoral vein: Fully compressible
- Superficial femoral vein: Fully compressible
- Popliteal vein: Non-compressible with visible intraluminal echogenic thrombus
- Augmentation absent in right popliteal vein

The candidate must demonstrate 2-point or 3-point compression technique: apply firm downward pressure with the probe until the adjacent artery deforms slightly. A normal vein collapses completely; a non-compressible vein confirms DVT.

- ECG: Sinus tachycardia at 118 bpm, S1Q3T3 pattern, T-wave inversions in V1-V4 (RV strain pattern)
- CBC: WBC 10.2, Hgb 13.8, Plt 256
- BMP: Na 140, K 4.2, BUN 16, Cr 0.9
- Troponin I: 0.18 ng/mL (elevated — indicates RV myocardial injury)
- BNP: 580 pg/mL (elevated — RV strain)
- D-dimer: Not required when clinical probability is high and bedside US confirms DVT with RV strain

Management

- Submassive PE: Confirmed by RV strain on echo (McConnell's sign, D-sign, dilated IVC), elevated troponin and BNP, hemodynamic stability (SBP >90), and proximal DVT on compression US.
- Anticoagulation: Unfractionated heparin 80 units/kg IV bolus followed by 18 units/kg/hour infusion (preferred over LMWH in submassive PE for titrability if clinical deterioration occurs)
- Discontinue oral contraceptives
- Risk-stratify using PESI score and RV function: this patient has submassive (intermediate-risk) PE with RV dysfunction and biomarker elevation
- Consult Pulmonary/Critical Care for ICU admission and monitored anticoagulation
- Systemic thrombolysis (tPA 100 mg IV over 2 hours) is NOT indicated at this time — reserved for massive PE with hemodynamic instability (SBP <90 for >15 minutes, cardiac arrest, or clinical deterioration despite anticoagulation)
- Prepare for thrombolysis if patient decompensates: have tPA drawn up and available at bedside
- Consider CT pulmonary angiography to define clot burden if patient is stable enough for transport, though bedside findings are sufficient to initiate treatment

Reassessment

One hour after heparin initiation: BP drops to 78/44, HR 132, SpO_2 86% on 15L NRB, altered mental status. Repeat bedside echo shows worsening RV dilation with interventricular septal bowing.

- Patient has progressed from submassive to massive PE with hemodynamic collapse
- Administer IV NS 500 mL bolus (avoid excessive volume — RV is already failing and volume overload worsens septal bowing)
- Initiate vasopressors: norepinephrine preferred (supports SVR without increasing pulmonary vascular resistance)
- Administer systemic thrombolysis: tPA (alteplase) 100 mg IV over 2 hours; continue heparin infusion during administration
- If cardiac arrest occurs, administer tPA 50 mg IV bolus with ongoing CPR; continue CPR for at least 60-90 minutes after thrombolytic administration
- Monitor for bleeding complications; type and crossmatch 2 units PRBCs

Patient Communication

- Explain that a large blood clot traveled from the leg to the lungs and is straining the heart
- Discuss risk-benefit of thrombolysis: significant bleeding risk (including intracranial hemorrhage 1-3%) vs. mortality benefit in hemodynamically unstable PE
- Recent knee surgery (14 days prior) is a relative contraindication to thrombolysis — discuss with patient and surgical team; benefit outweighs risk in life-threatening PE
- If patient unable to consent due to altered mental status, proceed under emergency doctrine

Critical Actions

- Recognize high pretest probability for PE (recent surgery, immobilization, OCP use, unilateral leg swelling, acute dyspnea)
- Perform bedside echocardiography and identify RV strain markers: RV dilation, D-sign, McConnell's sign, dilated IVC
- Perform lung ultrasound to rule out alternative diagnoses (pulmonary edema, pneumothorax, consolidation)
- Perform lower extremity compression ultrasound and identify non-compressible popliteal vein DVT

- Integrate multi-organ POCUS findings to confirm PE diagnosis at the bedside without delaying treatment
- Risk-stratify PE as submassive (RV strain with hemodynamic stability) and initiate heparin
- Recognize clinical deterioration to massive PE and escalate to systemic thrombolysis
- Discontinue OCP and address modifiable risk factors

Chest Tube Insertion

Opening Scenario

EMS arrives with a 35-year-old male involved in a motorcycle crash at approximately 40 mph. He was wearing a helmet but was thrown from the bike and landed on his left side. He is alert and complaining of severe left chest pain and progressive difficulty breathing.

EMS Report:

- GCS 15, alert and oriented
- BP 128/82, HR 104, RR 26, SpO_2 92% on 15L NRB
- Left chest wall tenderness with crepitus on palpation
- IV established, C-collar in place

Initial Assessment

Vitals: BP 124/78, HR 108, RR 28, SpO_2 91% on 15L NRB, T 36.8°C

- Airway: Patent, speaking in full sentences with effort
- Breathing: Tachypneic, decreased breath sounds on left, subcutaneous crepitus over left lateral chest
- Circulation: Tachycardic, regular, strong radial pulses, cap refill 2 seconds
- Disability: GCS 15, moving all extremities
- Exposure: Left lateral chest wall ecchymosis, road rash to left shoulder and hip

Immediate actions: Supplemental oxygen, continuous monitoring, two large-bore IVs, chest X-ray, FAST exam, T&C, trauma panel.

History

- HPI: Motorcycle crash 30 minutes ago, left-side impact. Wearing helmet with no LOC. Progressive dyspnea since the crash. Denies abdominal pain. No other vehicles involved.
- PMHx: None
- Medications: None
- Allergies: NKDA
- Social: No alcohol today, no drugs

Physical Examination

- General: Alert, in moderate respiratory distress, splinting left chest
- HEENT: Helmet removed, no scalp lacerations, no facial trauma
- Neck: C-collar in place, no tracheal deviation, no JVD
- Cardiovascular: Tachycardic, regular, no murmurs
- Pulmonary: Decreased breath sounds on left with dullness at left base and hyperresonance at left apex; subcutaneous crepitus from left axilla to nipple line; right lung clear
- Abdomen: Soft, nontender, no distension
- Pelvis: Stable
- Extremities: Road rash left shoulder and hip, no deformity, no long bone tenderness
- FAST: Negative
- Neurological: GCS 15, no focal deficits

Diagnostic Studies

- CXR (upright AP): Left-sided pneumothorax with approximately 30% lung collapse, associated left 4th-6th rib fractures laterally, no mediastinal shift, no hemothorax visible
- CBC: WBC 12.4, Hgb 14.2, Hct 42%, Plt 278
- BMP: Na 140, K 4.0, Cl 104, HCO_3 22, BUN 15, Cr 1.0
- Lactate 1.8
- CXR confirms indication for tube thoracostomy: traumatic pneumothorax with respiratory distress, subcutaneous emphysema suggesting ongoing air leak

Management

Indication and Consent:

- Traumatic pneumothorax with respiratory compromise and subcutaneous emphysema requires tube thoracostomy
- Explain the procedure, risks (bleeding, infection, organ injury, pain), benefits (lung re-expansion, improved breathing), and alternatives (observation is not appropriate given progressive symptoms)
- Obtain verbal consent from patient

Reassessment

Post-procedure CXR shows the tube in good position with improved but incomplete lung re-expansion. Persistent bubbling in the water seal chamber. One hour later: worsening subcutaneous emphysema extending from left chest to neck and face. Chest tube is draining air continuously with vigorous bubbling.

- Verify all tube connections are tight and airtight
- Ensure all drainage holes are within the pleural space (if a side hole is external, air entrains through the hole — requires repositioning or replacement)
- Apply additional suction (-20 cm H_2O) to the drainage system
- If persistent large air leak despite properly positioned tube, consider bronchopleural fistula from tracheobronchial injury (rare but associated with high-energy blunt trauma)
- Consult Thoracic Surgery and Trauma Surgery for bronchoscopy to evaluate for airway injury
- CT chest to evaluate for tube malposition, additional pneumothorax, or parenchymal injury
- Consider placing a second chest tube if drainage is inadequate
- Monitor for tension physiology: if tracheal deviation, hypotension, or worsening hypoxia develop, this is a surgical emergency

Patient Communication

The patient's partner arrives and is visibly upset, demanding to know why a "tube in the chest" is necessary and whether this means the injury is life-threatening.

- Acknowledge the partner's fear and validate that this is frightening
- Explain in plain language: "Air is leaking from his lung into his chest, which makes it hard to breathe. The tube lets the trapped air drain out so the lung can re-expand. Without it, the air buildup could become dangerous."
- Clarify that while the injury is serious, chest tubes are a standard and effective treatment for this type of injury
- Provide realistic expectations: the tube will remain in place for days, and the patient will need hospital admission
- Offer to answer specific questions and provide updates as care progresses

Critical Actions

- Recognize traumatic pneumothorax requiring tube thoracostomy based on imaging, respiratory distress, and subcutaneous emphysema
- Identify the triangle of safety and correct interspace (4th-5th ICS, mid-axillary line, superior border of the rib)
- Maintain strict sterile technique throughout the procedure
- Perform digital exploration (finger sweep) before inserting the tube to confirm pleural entry and rule out adhesions or abdominal organs
- Connect to closed drainage system and confirm function (tidaling, air leak assessment)
- Obtain post-procedure CXR to verify tube position and lung re-expansion
- Recognize persistent air leak and worsening subcutaneous emphysema as potential tube malposition or bronchopleural fistula
- Troubleshoot systematically: check connections, verify tube position, escalate to surgical consultation
- Communicate effectively with patient's partner using clear, non-medical language

Emergent Pericardiocentesis

Opening Scenario

A 62-year-old male with known metastatic non-small cell lung cancer presents with progressive dyspnea over 3 days, now acutely worsened with near-syncope. He arrives sitting bolt upright on the stretcher, unable to lie flat.

Initial Assessment

Vitals: BP 78/50, HR 124, RR 30, SpO_2 93% on RA, T 36.4°C

- Airway: Patent, speaking in short phrases
- Breathing: Tachypneic, clear lung fields bilaterally
- Circulation: Tachycardic, muffled heart sounds, JVD to the angle of the jaw, weak thready pulses, cool extremities, cap refill 5 seconds
- Disability: GCS 15, anxious and diaphoretic
- Exposure: Cachectic, port-a-cath right chest

Immediate actions: Two large-bore IVs, 500 mL NS bolus, continuous monitoring, bedside echocardiography, ECG. Recognize Beck's triad (hypotension, JVD, muffled heart sounds) — prepare for emergent pericardiocentesis.

History

- HPI: 3-day history of worsening dyspnea, initially with exertion, now at rest. Orthopnea for 2 days. Near-syncopal episode today prompting 911 call. Chest pressure described as "fullness" rather than sharp pain. No fever, cough, or hemoptysis. Last oncology visit 3 weeks ago; CT showed progressive disease with new pericardial metastases.
- PMHx: Non-small cell lung cancer (stage IV, diagnosed 14 months ago, on pembrolizumab, last dose 4 weeks ago), COPD, hypertension
- Medications: Pembrolizumab (immunotherapy), albuterol inhaler, lisinopril
- Allergies: NKDA
- Social: Former smoker (40 pack-years, quit at diagnosis), lives with wife and adult daughter, full code status per chart (last documented 3 months ago)
- Advance Directives: POLST form on file indicating full treatment measures; however, this was completed prior to most recent disease progression

Physical Examination

- General: Cachectic male sitting upright, anxious, diaphoretic, in acute distress
- HEENT: No facial edema, oropharynx clear
- Neck: JVD present and distending further with inspiration (Kussmaul's sign); no lymphadenopathy
- Cardiovascular: Tachycardic, muffled heart sounds, no friction rub, weak peripheral pulses; pulsus paradoxus present (>20 mmHg drop in systolic BP with inspiration)
- Pulmonary: Clear bilaterally — absence of crackles is important (fluid is in the pericardium, not the lungs)
- Abdomen: Soft, nontender, hepatomegaly 3 cm below costal margin
- Extremities: Cool, mottled, no edema
- Port-a-cath: Right subclavian, no erythema

Diagnostic Studies

Bedside Echocardiography:

- Subxiphoid view: Large circumferential pericardial effusion with fibrinous stranding. RV diastolic collapse present — the RV free wall inverts inward during diastole, confirming tamponade physiology. Swinging heart motion visible.
- Parasternal long axis: Confirms large effusion (>2 cm posterior to LV, >1 cm anterior to RV). RV compression evident.
- Apical 4-chamber: Bi-atrial compression with RA systolic inversion >1/3 of the cardiac cycle. LV cavity is small with hyperdynamic function (underfilled).
- IVC: Plethoric (>2.1 cm) with no respiratory variation, consistent with elevated right-sided pressures.
- ECG: Low-voltage QRS complexes diffusely, electrical alternans (beat-to-beat variation in QRS amplitude — classic for large effusion with swinging heart), sinus tachycardia
- CXR: Enlarged cardiac silhouette with "water bottle" configuration, clear lung fields, port-a-cath in place
- CBC: WBC 6.4, Hgb 10.2, Plt 142
- BMP: Na 136, K 5.1, Cl 100, HCO_3 20, BUN 38, Cr 1.6, Glucose 102
- Troponin: 0.04 ng/mL (normal)
- Lactate: 4.2

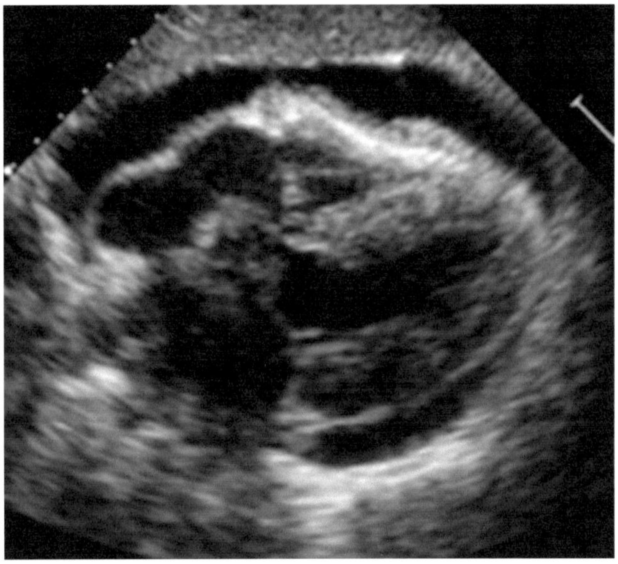

Management

Cardiac tamponade with hemodynamic compromise — emergent pericardiocentesis required. This is not a condition that responds to volume resuscitation or vasopressors alone; definitive treatment is drainage.

- Administer 500 mL NS bolus as temporizing bridge (increases preload to partially compensate for impaired filling)
- Avoid intubation if possible — positive pressure ventilation further reduces preload and can precipitate cardiac arrest in tamponade
- Do NOT delay pericardiocentesis for CT or cardiology consultation in hemodynamically unstable tamponade

Reassessment

After removing 60 mL of serosanguinous fluid: BP improves from 78/50 to 105/68, HR decreases from 124 to 94, patient reports immediate improvement in dyspnea. Repeat bedside echo shows decreased effusion size with resolution of RV diastolic collapse.

- Continue drainage until no further fluid aspirated or hemodynamics normalize; total aspirated volume: 450 mL
- If pigtail catheter placed, leave to gravity drainage and reassess for re-accumulation
- Send pericardial fluid for cytology, cell count, protein, LDH, glucose, culture, and AFB
- Consult Cardiothoracic Surgery for ICU admission
- Consult Oncology regarding disease trajectory and treatment options
- Admit to ICU for hemodynamic monitoring

Patient Communication

After stabilization, the patient asks "Does this mean my cancer is getting worse?" His wife and daughter are present.

- Acknowledge the question directly and honestly: the pericardial effusion is related to disease progression to the pericardium
- Explore the patient's understanding of his prognosis and current goals
- Clarify current code status: the POLST was completed before recent progression. Ask whether his goals have changed — "Given what has happened today, I want to make sure we understand what matters most to you."
- Discuss that while pericardiocentesis treated today's emergency, the effusion is likely to recur without a pericardial window or changes in cancer treatment
- Offer palliative care consultation for symptom management and goals-of-care planning regardless of whether the patient pursues further cancer-directed therapy
- Do not force a code status decision in the acute setting, but ensure the conversation is initiated and documented

Critical Actions

- Recognize Beck's triad (hypotension, JVD, muffled heart sounds) and pulsus paradoxus as tamponade physiology
- Perform bedside echocardiography and identify large pericardial effusion with RV diastolic collapse, RA compression, plethoric IVC, and electrical alternans on ECG
- Avoid intubation and positive pressure ventilation in tamponade unless absolutely necessary
- Perform ultrasound-guided pericardiocentesis using subxiphoid approach with real-time needle visualization — do not perform blind pericardiocentesis
- Monitor for procedural complications including RV perforation, pneumothorax, and arrhythmia
- Demonstrate clinical improvement after fluid removal and confirm with repeat echocardiography
- Initiate goals-of-care conversation in a patient with stage IV malignancy, addressing prognosis, code status, and palliative care referral
- Consult appropriate services: Cardiothoracic Surgery for pericardial window, Oncology for treatment planning

Difficulty Speaking

Opening Scenario

A 58-year-old right-handed woman is brought in by her husband because she suddenly stopped speaking and developed right-sided weakness at the breakfast table 50 minutes ago. He witnessed the onset at 08:10 and drove her straight in. You are working at a community hospital that administers thrombolytics but has no neurointerventional (thrombectomy) capability. The husband is at the bedside and able to give history.

Initial Assessment

Vitals: BP 196/104, HR 88 irregularly irregular, RR 16, SpO_2 98% RA, T 36.9°C, glucose 132

- Airway: Patent, handling secretions
- Breathing: Unlabored
- Circulation: Irregularly irregular rhythm on the monitor (atrial fibrillation)
- Disability: Awake, globally aphasic, follows no commands, leftward gaze deviation, dense right hemiparesis
- Exposure: No trauma

Immediate actions: Activate a stroke alert. Confirm the last-known-well time (08:10, witnessed), check point-of-care glucose, obtain IV access and an accurate weight, and move directly to noncontrast head CT with CT angiography of the head and neck. Perform the NIHSS en route or immediately after imaging. Door-to-imaging goal is under 20 minutes; door-to-needle goal is under 60 minutes.

History

- HPI (from the husband): Sudden onset of mutism and right-sided weakness at 08:10, witnessed, without seizure activity, head trauma, or preceding headache
- PMHx: Paroxysmal atrial fibrillation diagnosed last year and hypertension. She was prescribed apixaban but stopped taking it about three months ago because of cost. Ask specifically when the last dose of any anticoagulant was taken — a DOAC dose within 48 hours excludes thrombolysis; three months off therapy does not.
- Meds: Lisinopril (note: ACE inhibitor use is relevant if orolingual angioedema develops after thrombolysis)
- No recent surgery, GI bleeding, or prior intracranial hemorrhage; no prior stroke
- Allergies: NKDA

Physical Examination

- General: Anxious-appearing woman, awake, unable to speak
- Neurologic: NIHSS 18 — global aphasia, leftward gaze deviation, right homonymous hemianopia, right facial palsy, right arm and leg with no effort against gravity, right-sided sensory loss
- Cardiovascular: Irregularly irregular, no murmur; Lungs: clear

Diagnostic Studies

- Noncontrast head CT: No hemorrhage, no established infarct, hyperdense left MCA sign
- CTA head and neck: Left M1 middle cerebral artery occlusion with good collateral filling; no cervical dissection or high-grade stenosis
- Labs: Point-of-care glucose 132; CBC, BMP, INR/PTT, troponin sent — do not wait for results to treat unless coagulopathy is suspected
- ECG: Atrial fibrillation, rate-controlled, no acute ischemic changes

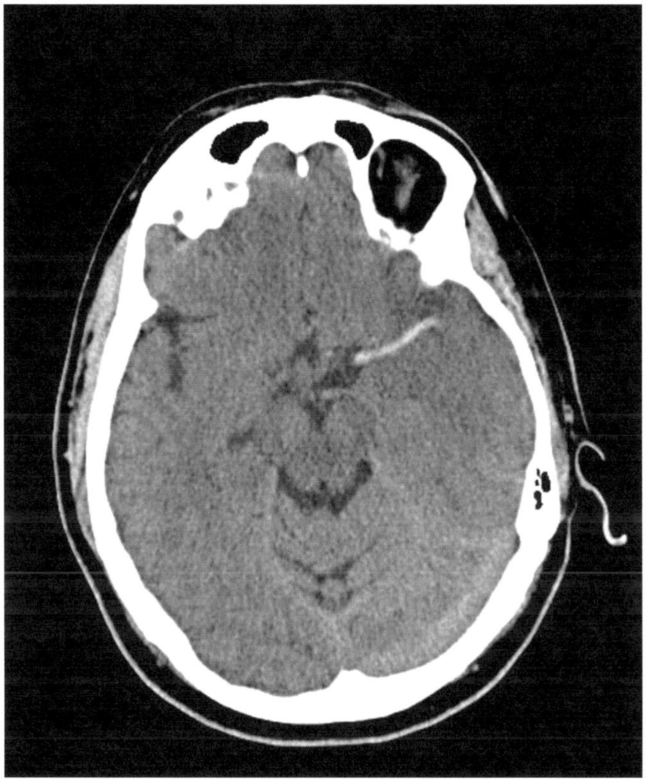

Management

- Lower the blood pressure below 185/110 before thrombolysis: labetalol 10–20 mg IV push, repeated, or a nicardipine infusion titrated to effect. Recheck and document the pressure before the bolus.
- Administer thrombolysis within the 4.5-hour window after verbally reviewing inclusion and exclusion criteria: tenecteplase 0.25 mg/kg IV bolus (maximum 25 mg) or alteplase 0.9 mg/kg (maximum 90 mg, 10% bolus then 60-minute infusion).
- Obtain emergency consent pragmatically: the patient is aphasic, so explain the risks (including a roughly 2–6% risk of symptomatic intracranial hemorrhage) and benefits to the husband, document the discussion, and do not delay treatment — thrombolysis is standard emergency care.
- Consult neurology (telestroke) in parallel. Neurology agrees with thrombolysis and, because she has a large-vessel occlusion with NIHSS 18, requests immediate transfer to the regional comprehensive stroke center for endovascular thrombectomy (intra-arterial clot retrieval).
- Initiate the transfer in parallel with thrombolysis ("drip and ship") — do not wait to observe a response to the lytic. Call the transfer center, arrange physician-to-physician acceptance with the neurointerventional team, and push the CT and CTA images electronically.
- Request a critical care transport team for post-thrombolytic monitoring en route (blood pressure and neuro checks every 15 minutes, nicardipine infusion capability). Door-in-door-out goal is under 60–90 minutes.

Reassessment

Twenty minutes after the tenecteplase bolus she squeezes with the right hand but remains aphasic with a dense hemiparesis (NIHSS 15), and her blood pressure rises to 204/108.

- Titrate the nicardipine infusion to keep the post-thrombolytic pressure below 180/105

- Recheck the airway, tongue, and lips for = angioedema (she takes an ACE inhibitor) — none is present
- Partial improvement does not cancel the thrombectomy: a persistent large-vessel occlusion with a disabling deficit still needs endovascular therapy — keep the transfer moving
- Hold all antiplatelet agents and anticoagulants for 24 hours after thrombolysis; her atrial fibrillation can be addressed after the acute period

Patient Communication

The husband asks, "You already gave the clot-busting drug — why does she still need to go somewhere else?" Explain in plain language: the medication alone reopens large blocked arteries in only a minority of cases; at the other hospital a specialist can thread a catheter to the clot and pull it out, which substantially improves the chance she will walk and talk again; the risks of transfer are far outweighed by the benefit; and the receiving team is already expecting her. Give him the destination, directions, and a realistic timeline, and let him see her before the transport team departs.

Disposition

Transfer emergently by critical care transport to the comprehensive stroke center for endovascular thrombectomy, with thrombolysis given, blood pressure controlled on a titratable infusion, images transmitted, records and a completed transfer form (risks, benefits, accepting physician) accompanying the patient, and a direct handoff to the accepting stroke team.

Critical Actions

- Establish the witnessed last-known-well time and check a point-of-care glucose
- Activate a stroke alert and obtain noncontrast CT plus CTA within door-to-imaging targets
- Perform and document an NIHSS
- Ask specifically about anticoagulant use and the timing of the last DOAC dose
- Lower the blood pressure below 185/110 with titratable agents before thrombolysis
- Administer tenecteplase or alteplase within the window after a documented risk–benefit discussion
- Identify the M1 occlusion on CTA and recognize endovascular thrombectomy candidacy
- Consult neurology and initiate the transfer in parallel with thrombolysis, not after it
- Arrange critical care transport with post-lytic blood pressure and neurologic monitoring and image transfer
- Maintain post-thrombolytic blood pressure below 180/105
- Communicate the rationale for transfer clearly to the family

Fever and Flank Pain in Pregnancy

Opening Scenario

A 26-year-old G1P0 woman at 26 weeks' gestation presents with two days of urinary frequency and burning, followed today by fever, shaking chills, right flank pain, and repeated vomiting. She has been unable to keep fluids down since last night. She has had routine prenatal care and an uncomplicated pregnancy. She is worried she is losing the baby.

Initial Assessment

Vitals: T 39.2°C, HR 122, BP 98/58, RR 22, SpO_2 97% RA

- Airway: Patent
- Breathing: Mildly tachypneic, lungs clear
- Circulation: Tachycardic, warm, mucous membranes dry
- Disability: Alert and oriented, uncomfortable
- Exposure: Gravid abdomen, right costovertebral angle tenderness

Immediate actions: Cardiac monitor, IV access, and a sepsis workup — lactate, blood cultures, urinalysis with culture — with intravenous crystalloid and antibiotics started within the first hour. Position her in the left lateral tilt, give an antipyretic, check fetal heart tones by Doppler early (150s, reassuring), and notify obstetrics of a septic patient at a viable gestational age.

History

- HPI: Two days of dysuria and frequency, now fever, rigors, right flank pain, and vomiting. Mild intermittent lower abdominal cramping. Normal fetal movement. No vaginal bleeding, fluid leakage, or contractions in a regular pattern.
- OB history: G1P0 at 26w2d by dating ultrasound; routine prenatal care; no infections or complications this pregnancy
- PMHx: None; Meds: Prenatal vitamins; Allergies: NKDA
- Physical Examination
- General: Ill-appearing, flushed, shivering
- Abdomen: Gravid, fundal height consistent with dates, mild diffuse tenderness without peritonitis; right costovertebral angle tenderness
- Lungs: Clear bilaterally — document a baseline, because pregnant patients with pyelonephritis are at particular risk of pulmonary edema and ARDS
- Fetal heart tones by Doppler: 155 beats per minute

Diagnostic Studies

- Urinalysis: Positive nitrites and leukocyte esterase, WBC too numerous to count, bacteriuria; urine culture sent
- Labs: WBC 18.4 with left shift, lactate 2.8, creatinine 0.9, potassium 3.3; blood cultures sent
- Renal ultrasound: Mild-to-moderate right hydronephrosis without a visualized stone — interpret in context, because mild right-sided hydronephrosis is a normal physiologic finding in late pregnancy and does not by itself indicate obstruction
- Continuous fetal monitoring and tocometry once obstetrics is at the bedside

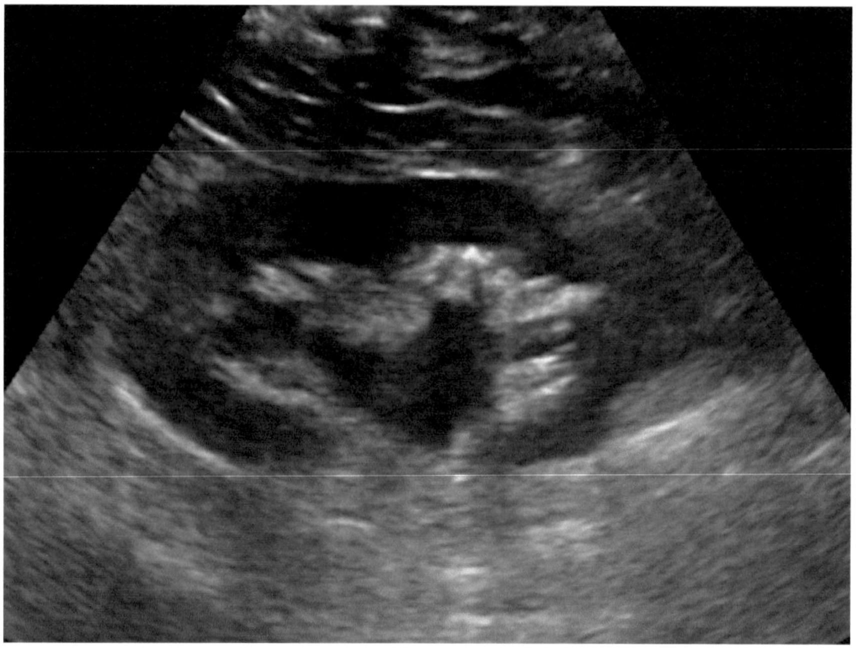

Management

- Give ceftriaxone 1 g IV (2 g is reasonable) within the first hour. Avoid fluoroquinolones and tetracyclines in pregnancy; nitrofurantoin and fosfomycin do not achieve adequate tissue levels for pyelonephritis.
- Resuscitate with crystalloid in weight-based boluses with frequent reassessment of the lungs and oxygen saturation — treat the sepsis, but do not volume-overload a patient at high risk of pulmonary edema
- Treat the fever aggressively with acetaminophen (maternal fever produces fetal tachycardia and distress) and control nausea (ondansetron or metoclopramide)
- Repeat the lactate and vital signs after the initial resuscitation

Reassessment

After two liters of lactated Ringer's and antibiotics: T 38.1°C, HR 104, BP 108/66, lactate 1.9. Fetal monitoring shows a reassuring tracing with occasional contractions, one to two per ten minutes, without a regular pattern. Obstetrics performs a cervical assessment: the cervix is closed and long. No tocolysis or steroids are indicated at this time, but she needs continued monitoring for preterm labor.

Managing Conflict

You call obstetrics to admit her. The obstetrician responds: "This is urosepsis — a medical problem. She should go to medicine or the ICU and we'll follow along." You call the medicine hospitalist, who responds: "She's 26 weeks and possibly contracting. She needs continuous fetal monitoring, and the only place that can do that is Labor and Delivery. This is an OB admission." Neither service will take her.

- Stay professional and keep the patient's needs at the center: she is a septic pregnant woman at a viable gestational age who needs IV antibiotics, sepsis monitoring, and continuous fetal monitoring — the last of which exists only on the antepartum/L&D unit
- Do not relay messages back and forth. Arrange a direct attending-to-attending conversation (a three-way call with you facilitating) so the two services talk to each other rather than through you.
- Offer the standard solution: pyelonephritis is among the most common non-obstetric reasons for antepartum admission, and the usual arrangement is admission to obstetrics/antepartum with medicine or infectious disease consultation for the sepsis

- Set escalation criteria everyone agrees on: worsening hemodynamics, rising lactate, or hypoxemia prompts ICU evaluation
- If the impasse persists, escalate through your chain of command (ED attending to department chair or chief medical officer) — but do not let the dispute delay antibiotics, monitoring, or nursing care, and do not board her without a plan. She remains your patient until she is admitted.
- After the two attendings speak directly, obstetrics admits her to the antepartum unit with internal medicine consulting on the sepsis.

Patient Communication

She asks whether the infection or the antibiotics will hurt the baby. Reassure her specifically: ceftriaxone is safe in pregnancy; treating the infection and the fever is protecting the baby; the baby's heart tracing is reassuring; and she will be on a unit where the baby is monitored continuously. Kidney infections are more serious in pregnancy, which is why she is being admitted rather than sent home on pills.

Disposition

Admit to the antepartum unit under obstetrics with medicine consultation, on IV ceftriaxone, with continuous fetal monitoring, serial lung examinations, and culture follow-up. Anticipate transition to oral therapy after 24–48 hours afebrile and suppressive therapy for the remainder of the pregnancy.

Critical Actions

- Recognize sepsis in pregnancy: lactate, blood and urine cultures, and antibiotics within the first hour
- Choose a pregnancy-safe antibiotic (ceftriaxone) and avoid fluoroquinolones
- Assess fetal well-being early (Doppler heart tones) and arrange continuous fetal monitoring at a viable gestational age
- Involve obstetrics early for a septic patient at 26 weeks
- Resuscitate with crystalloid while monitoring for pulmonary edema and ARDS, a particular risk of pyelonephritis in pregnancy
- Treat maternal fever and nausea
- Interpret right hydronephrosis in light of physiologic hydronephrosis of pregnancy
- Admit the patient — pyelonephritis in pregnancy is not managed as an outpatient
- Mediate the interservice dispute by facilitating a direct attending-to-attending conversation, proposing OB admission with medicine consultation, and escalating through the chain of command if needed
- Do not allow the admission dispute to delay antibiotics, monitoring, or disposition planning
- Monitor for preterm labor (tocometry and cervical assessment by obstetrics)

LVAD Alarm

Opening Scenario

A 61-year-old man with dilated cardiomyopathy and a continuous-flow left ventricular assist device implanted 14 months ago as destination therapy presents with three days of fatigue and exertional lightheadedness, and dark, tea-colored urine since this morning. His controller has been intermittently alarming "low flow." His wife, his trained device caregiver, is with him and has brought his backup controller and spare batteries. His LVAD was implanted at a tertiary center 90 miles away; your community hospital has cardiology coverage but no VAD program and no cardiothoracic surgery.

Initial Assessment

Vitals: No palpable pulse (expected with a continuous-flow device); Doppler opening (mean arterial) pressure 62 mmHg; HR 96 on the monitor, sinus; RR 18; SpO_2 unreliable due to low pulsatility, no cyanosis; T 37.1°C

- Airway: Patent
- Breathing: Unlabored, lungs clear
- Circulation: No palpable radial pulse — normal for the device; a steady pump hum is audible on precordial auscultation; extremities warm; capillary refill 3 seconds
- Disability: Alert, GCS 15
- Exposure: Driveline exit site clean, dry, and non-tender; controller displays a low-flow alarm with intermittent power spikes

Immediate actions: Cardiac monitor and ECG, IV access, assess perfusion with a Doppler MAP rather than a cuff, auscultate for the pump hum, examine the driveline site, interrogate the controller readings (flow, power, pulsatility), give a small crystalloid bolus (250–500 mL) for preload, send labs including a hemolysis panel, and call the patient's VAD coordinator at the implanting center immediately. Do not perform chest compressions on an awake, perfusing LVAD patient.

History

- HPI: Three days of fatigue and lightheadedness with exertion, now dark tea-colored urine. No fever, chest pain, melena, or driveline trauma.
- Device history (from the patient and wife): Baseline pump flow around 4.5 L/min; the controller now reads 2.8–3.2 L/min with intermittent power spikes. No recent speed changes.
- Meds: Warfarin and aspirin — but he has missed his warfarin for about a week because of an insurance lapse at the pharmacy
- PMHx: Dilated cardiomyopathy, atrial fibrillation, CKD stage 2
- Allergies: NKDA

Physical Examination

- General: Fatigued but conversant
- Cardiovascular: Continuous machine hum, no palpable pulse, mild jugular venous distension
- Lungs: Clear; Abdomen: soft, driveline exit site without erythema, induration, or discharge
- GU: Dark, tea-colored urine in the specimen container

Diagnostic Studies

- ECG: LVAD motor artifact with ventricular fibrillation (ventricular arrhythmias are both a cause and a consequence of low-flow states in LVAD patients)

- Labs: Hgb 11.2 (baseline 13), LDH 1,650 (baseline ~250; a value more than 2.5–3 times the upper limit of normal strongly suggests pump thrombosis), plasma free hemoglobin elevated, haptoglobin undetectable, creatinine 1.6 (baseline 1.0), potassium 4.8, INR 1.4 (goal 2–3)
- Urinalysis: Large blood on dipstick with few red cells microscopically — hemoglobinuria
- Bedside echocardiogram: Dilated, poorly decompressed left ventricle with the inflow cannula in place; no pericardial effusion

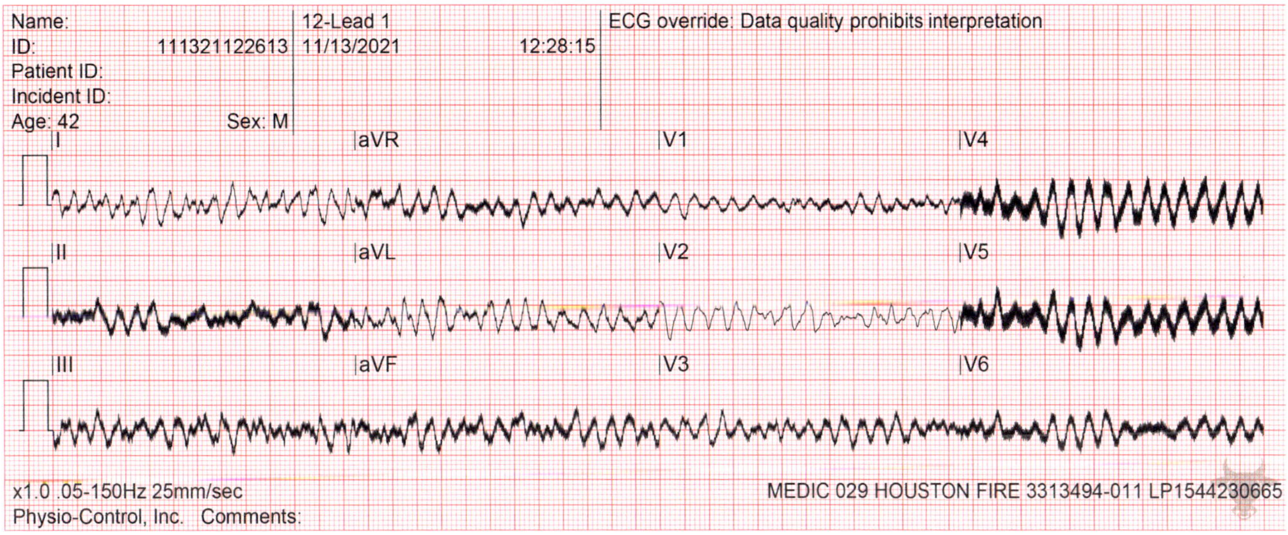

- Chest X-ray: Device components in expected position, clear lungs

Working diagnosis: LVAD pump thrombosis with intravascular hemolysis, precipitated by a week of subtherapeutic anticoagulation.

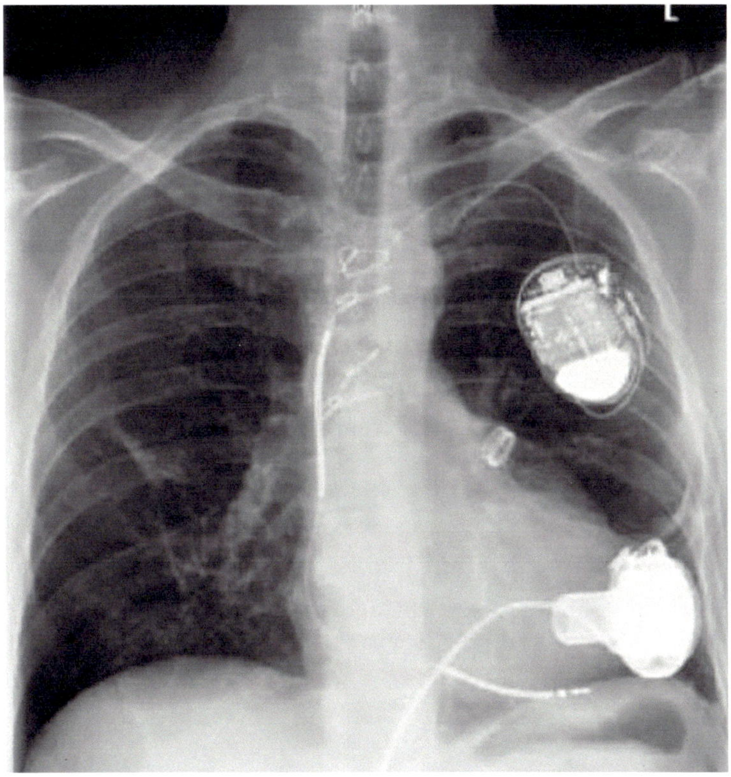

Management

- Keep the VAD coordinator and the implanting center's advanced heart failure team on the line and involve them in every device decision. Do not change pump speed except at their direction.
- Start intravenous unfractionated heparin (bolus and infusion) in consultation with the VAD team to limit thrombus propagation
- Optimize preload gently and avoid hypotension; recheck the Doppler MAP after each intervention (target roughly 70–90 mmHg)
- Type and screen; send blood cultures only if infection is suspected (the driveline site is clean and he is afebrile)
- Keep the backup controller, spare batteries, and power module physically with the patient at all times

Managing Conflict

The implanting center accepts the patient for possible pump exchange. The local EMS crew that responds for the interfacility transfer is uncomfortable: "We've never transported a VAD. He has no pulse and no blood pressure we can measure — our protocols don't cover this device, and 90 miles is a long way." Their concern is legitimate; do not pressure an untrained crew into transporting a patient with a failing pump, and do not let the transfer stall.

- Call the regional transfer center and request a dedicated critical care transport team (ground critical care or helicopter) with a nurse/paramedic crew, infusion capability for the heparin, and Doppler or arterial MAP monitoring
- Ask specifically for VAD-trained personnel, or arrange real-time telephone access to the VAD coordinator for the transport team en route
- When the transfer center offers a basic ambulance in three hours, escalate: state the clinical urgency plainly — pump thrombosis can progress to complete pump failure, refractory heart failure, or stroke — and request air medical transport if ground critical care is unavailable; ask the implanting center whether their own retrieval team can respond
- Confirm the backup controller, charged spare batteries, and power module travel with the patient, and that his trained caregiver accompanies him if the service allows
- Complete the transfer properly: named accepting physician, physician-to-physician handoff, copies of the ECG, labs, echocardiogram, and the controller's displayed parameters, and documentation that the benefits of transfer outweigh the risks

Reassessment

While awaiting the critical care team, he becomes more fatigued and the Doppler MAP falls to 58 mmHg. Give another small crystalloid bolus and reassess — the MAP improves to 66 mmHg and his mentation remains normal. Discuss inotropic support (dobutamine) with the VAD team should he deteriorate further; if he loses responsiveness and the pump stops, confirm true arrest before beginning chest compressions, and only per the VAD team's guidance. The heparin infusion is running, and repeat labs are drawn for the receiving team.

Patient Communication

The patient is anxious about being far from his family, and his wife is afraid the batteries will die on the road. Address both concretely: the spare batteries and power module travel with him, the transport team can run the device off its own power supply, his wife may follow (or accompany him if the service permits), and the team taking him is trained in critical care with his VAD team on the phone the entire way. Explain why the implanting center is the right place: the surgeons who know his pump can exchange it if needed.

Disposition

Emergent transfer by critical care transport to the implanting tertiary center's advanced heart failure service for management of pump thrombosis, on a heparin infusion, with device equipment and trained caregiver accompanying, and complete records and direct physician handoff.

Critical Actions

- Recognize that an absent palpable pulse and unreliable cuff pressures are expected with a continuous-flow LVAD; obtain a Doppler MAP
- Auscultate for the pump hum and interrogate the controller alarms and parameters
- Examine the driveline exit site
- Contact the VAD coordinator and implanting center early and involve them in every device decision
- Send a hemolysis panel (LDH, plasma free hemoglobin, haptoglobin, urinalysis) and recognize the pump thrombosis picture
- Identify subtherapeutic anticoagulation as the precipitant and start IV heparin in consultation with the VAD team
- Do not perform chest compressions on a perfusing LVAD patient
- Recognize the EMS crew's legitimate limitations and secure critical care transport rather than pressuring an untrained crew or accepting an unsafe delay
- Ensure the backup controller, batteries, and power module travel with the patient
- Complete an appropriate interfacility transfer: accepting physician, physician-to-physician handoff, records and images sent
- Reassess perfusion (Doppler MAP, mentation, urine output) while awaiting transport and respond to deterioration

PROCEDURES

Airway Techniques

Endotracheal Intubation — Direct and Video-Assisted Laryngoscopy

Indications:

- Failure to maintain or protect the airway (depressed mental status, absent gag with vomiting, airway edema or burns, expanding neck hematoma)
- Failure of oxygenation or ventilation despite noninvasive support
- Anticipated clinical deterioration requiring a secured airway (transport, combativeness with critical illness, progressive airway compromise)

Contraindications:

- No absolute contraindications in a patient who needs an emergency airway
- Relative: anticipated impossible laryngoscopy where an awake technique or primary surgical airway is safer (severe airway distortion, fixed cervical flexion)
- Total upper airway obstruction or transected trachea favors a surgical airway from the outset

Steps:

1. Perform pre-procedure timeout and confirm indication; assess for difficult airway predictors (LEMON or HEAVEN criteria)
2. Prepare equipment: laryngoscope handle with appropriate blade (Macintosh Miller 2-4 or video device), endotracheal tube (ETT) 7.0-8.0 mm ID for adult females, 8.0-8.5 mm for males, stylet shaped to 35-degree angle, 10 mL syringe, suction catheter (Yankauer and flexible), bag-valve-mask (BVM) with PEEP valve, capnography, and backup airway devices (LMA, bougie, scalpel)
3. Pre-oxygenate with 100% oxygen for 3 minutes or 8 vital capacity breaths; apply nasal cannula at 15 L/min for apneic oxygenation during intubation
4. Position patient in sniffing position: elevate head 8-10 cm and align external auditory meatus with sternal notch; use ramping for obese patients
5. Decide on intubation strategy: rapid sequence intubation (RSI) vs. awake intubation; ensure aspiration risk assessment complete
6. Induction: etomidate 0.3 mg/kg IV or ketamine 1-2 mg/kg IV or propofol 1.5-2.5 mg/kg IV
7. Paralysis: succinylcholine 1.5 mg/kg IV or rocuronium 1.2 mg/kg IV (dose 1.2 mg/kg if using for RSI to ensure rapid onset)
8. Wait 45 seconds (succinylcholine) or 60 seconds (rocuronium 1.2 mg/kg) for optimal intubating conditions
9. Perform laryngoscopy: hold scope in left hand, insert blade right side of mouth, sweep tongue left, advance to epiglottis or vallecula depending on blade type
10. Visualize vocal cords (Cormack-Lehane grade I or II); external laryngeal manipulation (BURP maneuver) if needed
11. Insert ETT from right side of mouth; pass through cords to 22 cm at lips for females, 23 cm for males (adjust for height: height in cm/10 + 3 for nasal intubation)
12. Inflate cuff to 20-30 cm H2O pressure (minimum occluding volume)
13. Confirm placement: continuous quantitative waveform capnography (gold standard), auscultate bilateral breath sounds and absent epigastric sounds, rising SpO_2, misting of tube, and chest rise
14. Secure ETT with adhesive tape or commercial holder; mark depth at teeth/lips
15. Order post-intubation chest X-ray to confirm tip position 3-5 cm above carina
16. Initiate post-intubation sedation (propofol infusion or dexmedetomidine) and analgesia (fentanyl); maintain paralysis if indicated

17. Document intubation time, attempts, Cormack-Lehane grade, and any complications

Airway Adjuncts — Laryngeal Mask Airway (LMA)

Indications:

- Rescue oxygenation after failed intubation attempts (a can't-intubate, can-oxygenate bridge)
- Primary airway during cardiac arrest when intubation is not immediately achievable
- Bridge device while preparing for a surgical airway or fiberoptic technique

Contraindications:

- Intact gag reflex or responsive patient
- High aspiration risk (active vomiting, massive hemorrhage) — the LMA does not protect the airway
- Upper airway obstruction at or below the glottis (the LMA sits above the obstruction and will not bypass it)
- Severely limited mouth opening

Steps:

1. Select appropriate size: Size 3 for 30-50 kg, Size 4 for 50-70 kg, Size 5 for 70-100 kg
2. Check cuff integrity by inflating with maximum recommended air volume (Size 3: 20 mL, Size 4: 30 mL, Size 5: 40 mL) then deflate completely leaving slight roundness
3. Lubricate posterior surface with water-soluble gel sparingly to avoid cuff obstruction
4. Position patient supine with head extended and neck flexed (sniffing position)
5. Hold LMA like a pen; press mask tip against hard palate
6. Advance following palate curvature with index finger until resistance encountered at hypopharynx
7. Inflate cuff with appropriate volume; do not overinflate
8. Remove hand without pushing LMA deeper
9. Confirm position: chest rise, bilateral breath sounds, capnography waveform, and minimal leak at 20 cm H_2O ventilation pressure
10. Secure with tape or dedicated holder; mark insertion depth

Surgical Airway — Cricothyrotomy

Indications:

- Can't intubate, can't oxygenate after failed maximal attempts at intubation and rescue ventilation
- Complete upper airway obstruction (foreign body, angioedema, mass, trauma) not bypassable from above
- Massive facial or oropharyngeal trauma or hemorrhage precluding laryngoscopy

Contraindications:

- No absolute contraindications when it is the only route to oxygenation
- Relative: age under approximately 10–12 years (needle cricothyrotomy with jet oxygenation preferred)
- Relative: laryngotracheal disruption or fracture (may require tracheostomy below the injury)
- Relative: distorted anterior neck anatomy (hematoma, tumor, prior surgery, obesity) — proceed, but anticipate difficulty

Steps:

1. Identify CICV (Can't Intubate, Can't Ventilate) situation; ensure failed facemask ventilation and failed intubation attempts
2. Position patient supine with neck extended; hyperextend if no cervical spine concern
3. Palpate landmarks: thyroid cartilage, cricoid cartilage, cricothyroid membrane (depression between)

4. Clean neck with antiseptic; infiltrate local anesthetic with epinephrine if patient conscious
5. Stabilize larynx with non-dominant hand between thumb and fingers
6. Make vertical midline incision 3-4 cm over cricothyroid membrane through skin and subcutaneous tissue
7. Make horizontal stab incision through cricothyroid membrane; keep blade perpendicular to skin
8. Rotate blade 90 degrees or use dilator to open membrane
9. Insert tracheal hook to stabilize inferior aspect of thyroid cartilage; lift upward
10. Insert bougie through incision into trachea directed caudally
11. Railroad 6.0 cuffed ETT or tracheostomy tube (size 6 Shiley) over bougie into trachea
12. Remove bougie; inflate cuff
13. Confirm placement with capnography and bilateral breath sounds
14. Secure tube; obtain chest X-ray

Non-Invasive Ventilatory Management

CPAP/BiPAP

Indications:

- Acute cardiogenic pulmonary edema
- COPD exacerbation with hypercapnic respiratory failure
- Hypoxemic respiratory failure in an awake, cooperative patient (including immunocompromised patients, to avoid intubation)
- Preoxygenation before intubation in the hypoxemic patient

Contraindications:

- Apnea, respiratory arrest, or need for immediate intubation
- Depressed mental status or inability to protect the airway
- Active vomiting, upper GI bleeding, or high aspiration risk
- Facial trauma, burns, or deformity preventing mask seal
- Untreated pneumothorax
- Hemodynamic instability or life-threatening arrhythmia

Steps:

1. Assess indication: COPD exacerbation, pulmonary edema, hypoxemic respiratory failure without impending respiratory arrest
2. Ensure hemodynamic stability; exclude contraindications (facial trauma, vomiting, inability to protect airway, hemodynamic instability)
3. Select interface: nasal mask vs. oronasal mask vs. full face mask; check fit without leaks
4. Initiate settings: CPAP 5-10 cm H2O or BiPAP IPAP 10-15 cm H2O, EPAP 5 cm H2O
5. Titrate: increase IPAP by 2 cm H2O every 5 minutes to achieve tidal volume 6-8 mL/kg and respiratory rate <25
6. Monitor SpO_2, respiratory rate, accessory muscle use, mental status, and blood gases
7. Check for gastric insufflation; consider nasogastric tube decompression if needed

High Flow Nasal Cannula (HFNC)

Indications:

- Hypoxemic respiratory failure (pneumonia, bronchiolitis) in a spontaneously breathing patient
- Preoxygenation and apneic oxygenation during intubation

- Patients intolerant of a noninvasive ventilation mask
- Support in patients with do-not-intubate goals of care

Contraindications:

- Apnea or need for immediate intubation
- Inability to protect the airway
- Complete nasal obstruction; severe midface trauma or recent skull base fracture (relative)
- It provides no meaningful ventilatory support — do not rely on it in primarily hypercapnic failure

Steps:

1. Set flow rate: start at 30-40 L/min, titrate to 60 L/min based on comfort and oxygenation
2. Set FiO2: blend to target SpO_2 88-92% (COPD) or 94-96% (other conditions)
3. Set temperature: 37°C (body temperature)
4. Ensure humidification chamber filled with sterile water
5. Assess work of breathing and oxygenation within 15-30 minutes; failure to improve suggests need for intubation

Bag Valve Mask Ventilation

Indications:

- Apnea or hypoventilation from any cause
- Rescue ventilation during and between intubation attempts
- Cardiac arrest
- Preoxygenation when spontaneous effort is inadequate

Contraindications:

- No absolute contraindications in the apneic patient
- Relative: unrepaired facial trauma preventing a seal, suspected active vomiting (suction first), and gastric insufflation with prolonged ventilation — use two-person technique, an airway adjunct, and slow, low-volume breaths

Steps:

1. Select appropriate mask size: bridge of nose to mentum of mandible
2. Position patient: ear-to-sternal notch alignment; jaw thrust or chin lift
3. Create seal using C-E technique: thumb and index finger form "C" on mask, remaining fingers form "E" under mandible (not under soft tissue)
4. Two-person technique recommended: one person secures mask with two hands performing jaw thrust, second person squeezes bag
5. Deliver tidal volume 6-7 mL/kg over 1 second at rate 10-12/minute; observe chest rise
6. Attach PEEP valve (10 cm H2O) if available
7. Use oropharyngeal or nasopharyngeal airway if obstruction persists

Procedural Sedation

Indications:

- Painful or anxiety-provoking procedures requiring analgesia, anxiolysis, or motion control (reductions, cardioversion, complex laceration repair, abscess drainage, imaging in children)

Contraindications:

- No absolute contraindications; risk is stratified and mitigated
- Relative: high aspiration risk (recent meal is not an absolute bar for emergency procedures — weigh urgency, depth, and agent)
- Relative: anticipated difficult airway or ASA class III or higher — consider location, backup, and agent choice
- Relative: hemodynamic instability — choose agents accordingly (ketamine, etomidate) and correct volume status first when possible

Steps:

1. Pre-sedation assessment: ASA classification, airway evaluation (Mallampati, thyromental distance), fasting status (2 hours clear liquids, 4 hours breast milk, 6 hours light meal, 8 hours fatty meal)
2. Obtain informed consent; ensure NPO status documented
3. Establish IV access; ensure continuous monitoring (ECG, pulse oximetry, non-invasive blood pressure, capnography)
4. Pre-oxygenate with 100% oxygen; ensure suction, airway equipment, and reversal agents (naloxone, flumazenil) immediately available
5. Ketamine: 1-2 mg/kg IV push over 60 seconds or 4-5 mg/kg IM; maintain with 0.5 mg/kg IV q10-15min
6. Propofol: 1-2 mg/kg IV bolus followed by 0.5 mg/kg q2-3 minutes as needed
7. Etomidate: 0.1-0.2 mg/kg IV for brief procedures (CT scans)
8. Midazolam/Fentanyl: Midazolam 0.05 mg/kg IV (max 4 mg) plus Fentanyl 1-2 mcg/kg IV (max 100 mcg)
9. Monitor for respiratory depression, hypoxia, apnea, and laryngospasm; maintain verbal contact with patient
10. Document vital signs every 5 minutes and level of sedation (Observer's Assessment of Alertness/ Sedation scale)
11. Recovery: patient awake, protective reflexes intact, able to maintain airway, hemodynamically stable; Aldrete score ≥9
12. Discharge criteria: return to baseline mental status, tolerating oral intake (if required), responsible adult present for transport

Vascular Access

Arterial Line Placement

Indications

- Continuous blood pressure monitoring in shock, on vasoactive infusions, or during controlled blood pressure titration (e.g., ICH, aortic dissection)
- Frequent arterial blood gas sampling (ventilated patients, severe acid-base disturbances)
- Unreliable noninvasive pressures (obesity, arrhythmia, LVAD)

Contraindications

- Absent collateral circulation to the distal limb (e.g., abnormal perfusion assessment) — choose another site
- Infection, burn, or vascular graft at the insertion site
- Severe peripheral vascular disease or prior surgery compromising the vessel (relative)
- Coagulopathy is a relative contraindication at compressible sites (radial preferred over femoral)

Steps:

1. Select site: radial artery (preferred), dorsalis pedis, femoral, or brachial; Allen's test mandatory for radial approach (<5 seconds return is normal)
2. Prepare sterile field; use full sterile barrier
3. Anesthetize skin and periarterial tissue with 1% lidocaine
4. Palpate artery with non-dominant hand; keep fingers on either side to guide but do not compress
5. Insert 20-gauge arterial catheter at 30-45 degree angle until flashback observed
6. Advance catheter while withdrawing needle; if resistance met, withdraw slightly and advance again
7. Confirm pulsatile blood return; attach pressure tubing primed with heparinized saline
8. Connect to transducer zeroed at phlebostatic axis (4th intercostal space, mid-axillary line)
9. Secure with suture or arterial line device; apply transparent dressing
10. Check waveform and confirm arterial pressure tracing distinct from venous

Central Venous Catheterization

Indications

- Vasopressor or caustic infusions requiring central delivery
- Inadequate peripheral access after reasonable attempts (including ultrasound-guided peripheral and IO alternatives)
- Specific therapies: transvenous pacing, emergent dialysis catheter, massive transfusion with inadequate access, central venous monitoring

Contraindications

- No absolute contraindications in an emergency; site selection mitigates risk
- Relative: infection, burn, or distorted anatomy at the chosen site — pick another
- Relative: severe coagulopathy — prefer a compressible site (femoral or ultrasound-guided IJ over subclavian)
- Relative: contralateral pneumothorax risk (avoid subclavian opposite an existing chest injury); thrombus at the target vein

Steps:

1. Select site: internal jugular (preferred for ultrasound), subclavian (lowest infection risk), or femoral

2. Ultrasound guidance recommended for IJ and femoral; identify vein (compressible, non-pulsatile) vs. artery
3. Position patient: Trendelenburg 15 degrees for IJ, supine for femoral, 15-20 degrees Trendelenburg with towel roll under spine for subclavian
4. Full sterile prep: chlorhexidine scrub, sterile drapes, mask, cap, sterile gown and gloves
5. Local anesthetic: 1% lidocaine with 25-gauge needle
6. Micropuncture technique or standard Seldinger:
7. IJ: apex of triangle between sternal and clavicular heads of sternocleidomastoid, lateral to carotid, 45-degree angle toward ipsilateral nipple
8. Subclavian: 1 cm inferior to clavicle at junction of middle and medial thirds, needle directed toward sternal notch
9. Femoral: 1-2 cm medial to femoral artery, 45-degree angle cephalad
10. Advance needle while aspirating; observe for venous return (dark, non-pulsatile)
11. Remove syringe; insert guidewire through needle; never let go of wire
12. Confirm wire position: should pass easily without resistance; ECG monitoring for arrhythmias
13. Remove needle; make skin nick with scalpel
14. Pass dilator over wire with gentle twisting motion; remove dilator
15. Pass catheter (triple lumen or introducer) over wire; remove wire when tip visible at hub
16. Aspirate and flush all ports
17. Suture catheter; apply sterile dressing
18. Confirm placement: chest X-ray for IJ/subclavian (tip at cavoatrial junction, superior vena cava); ultrasound or pressure transducer for femoral

Intraosseous Line Placement

Indications:

- Emergency vascular access when peripheral IV attempts fail or would cause unacceptable delay (arrest, shock, status epilepticus) in adults or children

Contraindications:

- Fracture of the target bone or vascular injury proximal to the site
- Previous IO attempt in the same bone (extravasation risk)
- Infection or burn overlying the insertion site
- Bone disease at the site (osteogenesis imperfecta, tumor) and inability to identify landmarks (relative)

Steps:

1. Select site: proximal tibia (2 cm medial and 1 cm proximal to tibial tuberosity), distal tibia (2 cm proximal to medial malleolus), or humeral head (greater tubercle)
2. Use EZ-IO device or manual Jamshidi needle; select appropriate needle length based on patient habitus
3. Clean site with antiseptic; local anesthetic if conscious (2% lidocaine without epinephrine)
4. Needle perpendicular to bone surface (90 degrees)
5. Advance with firm pressure and twisting motion until decrease in resistance ("pop" or give) felt
6. Remove stylet; confirm position: needle stands upright without support, flushable without extravasation, fluids flow freely under gravity
7. If conscious patient, infuse 2% lidocaine 0.5 mg/kg (max 50 mg) slowly through IO before fluid bolus to reduce pain
8. Secure with commercial device or gauze and tape; immobilize extremity

9. Label as IO access; all medications/fluids safe via IO route

Umbilical Vessel Catheterization

Indications

- Emergency vascular access in the neonate (generally under 7–14 days of life) for resuscitation medications, fluids, and blood sampling when peripheral access fails or during active resuscitation

Contraindications

- Omphalitis (infected cord or periumbilical tissue)
- Abdominal wall defects involving the cord (omphalocele, gastroschisis)
- Peritonitis or necrotizing enterocolitis
- Vascular compromise of the lower limbs or buttocks (for arterial catheters)

Steps:

1. Prepare umbilical cord: sterile field, sterile gloves, povidone-iodine prep of umbilical stump and 5 cm surrounding skin
2. Identify vessels: two thick-walled arteries (arise from internal iliacs) and one thin-walled vein (single lumen, larger)
3. Measure catheter length:
4. UVC: shoulder to umbilicus distance plus 2 cm, or (birth weight in kg × 3) + 9 cm + umbilical stump length; tip should be at T8-T9 (just above diaphragm, below LA)
5. UAC: (birth weight in kg × 4) + 10 cm; high position T6-T9, low position L3-L4 (below L3 to avoid mesenteric artery)
6. Cut cord with scalpel 1-2 cm from base to expose vessels; place umbilical tape around base to prevent bleeding
7. Grasp artery with fine forceps; gently dilate vessel with curved hemostat or dilator
8. Advance catheter (3.5 Fr for <1.5 kg, 5 Fr for >1.5 kg) until measured length; should meet resistance at 2-3 cm if in artery
9. Confirm position: aspiration of blood (venous blood darker, arterial pulsatile), X-ray for tip location
10. Secure with suture or umbilical tie; apply sterile dressing

Regional Anesthesia

Contraindications common to all of the blocks below:

- Patient refusal
- Allergy to the local anesthetic class
- Infection or cellulitis over the injection site
- Inability to cooperate with the block.

Document a neurovascular examination before every block.
Where a specific concern exists it is listed with the individual block.

Hematoma Block

Indications:

- Analgesia for closed fracture reduction (classically distal radius) when procedural sedation is undesirable or unavailable

Contraindications:

- Open fracture or skin compromise over the fracture site
- Injury at high risk for compartment syndrome (the block can mask evolving symptoms)
- Overlying infection; significant coagulopathy is a relative concern

Steps:

1. Identify fracture site radiographically; locate point of maximal displacement
2. Sterile prep of skin over fracture site
3. Insert 18-22 gauge needle into fracture hematoma; confirm position by aspirating blood
4. Inject 10-20 mL of 1% lidocaine or 0.25% bupivacaine (without epinephrine) into hematoma cavity
5. Wait 5-10 minutes for anesthesia before manipulation

Penile Block (Dorsal Penile Nerve)

Indications

- Analgesia for paraphimosis reduction, dorsal slit, laceration repair, or release of entrapped skin (e.g., zipper injury)

Contraindications

- Infection at the injection site
- Do not use epinephrine-containing anesthetic
- Coagulopathy is a relative concern

Ultrasound-Guided Technique

1. Position the patient supine with the penis in anatomical position; perform sterile preparation with chlorhexidine or povidone-iodine.
2. Select a high-frequency linear probe (15—6 MHz); apply sterile gel and place the probe in a transverse orientation on the dorsal aspect of the penile shaft at the mid-shaft level.
3. Identify the midline septum (appearing as a hyperechoic line), paired dorsal arteries (lateral to midline, pulsatile with color Doppler), the dorsal vein (midline, compressible), and the paired dorsal nerves (lateral to the arteries at approximately the 11 and 1 o'clock positions).
4. Visualize Buck's fascia (deep hyperechoic line surrounding neurovascular bundle) and ensure differentiation from the superficial Dartos fascia.
5. Choose an in-plane approach from the ventral aspect (avoiding the urethra) or an out-of-plane approach from the dorsal aspect; insert a 25—27 gauge needle.
6. Advance the needle tip to penetrate Buck's fascia lateral to the midline septum, targeting the potential space deep to Buck's fascia but superficial to the tunica albuginea.
7. Aspirate to confirm extravascular placement; inject 2—5 mL of local anesthetic (1% lidocaine or 0.25% bupivacaine without epinephrine) per side, observing hydrodissection beneath Buck's fascia and spread around the neurovascular bundle.
8. Repeat on the contralateral side; optional ventral midline injection subcutaneously to block the perineal nerves.
9. Monitor for vascular injection (color Doppler) and ensure no intrafascicular injection (high resistance to injection).

Landmark-Based (Blind) Technique

1. Position the patient supine. Prep the base of the penis with antiseptic.
2. Palpate the symphysis pubis and identify the dorsal base of the penis at its junction with the pubic arch.
3. At the 10—11 o'clock and 1—2 o'clock positions at the base of the penis (just below the pubic symphysis), insert a 25—27 gauge needle perpendicular to the skin, angling slightly caudally.
4. Advance through the skin and Dartos fascia until a subtle "pop" or loss of resistance is felt as the needle penetrates Buck's fascia (typically 3—5 mm depth in adults).
5. Aspirate to confirm extravascular placement. Inject 2—5 mL of local anesthetic (1% lidocaine or 0.25% bupivacaine WITHOUT epinephrine) per side.
6. Repeat on the contralateral side. For complete anesthesia, add a subcutaneous ventral midline ring block at the base of the penis (1—3 mL) to cover perineal nerve branches (frenular innervation).

Penile Block — Cross-Sectional Anatomy

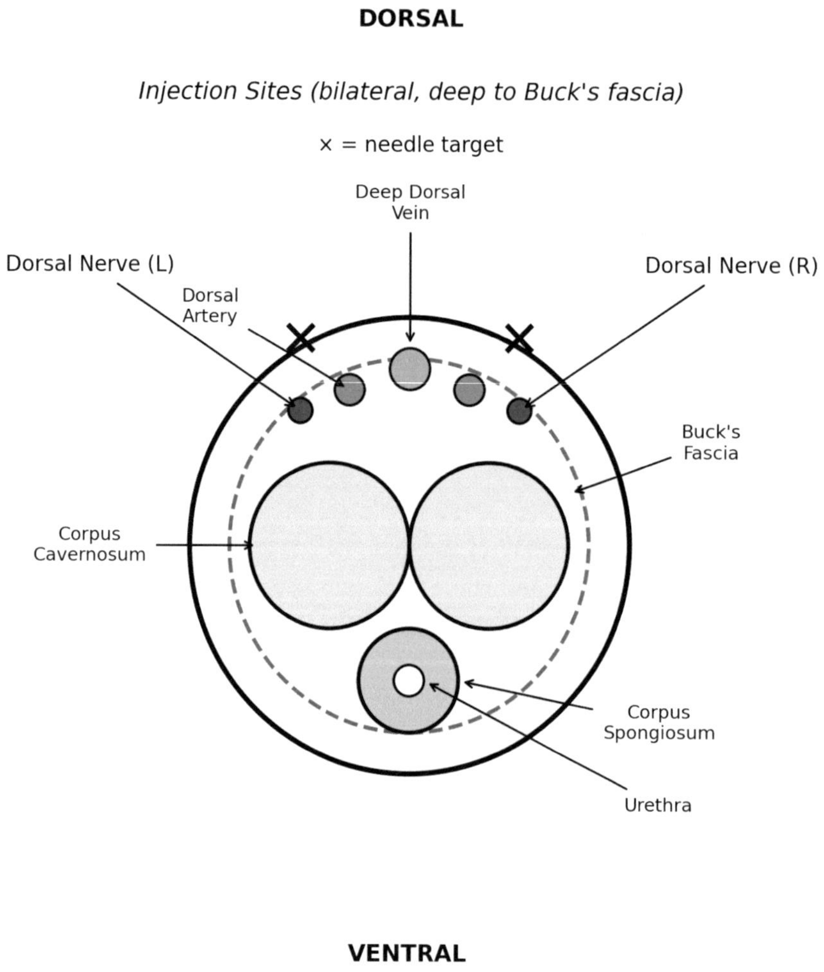

Supraorbital Nerve Block

Indications

- Anesthesia of the forehead and anterior scalp for laceration repair or wound care when local infiltration would distort tissue or require large volumes

Contraindications

- No absolute contraindications beyond those common to all blocks (site infection, anesthetic allergy, patient refusal).

Ultrasound-Guided Technique

1. Position the patient supine or semi-upright; prep the skin over the supraorbital ridge.
2. Select a high-frequency linear probe (15—8 MHz); place in a transverse orientation over the supraorbital margin at the junction of the medial one-third and lateral two-thirds.
3. Identify the supraorbital foramen (notch) as a bony discontinuity in the hyperechoic orbital rim; locate the supraorbital artery with color Doppler (medial to the nerve).
4. Visualize the supraorbital nerve exiting the foramen and coursing superiorly in the subcutaneous tissue (hyperechoic fibrillar structure).
5. Insert a 25—27 gauge needle using an in-plane approach from inferior to superior or out-of-plane from medial to lateral.
6. Target the perineural space at the level of the supraorbital notch; aspirate prior to injection.
7. Inject 1—3 mL of local anesthetic (1% lidocaine or 0.25% bupivacaine) observing spread around the nerve and into the foramen; avoid injection into the foramen itself to prevent bone pain.
8. Apply gentle pressure to prevent hematoma formation from the supraorbital artery.

Landmark-Based (Blind) Technique

1. With the patient looking straight ahead, draw an imaginary vertical line from the medial limbus (or pupil) superiorly to the supraorbital rim.
2. Palpate the supraorbital notch (or foramen) along the supraorbital rim at this point, approximately 2.5—2.7 cm from the midline. The patient will often feel tenderness or a tingling sensation confirming the nerve location.
3. Insert a 25—27 gauge needle perpendicular to the skin at the level of the supraorbital notch, directed toward the notch from just below the brow.
4. Aspirate and inject 1—2 mL of local anesthetic at the notch, fanning medially and laterally to ensure coverage of both the supraorbital and supratrochlear nerves (the supratrochlear nerve exits approximately 1 cm medial to the supraorbital notch).
5. Apply pressure for 2—3 minutes to minimize ecchymosis. Confirm anesthesia of the ipsilateral forehead to the vertex.

Supraorbital Nerve Block — Anatomy

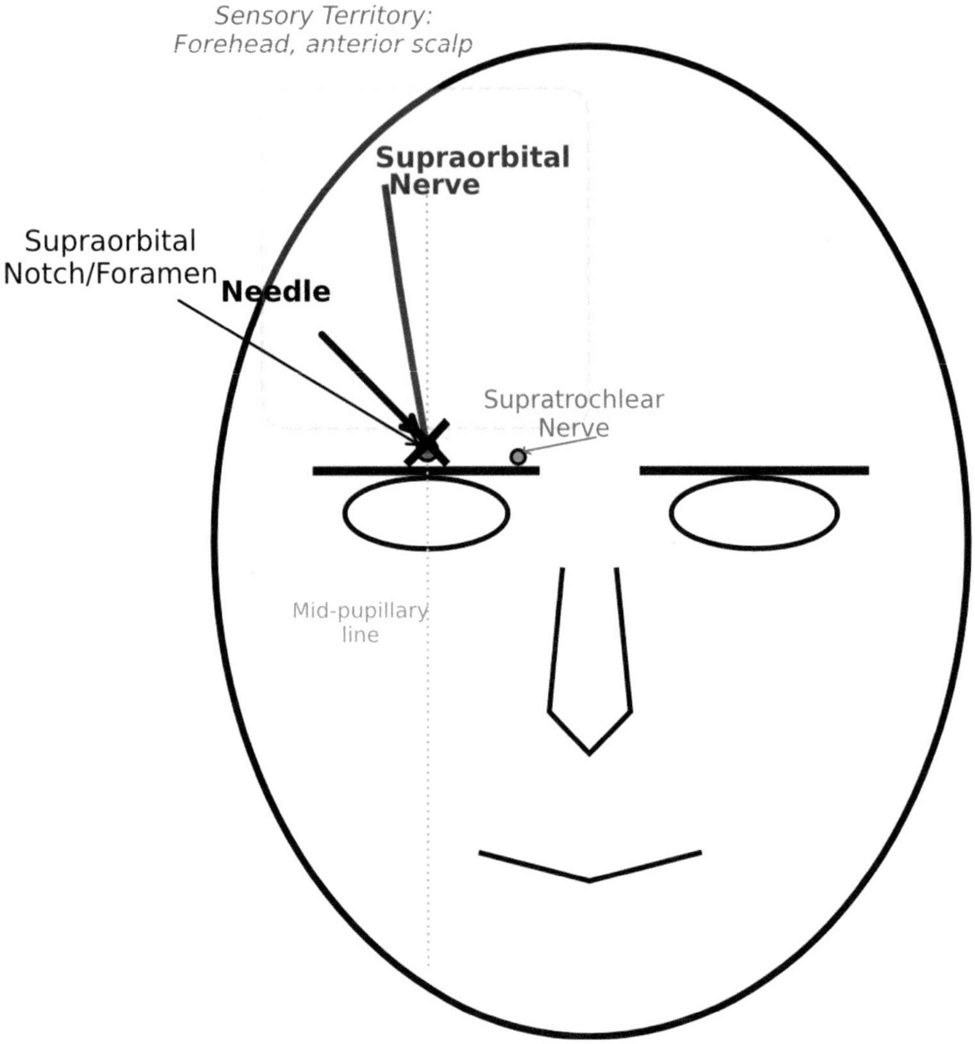

Infraorbital Nerve Block

Indications

- Anesthesia of the midface — lower eyelid, lateral nose, upper lip — for laceration repair, especially the vermilion border, where infiltration would distort landmarks

Contraindications

- No absolute contraindications beyond those common to all blocks.

Extraoral Approach

1. Palpate the infraorbital rim. The infraorbital foramen lies approximately 1 cm inferior to the infraorbital rim along the mid-pupillary line (with the patient looking straight ahead), or in line with the second premolar tooth.
2. Palpate the foramen directly — it is often felt as a subtle depression in the maxilla, and pressure over it will reproduce paresthesia in the nerve distribution.
3. Insert a 25—27 gauge needle perpendicular to the skin, directed slightly superiorly and laterally toward the foramen. Do not advance the needle into the canal.
4. Aspirate; inject 1—2 mL of local anesthetic at the foramen opening. Gently massage to promote spread into the canal.

Intraoral Approach

1. Retract the upper lip. Palpate the infraorbital foramen extraorally with the non-dominant hand to serve as a target.
2. Insert the needle through the buccal mucosa at the superior gingivobuccal sulcus above the second premolar, directing the needle superiorly toward the palpating finger over the foramen.
3. Advance approximately 1.5—2.5 cm until the needle tip is felt near the foramen (the palpating finger should feel the needle approaching). Do not enter the foramen.
4. Aspirate; inject 1—2 mL of anesthetic. Confirm anesthesia of the ipsilateral lower eyelid, lateral nose, and upper lip.

Infraorbital Nerve Block — Anatomy

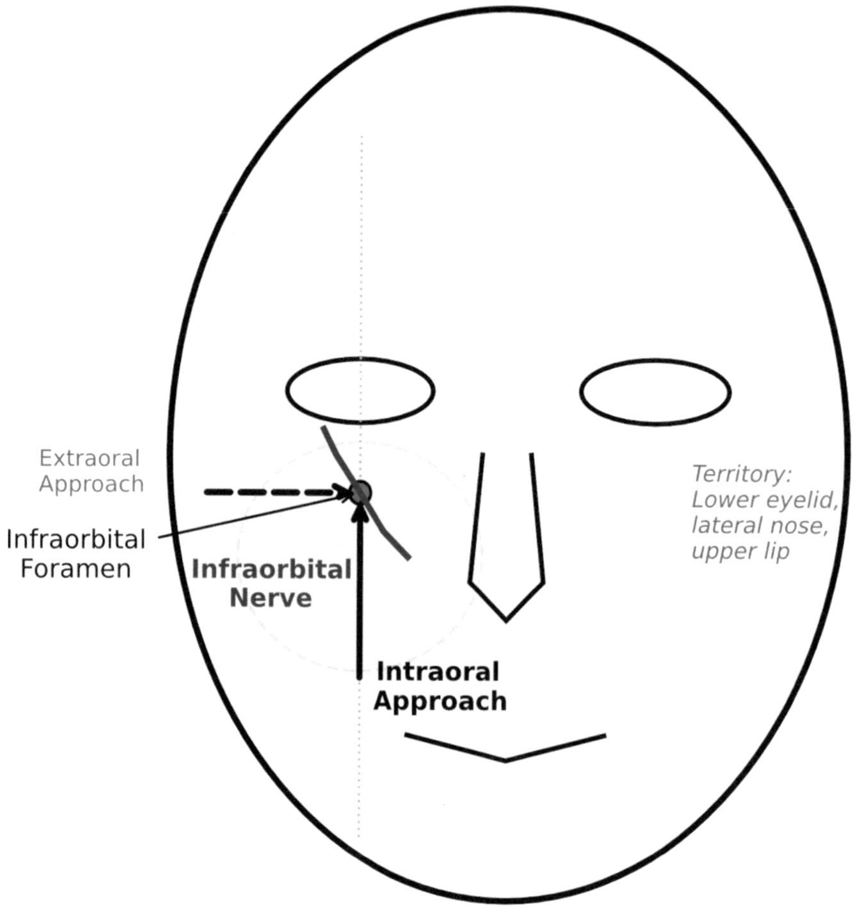

Mental Nerve Block

Indications

- Anesthesia of the lower lip and chin for laceration repair without tissue distortion

Contraindications

- No absolute contraindications beyond those common to all blocks.

Landmark-Based (Blind) Technique — Extraoral Approach

1. With the patient looking straight ahead, identify the mid-pupillary line. The mental foramen lies along this line on the mandible, between the apices of the first and second premolars.
2. Palpate the mandibular body at the level of the second premolar, approximately halfway between the inferior border and the alveolar crest. The foramen may be felt as a subtle depression, and digital pressure may elicit tenderness or paresthesia.
3. Insert a 25—27 gauge needle perpendicular to the mandible at this point; aspirate and inject 1—2 mL of anesthetic at the foramen.

Landmark-Based (Blind) Technique — Intraoral Approach

1. Retract the lower lip. Insert the needle through the buccal mucosa at the inferior gingivobuccal sulcus between the first and second premolars.
2. Direct the needle inferiorly toward the palpated foramen (approximately 1 cm depth). Aspirate and inject 1—2 mL. Gently massage to promote diffusion into the mental canal for incisive nerve coverage.

Mental Nerve Block — Anatomy

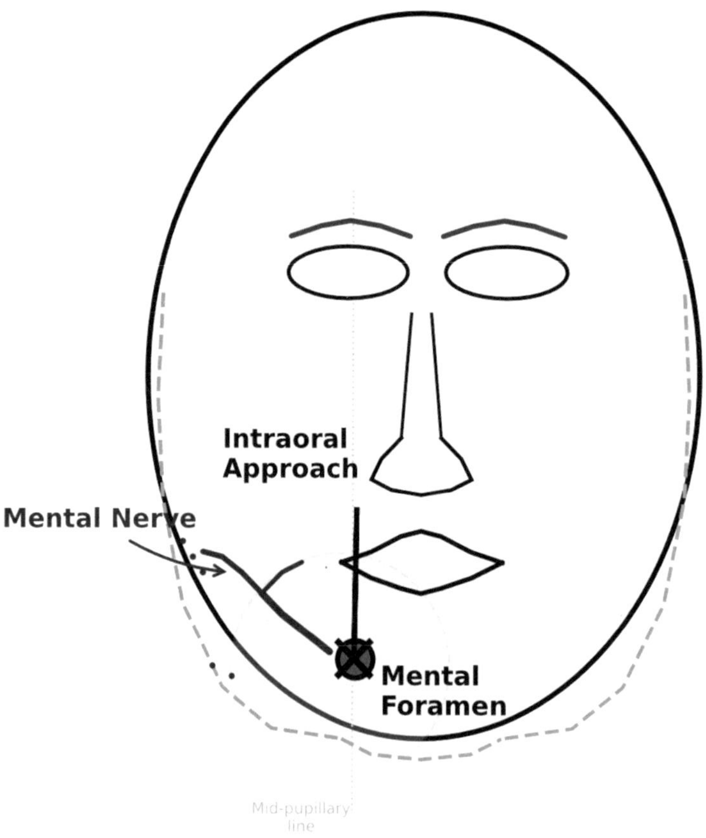

Retract lower lip → insert at mucobuccal fold above 2nd premolar → aim toward foramen → aspirate → inject 1-2 mL

Inferior Alveolar Nerve Block

Indications

- Dental pain of the mandibular teeth (pulpitis, fracture, dry socket) and anesthesia of the lower lip and chin via the mental branch

Contraindications

- Infection at the injection site (pterygomandibular space)
- Trismus limiting access (relative)
- Coagulopathy is a relative concern given the vascularity of the region

Intraoral Approach

1. Position the patient upright or semi-reclined, facing the operator. Ask the patient to open the mouth as wide as comfortable.
2. With the non-dominant hand, palpate the coronoid notch (the greatest concavity on the anterior border of the ramus) by placing the thumb intraorally on the anterior ramus. The pterygomandibular raphe runs vertically posterior to the last molar as a palpable ridge when the mouth is wide open.
3. The target is the mandibular foramen (sulcus) on the medial aspect of the ramus, located at the level of the occlusal plane of the mandibular teeth. In adults, this is approximately 1—1.5 cm above the occlusal surface of the inferior molars.
4. Position the syringe barrel over the contralateral premolars (the syringe crosses the midline). Insert a 25—27 gauge, 1.5-inch needle through the buccal mucosa lateral to the pterygomandibular raphe, at the level of the occlusal plane, approximately 1 cm posterior to the coronoid notch.
5. Advance the needle posterolaterally until bone is contacted (the medial aspect of the ramus), typically at a depth of 2—2.5 cm. Withdraw 1—2 mm from the periosteum.
6. Aspirate (the IAN block has the highest positive aspiration rate of any dental block, approximately 10—15). If negative, slowly inject 1.5—2 mL of anesthetic.
7. As the needle is withdrawn, inject an additional 0.5—1 mL to block the lingual nerve, which lies anterior and medial to the IAN in the pterygomandibular space.
8. Confirm anesthesia: the patient should report ipsilateral lip and tongue tingling within 3—5 minutes.

Inferior Alveolar Nerve Block — Intraoral Technique

(Patient's mouth — open view)

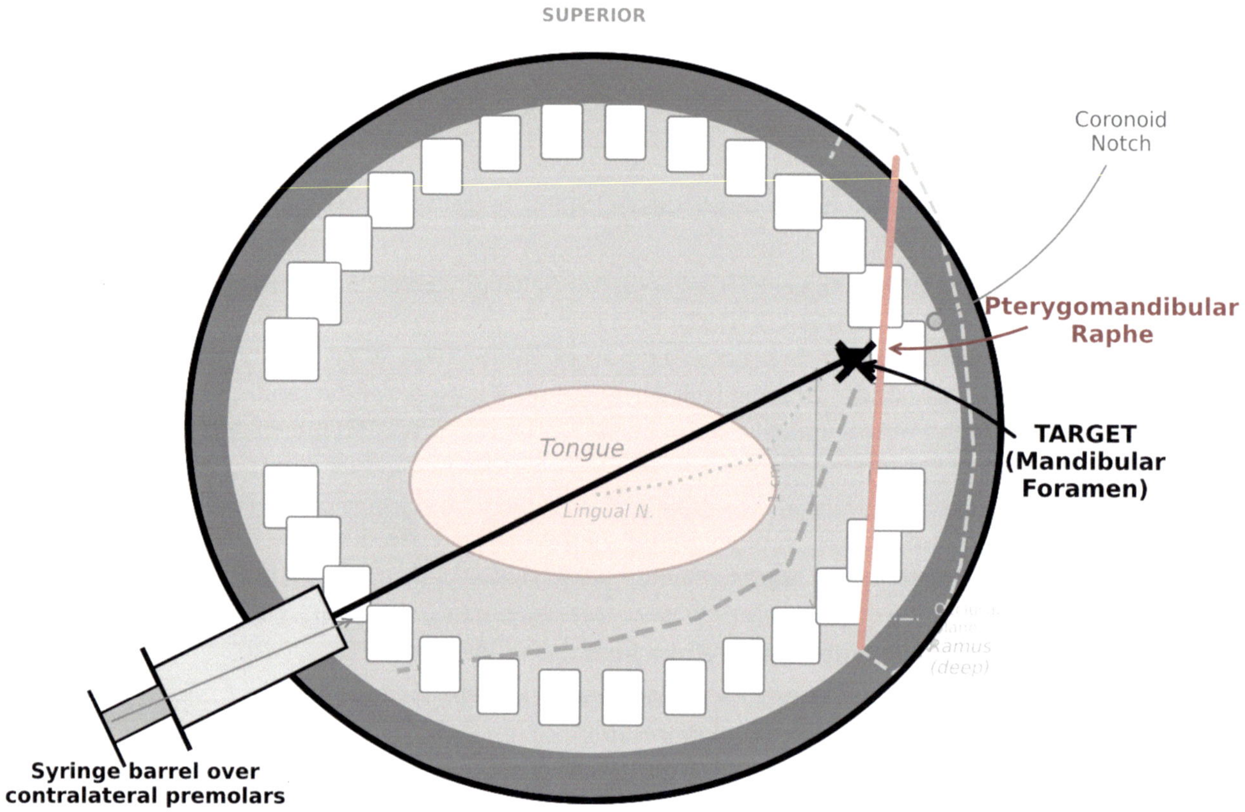

Inferior Alveolar nerve - innervates teeth, chin, lower lip

Palpate coronoid notch with index finger → identify raphe
Insert needle medial to raphe, 1 cm above occlusal plane
Syringe barrel over contralateral premolars → advance to bone
Withdraw 1 mm → aspirate → inject 1.5–2 mL
Blocks: IAN (teeth, chin, lower lip) + Lingual N. (anterior 2/3 tongue)

Auricular Field Block

Indications

- Anesthesia of the ear for laceration repair, hematoma drainage, or incision and drainage without distorting cartilage landmarks

Contraindications

- No absolute contraindications beyond those common to all blocks. Do not use epinephrine-containing anesthetic near the ear in classic teaching (largely theoretical, but avoid in compromised tissue).

Landmark-Based Technique

1. Prep the skin circumferentially around the ear base. Use a 25—27 gauge needle and 1% lidocaine with epinephrine (the epinephrine reduces bleeding and prolongs analgesia; the auricle is safe for epinephrine use).
2. Create a diamond-shaped or V-shaped subcutaneous infiltration around the ear base by injecting in four quadrants:
3. Anterior-superior: Inject 2—3 mL subcutaneously from the tragus superiorly along the root of the helix (blocks the auriculotemporal nerve, V3).
4. Anterior-inferior: Inject 2—3 mL from the tragus inferiorly along the preauricular crease to the lobule (blocks the great auricular nerve contribution).
5. Posterior-superior: Inject 2—3 mL posterior to the pinna along the mastoid process (blocks the lesser occipital nerve, C2).
6. Posterior-inferior: Inject 2—3 mL along the posterior auricular groove to the lobule (blocks the great auricular nerve, C2—C3).
7. Total volume is typically 8—12 mL. Note: The concha (bowl of the ear) is innervated by Arnold's nerve (CN X) and may require direct local infiltration if procedures involve this area.

Auricular Field Block — Ring Block Technique

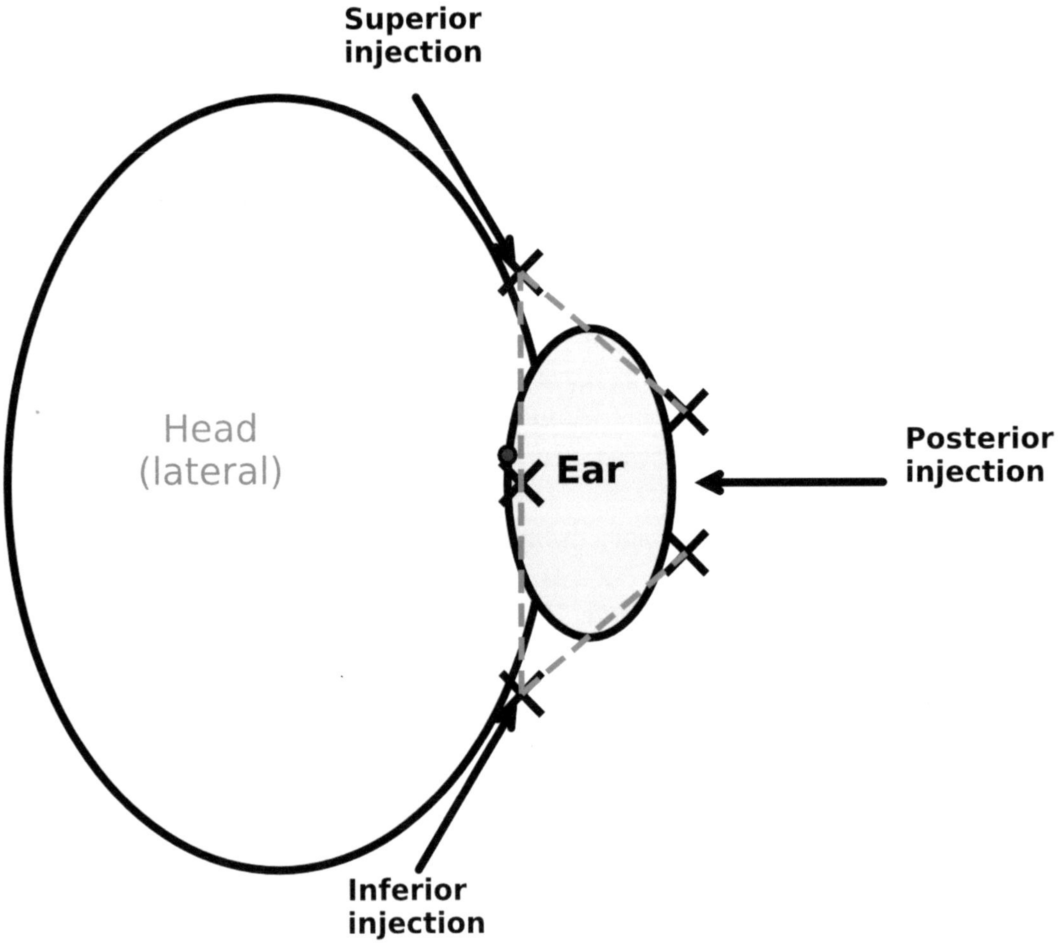

Inject subcutaneously in a V or diamond pattern around the ear base: anterior, posterior, superior, inferior
Total: 5-10 mL local anesthetic

Posterior Tibial Nerve Block

Indications

- Anesthesia of the plantar foot for foreign body removal, laceration repair, or abscess drainage — infiltrating the sole directly is painful and poorly effective

Contraindications

- Posterior tibial vascular compromise of the foot (relative)
- Otherwise, those common to all blocks

Ultrasound-Guided Technique

1. Position the patient supine with the leg externally rotated or prone; place a pillow under the ankle.
2. Select a high-frequency linear probe (15—6 MHz); place in a transverse orientation posterior to the medial malleolus.
3. Identify the tibia (medial), the flexor hallucis longus (posterior), and the flexor digitorum longus (anterior); locate the tarsal tunnel containing the tibial artery (pulsatile) and tibial nerve (posteromedial to artery, honeycomb appearance).
4. Identify the flexor retinaculum (superficial hyperechoic band) and the tibial nerve deep to it.
5. Insert a 25 gauge needle using an in-plane approach from anterior to posterior (medial approach) or posterior to anterior.
6. Target the perineural space around the tibial nerve; aspirate to avoid intravascular injection.
7. Inject 5—10 mL of local anesthetic (1% lidocaine or 0.25% bupivacaine) observing circumferential spread around the nerve (donut sign).
8. Confirm anesthesia of the sole of the foot (plantar aspect) and medial calcaneal region.

Landmark-Based (Blind) Technique

1. Position the patient supine with the leg externally rotated. Palpate the posterior tibial artery pulse in the groove between the medial malleolus and the Achilles tendon, approximately 1—2 cm posterior and inferior to the medial malleolus.
2. Insert a 25—27 gauge needle perpendicular to the skin immediately posterior to the palpated pulse (the nerve lies just posterior to the artery).
3. Advance until paresthesia is elicited to the sole of the foot (if no paresthesia, advance to the bone and withdraw 2—3 mm). Aspirate to rule out arterial puncture.
4. Inject 3—5 mL of local anesthetic. If the artery is not palpable, insert the needle midway between the posterior border of the medial malleolus and the Achilles tendon, advance to bone, withdraw slightly, and inject while fanning the needle.

Posterior Tibial Nerve Block — Probe Placement (Medial View)

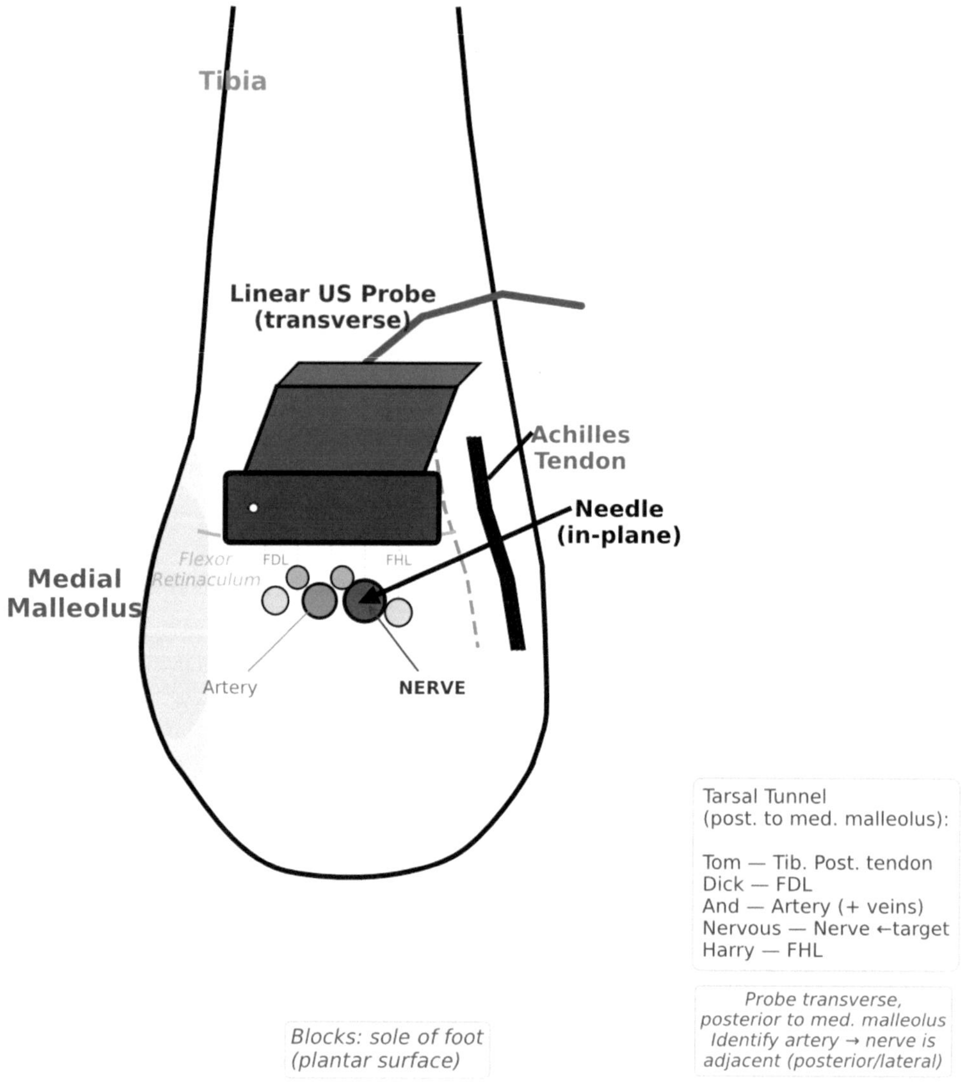

Posterior Tibial Block — Medial Ankle Anatomy

Tom, Dick, ANd Harry
(TP, FDL, Artery+Nerve, FHL)

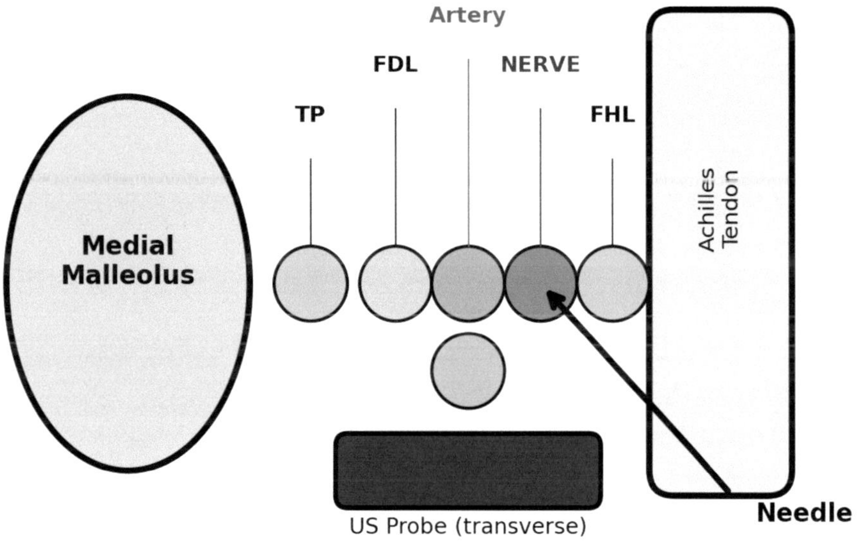

Target: posterior tibial nerve adjacent to artery
Probe transverse, posterior to medial malleolus
Blocks sole of foot (useful for plantar lacerations)

Axillary Nerve Block

Indications

- Anesthesia of the forearm and hand (median, ulnar, radial distributions) for fracture reduction, complex lacerations, or burns

Contraindications

- Injury at risk for forearm compartment syndrome (masks symptoms)
- Axillary adenopathy, infection, or vascular abnormality at the site
- Coagulopathy (relative; the transarterial approach is contraindicated with coagulopathy)

Ultrasound-Guided Technique

1. Position the patient supine with the arm abducted 90 degrees and externally rotated (exaggerated position); place the hand behind the head if possible.
2. Select a high-frequency linear probe (10—5 MHz); place in a transverse orientation in the axillary crease.
3. Identify the axillary artery (anechoic, pulsatile), axillary vein (medial, compressible), and the four terminal nerves:
    - Median nerve: Lateral and superficial to the artery (9—12 o'clock)
    - Ulnar nerve: Medial to the artery (2—3 o'clock)
    - Radial nerve: Posterior to the artery (deep, 5—6 o'clock)
    - Musculocutaneous nerve: Lateral cord, within the coracobrachialis muscle or between biceps and coracobrachialis (lateral to the artery)
4. Insert a 22 gauge needle using an in-plane approach from lateral to medial.
5. Target the musculocutaneous nerve first (within coracobrachialis) with 5 mL of local anesthetic.
6. Advance to target the radial nerve posterior to the artery with 5—10 mL.
7. Target the median and ulnar nerves with 5—10 mL each, ensuring circumferential spread around the artery (axillary sheath injection).
8. Alternatively, perform a perivascular injection of 30—40 mL total volume (0.5% ropivacaine or 0.25% bupivacaine) observing spread within the axillary sheath.
9. Compress the axillary vein during injection to reduce intravascular uptake; aspirate frequently.

Landmark-Based Technique — Transarterial Approach

1. Position as above. Palpate the axillary artery pulse as high in the axilla as possible (more proximal = better chance of blocking all four nerves within the axillary sheath).
2. Insert a 22—25 gauge, 1.5-inch needle directly into the axillary artery (confirmed by bright red blood on aspiration). Advance through the artery until blood can no longer be aspirated (posterior wall).
3. Inject 15—20 mL of local anesthetic posterior to the artery (this targets the radial nerve). Slowly withdraw the needle back through the artery until arterial blood returns, then continue withdrawing until blood stops again (anterior wall).
4. Inject 15—20 mL anterior to the artery (this targets the median and ulnar nerves).
5. The musculocutaneous nerve often travels outside the axillary sheath; supplement with 5 mL injected into the belly of the coracobrachialis muscle (palpated as a cord-like structure lateral to the artery).
6. Apply firm pressure over the injection site for 3—5 minutes to prevent hematoma and promote distal spread.

Axillary Block — Cross-Sectional Anatomy

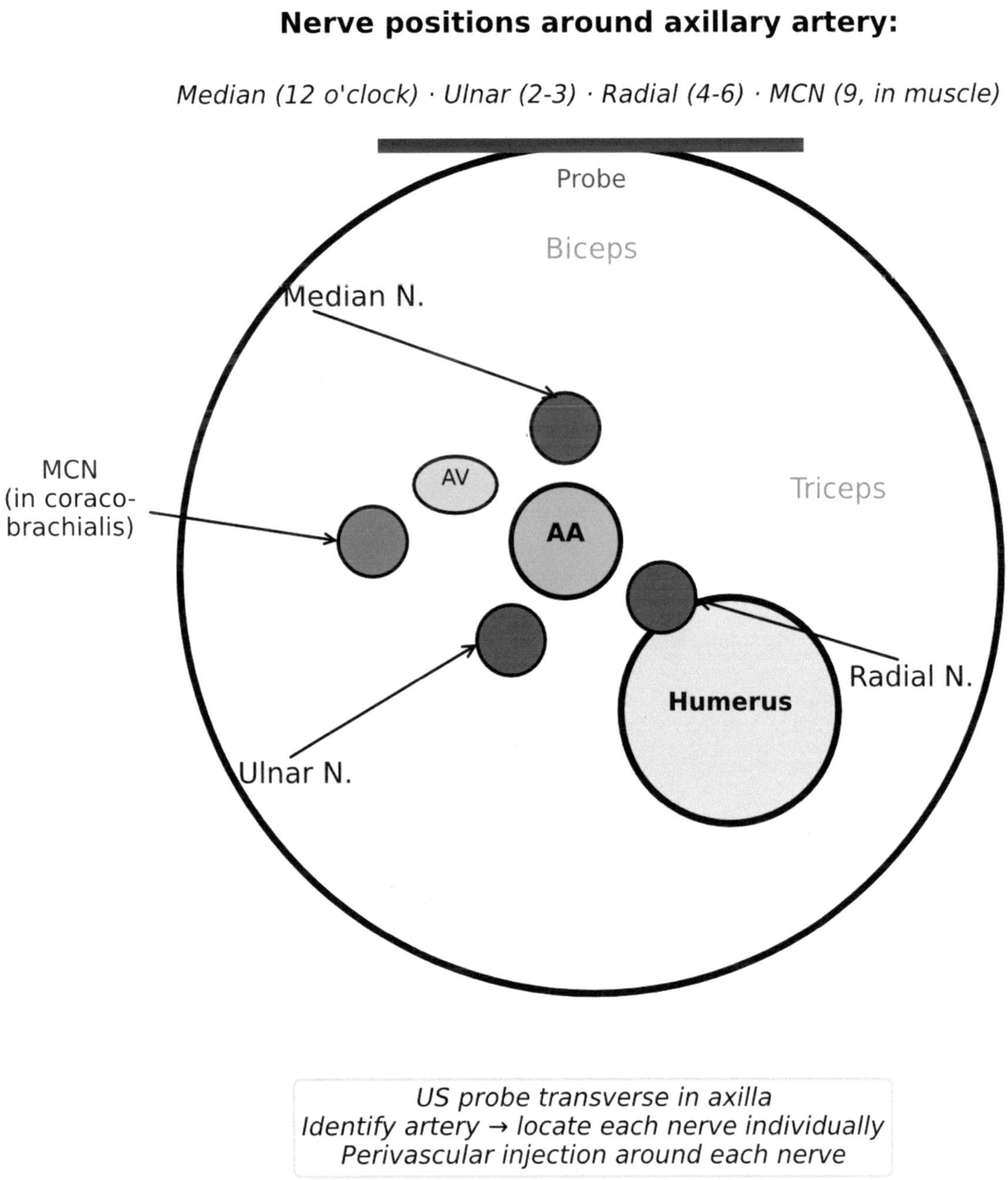

Distal Radial, Median, and Ulnar Nerve Block

Indications

- Anesthesia of the hand for laceration repair, fracture or dislocation reduction, burns, and complex wound care while preserving motor function proximally

Contraindications

- Concern for hand or forearm compartment syndrome

Ultrasound-Guided Technique

1. Position the patient supine with the arm supinated and wrist neutral; prep the volar and lateral forearm.
2. Select a high-frequency linear probe (15—6 MHz).

Radial Nerve:

- Place the probe in a transverse orientation at the distal third of the forearm between the brachioradialis and brachialis/brachioradialis tendon.
- Identify the superficial radial nerve (lateral to the radial artery, adjacent to the cephalic vein) or the deep radial nerve between the brachioradialis and extensor carpi radialis longus.
- Insert a 25 gauge needle in-plane; inject 3—5 mL of local anesthetic around the nerve.

Median Nerve:

- Move the probe to the mid-forearm between the flexor digitorum superficialis (medial) and flexor carpi radialis (lateral).
- Identify the median nerve (round, hyperechoic) medial to the radial artery and deep to the flexor digitorum superficialis.
- Insert the needle in-plane; inject 3—5 mL of local anesthetic observing spread around the nerve.

Ulnar Nerve:

- Place the probe medial to the flexor carpi ulnaris tendon at the mid-forearm level.
- Identify the ulnar nerve adjacent to the ulnar artery (more medial and superficial than the median nerve).
- Insert the needle in-plane; inject 3—5 mL of local anesthetic around the nerve.
- Confirm anesthesia of the radial dorsum (radial), palmar thumb/index/middle (median), and little finger/medial ring finger (ulnar).

Landmark-Based Wrist Block Technique

Median Nerve at the Wrist:

1. Identify the palmaris longus tendon by having the patient oppose the thumb and small finger while flexing the wrist. The median nerve lies immediately radial (lateral) to this tendon and deep to the flexor retinaculum. If the palmaris longus is absent (approximately 15 of patients), the nerve lies between the tendons of flexor carpi radialis and flexor digitorum superficialis.
2. At the level of the proximal wrist crease, insert a 25—27 gauge needle perpendicular to the skin between the palmaris longus and flexor carpi radialis tendons.
3. Advance 5—10 mm until the patient reports paresthesia to the thumb/index/middle fingers (if elicited, withdraw 1 mm). Aspirate and inject 3—5 mL of anesthetic.

Ulnar Nerve at the Wrist:

1. Identify the flexor carpi ulnaris (FCU) tendon at the wrist (most medial tendon, palpable with wrist flexion and ulnar deviation). The ulnar nerve lies immediately radial (lateral) to the FCU tendon and medial to the ulnar artery.
2. At the level of the proximal wrist crease, insert a 25—27 gauge needle just radial to the FCU tendon, directed toward the ulnar styloid.
3. Advance 5—10 mm. Aspirate (the ulnar artery is nearby). Inject 3—5 mL of anesthetic. For the dorsal sensory branch of the ulnar nerve, inject an additional 2—3 mL subcutaneously from the FCU tendon dorsally around the ulnar border of the wrist.

Radial Nerve at the Wrist:

1. The superficial branch of the radial nerve is purely sensory at the wrist and lies in the anatomical snuffbox region, lateral to the radial artery.
2. Palpate the radial artery at the wrist. Insert a 25—27 gauge needle at the level of the radial styloid, just lateral to the radial artery.
3. This nerve has multiple branches at the wrist and is best blocked as a field block: inject 3—5 mL subcutaneously in a band from the radial artery dorsally across the anatomical snuffbox to the mid-dorsum of the wrist. This ensures capture of all terminal branches.

Wrist Block — Cross-Sectional Anatomy at Distal Wrist Crease

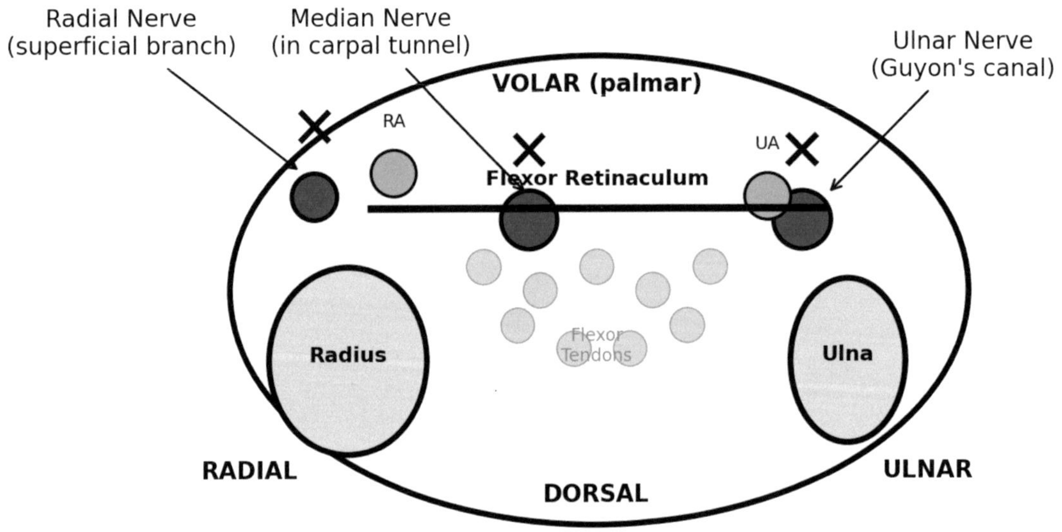

× = injection sites
Median: between PL & FCR tendons | Ulnar: lateral to FCU tendon
Radial: lateral to radial artery (subcutaneous "snuffbox" infiltration)

Serratus Anterior Plane Block

Indications

- Analgesia for multiple rib fractures (improves pulmonary mechanics and reduces opioid need), chest tube placement, and herpes zoster of the chest wall

Contraindications

- Coagulopathy or therapeutic anticoagulation (relative — weigh against the pulmonary benefit)
- Infection over the site; local anesthetic systemic toxicity risk with large volumes (calculate the maximum dose)

Ultrasound-Guided Technique

1. Position the patient supine or lateral decubitus (affected side up) with the arm abducted or overhead.
2. Select a high-frequency linear probe (10—5 MHz); place in a transverse orientation at the mid-axillary line at the level of the 4th or 5th rib.
3. Identify the latissimus dorsi (superficial, posterior), the serratus anterior (deep, anterior), and the ribs (hyperechoic with shadowing).
4. Identify the thoracodorsal artery (branch of subscapular) between the latissimus and serratus with color Doppler.
5. Insert a 20—22 gauge needle using an in-plane approach from posterior to anterior.
6. Target the plane between the serratus anterior and the intercostal muscles (or between serratus and latissimus); aspirate to avoid pneumothorax or vascular injection.
7. Inject 20—30 mL of local anesthetic (0.25% bupivacaine with 1:200,000 epinephrine) observing hydrodissection of the serratus anterior muscle away from the ribs.
8. Confirm spread craniocaudally over 3—4 rib spaces; multiple injections may improve spread.
9. Monitor for pneumothorax (pleural line identification is critical before injection).

Serratus Anterior Plane Block — Probe Placement (Lateral Chest Wall)

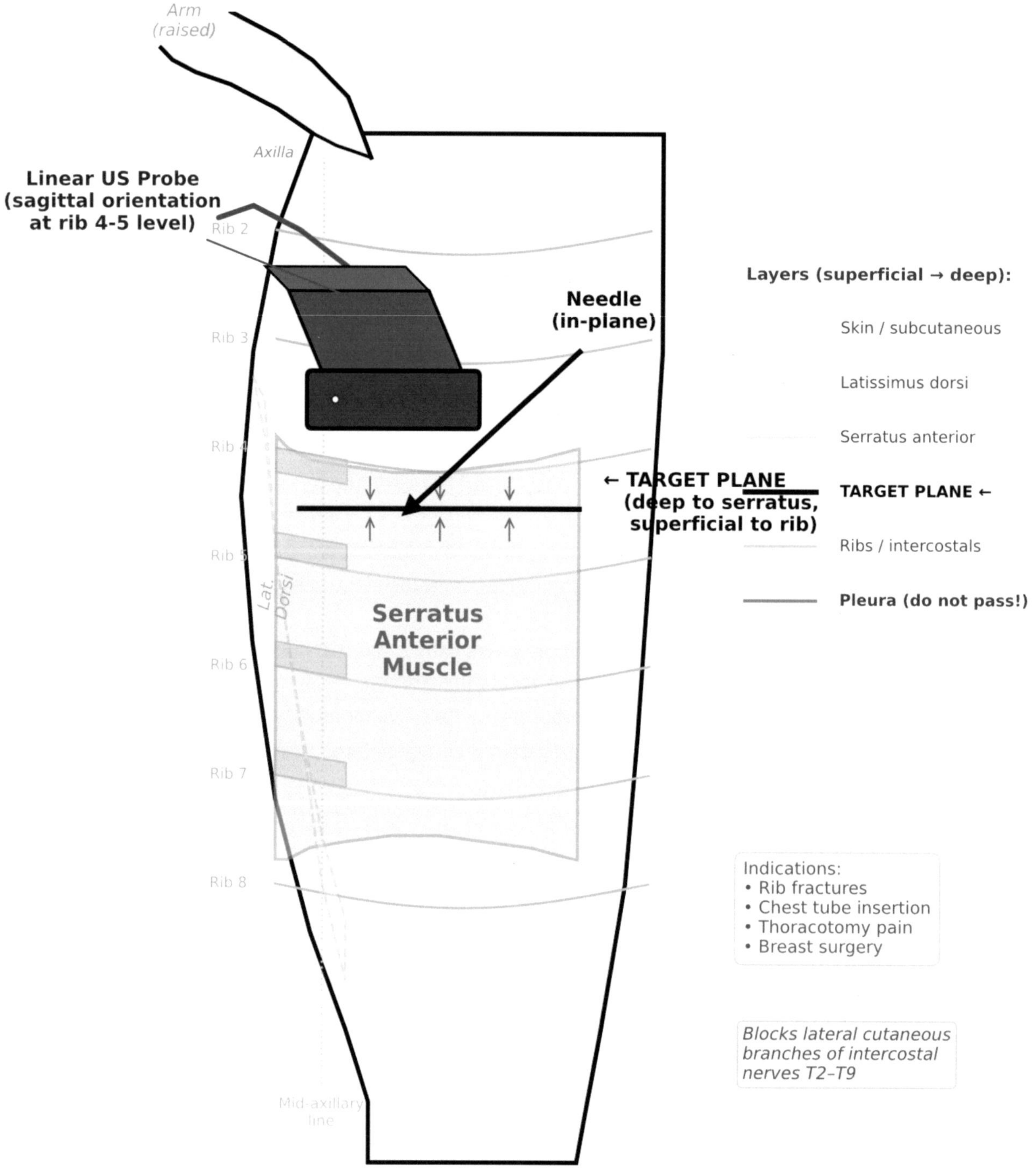

Serratus Anterior Plane Block — US View (Lateral Chest Wall)

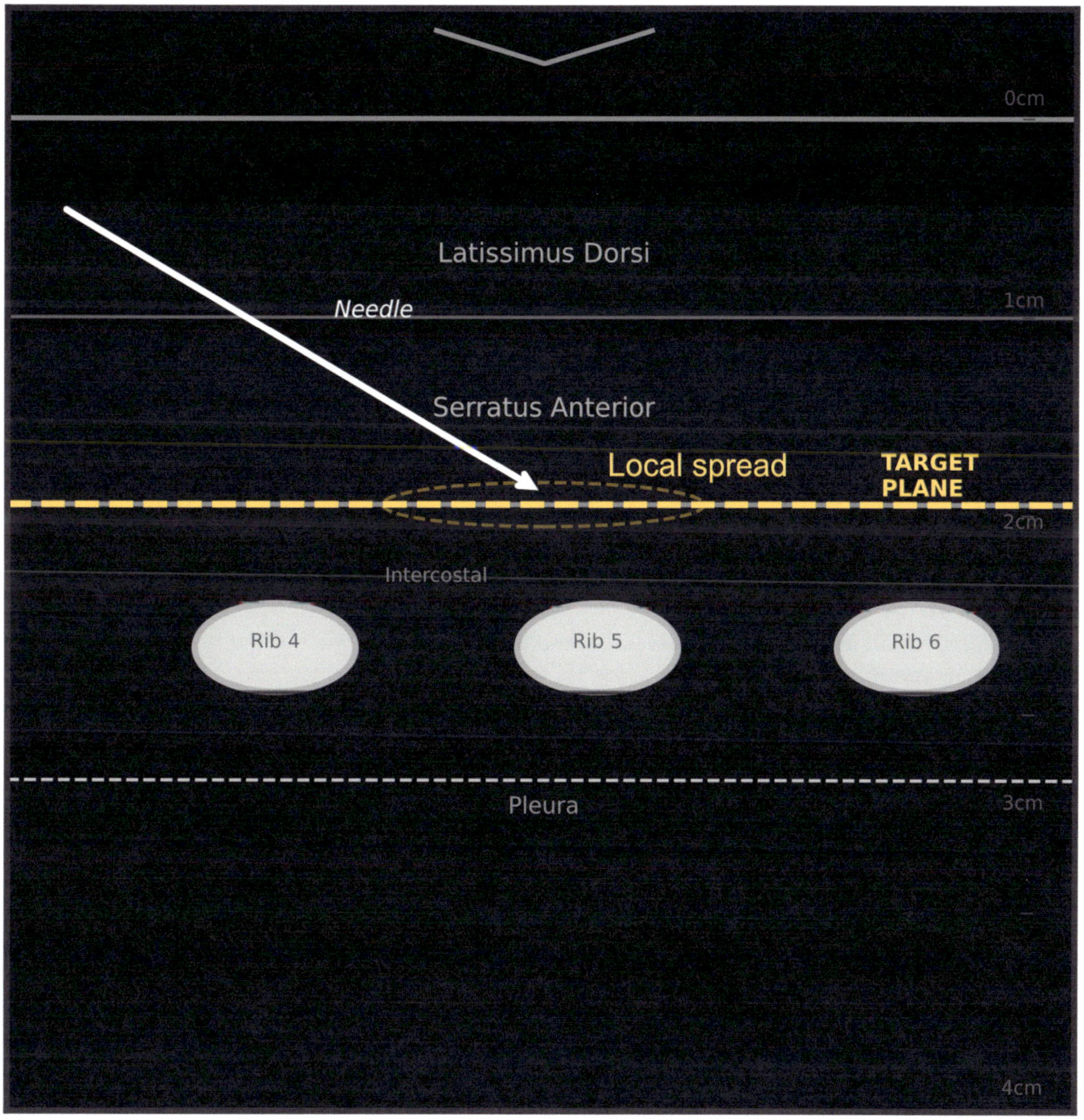

Femoral Nerve Block

Indications

- Analgesia for femoral neck and shaft fractures, especially in elderly patients where opioid-sparing matters

Contraindications

- Injury at risk for thigh compartment syndrome (masks symptoms)
- Femoral vascular graft or planned vascular access at the site
- 4Coagulopathy (relative); infection over the inguinal region

Steps:

1. Select linear probe (6—15 MHz) for superficial blocks (femoral, interscalene, axillary) or curvilinear (2—5 MHz) for deep blocks (sciatic, infraclavicular).
2. Identify target nerve: hyperechoic oval/round structure with internal fascicular ("honeycomb") pattern; distinguish from tendons (fibrillar, anisotropic) and vessels (compressible, pulsatile on color Doppler).
3. For femoral nerve: locate lateral to femoral artery, deep to fascia iliaca, superficial to iliopsoas muscle.
4. Sterile skin preparation; local anesthetic skin wheal.
5. In-plane approach: align probe parallel to nerve, insert needle at probe edge to visualize entire shaft approaching nerve.
6. Hydrodissection: inject 1—2 mL D5W or saline to confirm needle tip position (fluid spreads circumferentially around nerve).
7. Inject local anesthetic (20—30 mL for femoral, 15—20 mL for interscalene) observing spread around nerve (donut sign); avoid intraneural injection (high resistance, nerve swelling).
8. Assess for complications: intravascular injection (color Doppler), local anesthetic systemic toxicity.

Femoral Nerve Block — Short Axis View

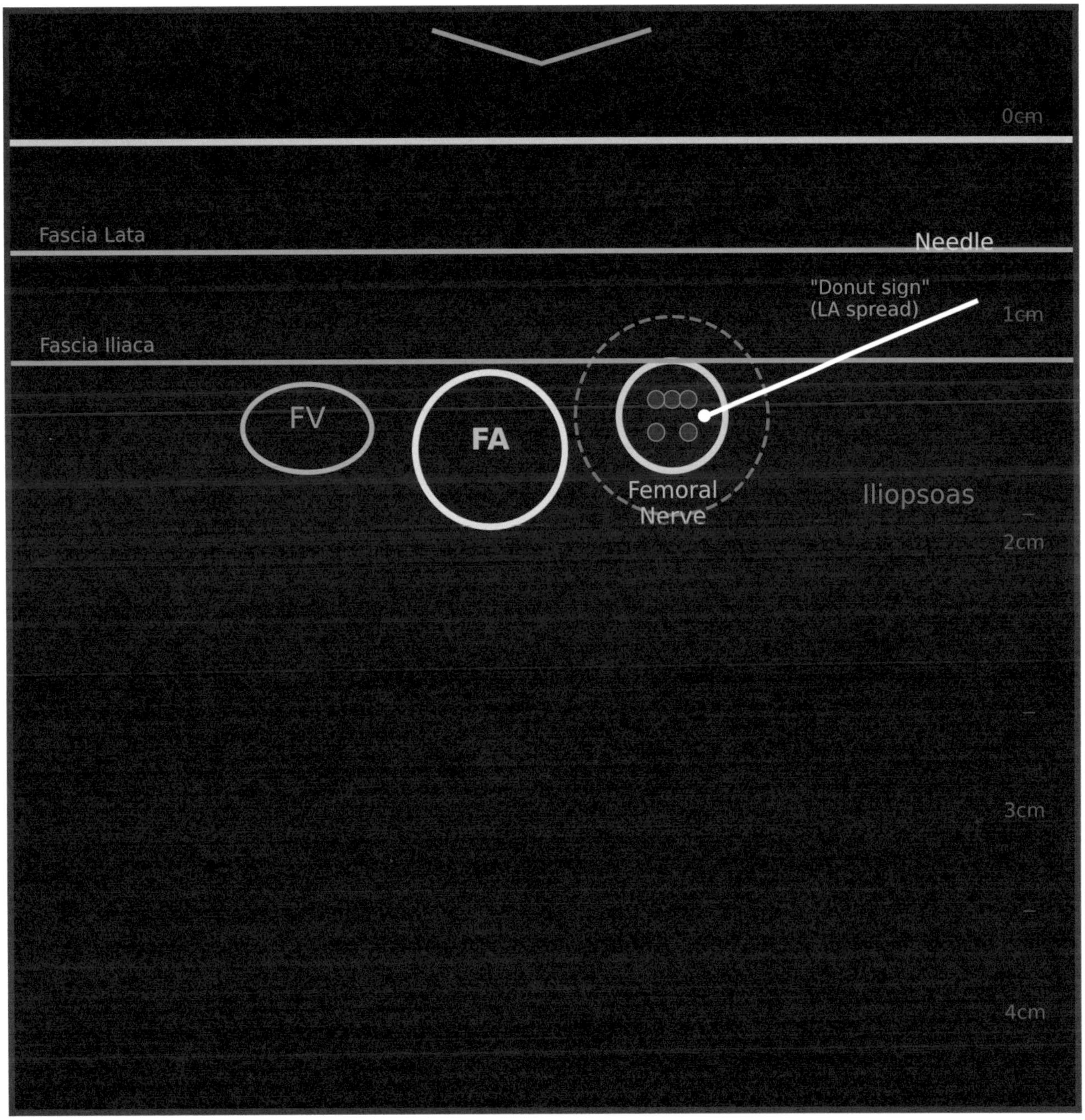

Femoral Nerve Block — Cross-Sectional Anatomy

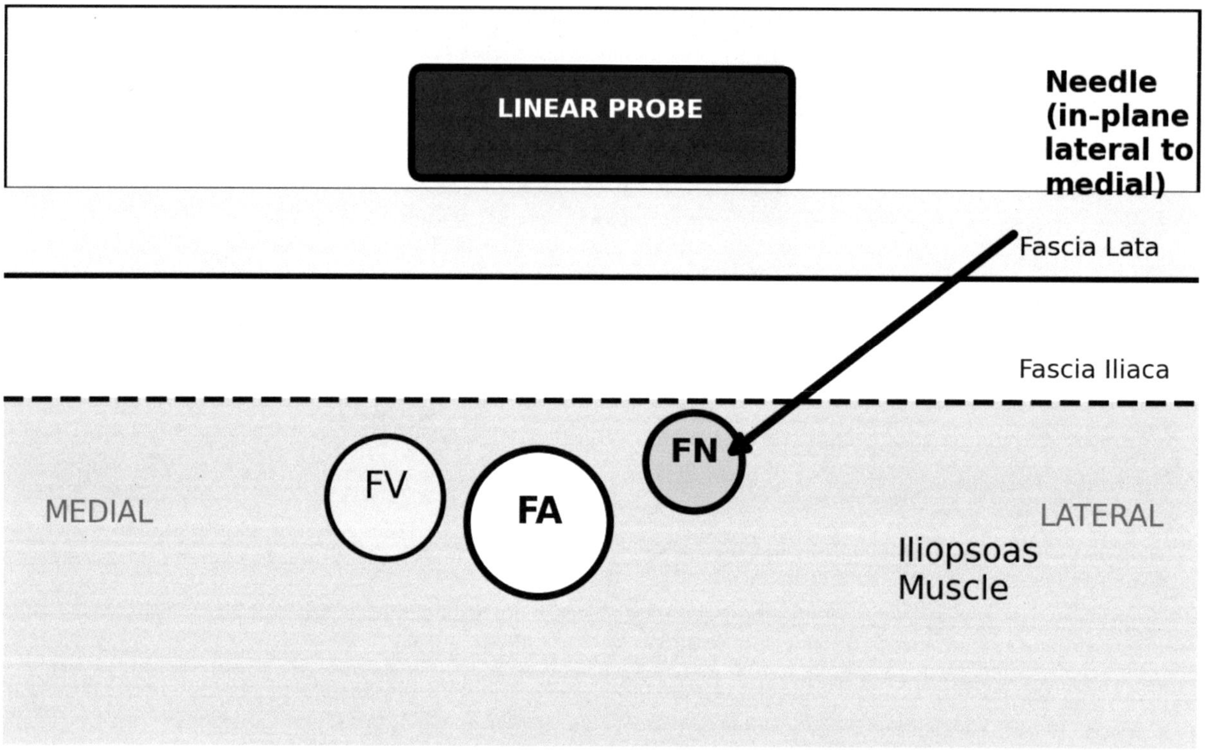

Mnemonic: VAN (Vein-Artery-Nerve)
Medial → Lateral

Fascia Iliaca Compartment Block

Indications

- Analgesia for hip, femoral neck, and proximal femur fractures; an anatomically safer alternative to the femoral block because the needle is remote from the vessels

Contraindications

- Same cautions as the femoral nerve block: compartment syndrome risk, overlying infection, prior femoral vascular surgery, and relative caution with coagulopathy
- Large-volume block — calculate the maximum local anesthetic dose, particularly in elderly, low-weight patients

Ultrasound-Guided Technique

1. Position the patient supine with the leg in a neutral position; identify the inguinal ligament and femoral pulse.
2. Select a curvilinear probe (5—2 MHz) or high-frequency linear (10—5 MHz); place in a transverse orientation 1—2 cm lateral to the femoral artery at the level of the inguinal ligament.
3. Identify the fascia lata (superficial hyperechoic line), the sartorius muscle (lateral, triangular), the iliacus muscle (deep, hypoechoic), and the fascia iliaca (deep hyperechoic line overlying iliacus).
4. Identify the femoral nerve (lateral to the artery, triangular, hyperechoic, deep to fascia iliaca) and the iliopsoas tendon (medial to the nerve).
5. Insert a 22 gauge block needle using an in-plane approach from lateral to medial (lateral approach) or lateral to medial but staying lateral to the nerve.
6. Penetrate the fascia lata and advance until a tactile "pop" is felt or visualized as the needle penetrates the fascia iliaca.
7. Confirm position by injecting 1—2 mL of normal saline or D5W; observe the fascia iliaca lifting off the iliacus muscle (bow tie or double-line sign).
8. Aspirate to rule out intravascular placement (femoral artery or lateral circumflex femoral artery branches).
9. Inject 30—40 mL of local anesthetic (0.25% bupivacaine or 0.2 ropivacaine) in 5 mL increments with aspiration, observing medial spread toward the femoral nerve and lateral spread beneath the fascia iliaca.
10. Ensure spread medially to the femoral nerve and laterally toward the lateral femoral cutaneous nerve; the obturator nerve may be blocked with sufficient medial spread.

Landmark-Based — Classic "Double-Pop" Approach

1. Position the patient supine. Identify the anterior superior iliac spine (ASIS) and the pubic tubercle. The inguinal ligament runs between these two landmarks.
2. Divide the inguinal ligament into thirds. Mark the junction of the lateral one-third and medial two-thirds. The injection site is 1—2 cm inferior (caudal) to this point.
3. Palpate the femoral artery pulse — the injection site should be approximately 2—3 cm lateral to the artery. This lateral positioning is key to avoiding the femoral neurovascular bundle.
4. Insert a 22 gauge, short-bevel or blunt-tip needle (blunt tip improves fascial pop detection) perpendicular to the skin.
5. Advance slowly. The first "pop" (loss of resistance) is felt as the needle penetrates the fascia lata. Continue advancing until a second "pop" is felt as the needle penetrates the fascia iliaca. This is the classic "double-pop" or "2-click" technique.

6. Aspirate to rule out intravascular placement. Inject 30—40 mL of local anesthetic (0.25% bupivacaine or 0.2 ropivacaine) slowly. Apply digital pressure distal to the injection site to promote cephalad and lateral spread beneath the fascia iliaca.
7. Confirm analgesia of the anterior thigh (femoral nerve) and lateral thigh (lateral femoral cutaneous nerve) within 15—20 minutes.

Fascia Iliaca Block — Inguinal Anatomy

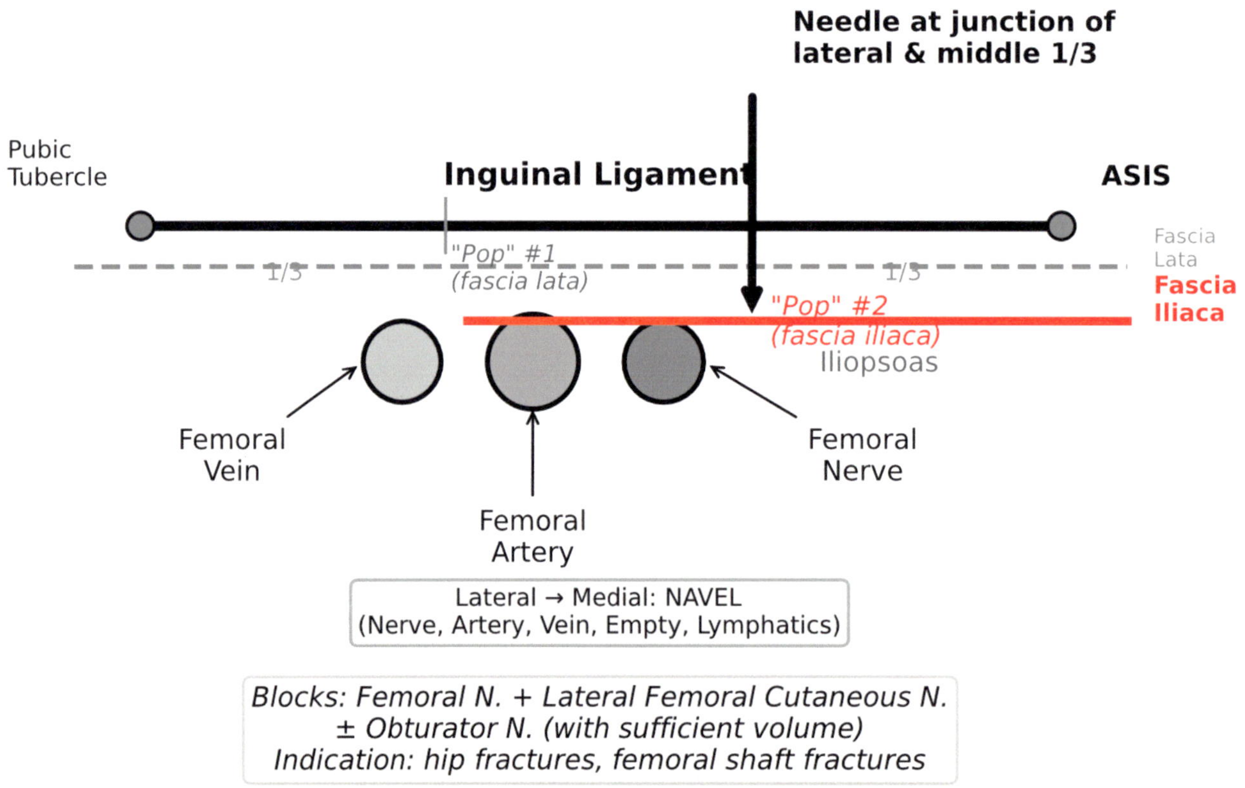

Cardiovascular and Thoracic

Transcutaneous Cardiac Pacing

Indications

- Symptomatic bradycardia with hypoperfusion unresponsive to atropine (high-grade AV block, sick sinus, drug toxicity) as a bridge to transvenous pacing or definitive therapy
- Bradyasystolic arrest immediately after witnessed onset (rarely effective; do not delay CPR)

Contraindications

- No contraindications in the unstable bradycardic patient
- Severe hypothermia is a relative contraindication (the bradycardia is physiologic and the irritable myocardium is prone to VF — rewarm first)

Steps:

1. Indications: symptomatic bradycardia unresponsive to atropine, high-grade AV block with hemodynamic compromise
2. Place pacing pads: anterior-posterior (preferred) with anterior pad at V3 position and posterior pad left infrascapular, or anterior-lateral
3. Set pacemaker to demand mode; initial rate 60-80 bpm
4. Start at 0 mA; increase until electrical capture (wide QRS complex after each pacer spike)
5. Confirm mechanical capture: palpable pulse corresponding to paced beats; check pulse distal to pacing site
6. Set 10 above capture threshold (typically 50-100 mA)
7. If conscious, administer analgesia/sedation (fentanyl 25-50 mcg IV, midazolam 2 mg IV)
8. Prepare for transvenous pacing if temporary pacing required >30 minutes

Cardioversion

Indications

- Unstable tachyarrhythmia with a pulse (hypotension, altered mentation, ischemic chest pain, acute pulmonary edema) — atrial fibrillation or flutter, SVT, or VT with a pulse
- Elective/urgent cardioversion of recent-onset atrial fibrillation per institutional practice

Contraindications

- Digoxin-toxic tachyarrhythmias (relative — high risk of refractory VF)
- Known atrial thrombus or nonanticoagulated atrial fibrillation over 48 hours for elective cardioversion (does not apply to the unstable patient)
- Do not synchronize-shock a pulseless rhythm — defibrillate
- Multifocal atrial tachycardia and sinus tachycardia will not respond — treat the underlying cause

Steps:

1. Indication: unstable tachyarrhythmia (AF with RVR, atrial flutter, SVT, VT with pulse)
2. Ensure synchronization mode ON to avoid shock during vulnerable period (R-wave)
3. Energy selection: start 120-200 J biphasic for AF, 50-100 J for atrial flutter, 100-200 J for VT
4. Apply conductive gel or pads in anterior-posterior or anterior-apex position
5. Conscious sedation: etomidate 0.1 mg/kg or propofol 1 mg/kg
6. Charge capacitor; ensure all personnel "clear" (no contact with patient, bed, or equipment)
7. Deliver shock; reassess rhythm immediately

8. If unsuccessful, increase energy by 100 J and repeat after 30-60 seconds
9. Post-cardioversion: monitor for bradycardia, embolic events, and recurrence

Defibrillation

Indications:

- Ventricular fibrillation
- Pulseless ventricular tachycardia

Contraindications:

- No contraindications in the pulseless patient with a shockable rhythm. Ensure scene and crew safety (dry patient, no contact during shock) and remove transdermal medication patches from pad sites.

Steps:

1. Indication: pulseless VT or VF
2. Immediate CPR while preparing defibrillator; minimize interruptions to <10 seconds
3. Biphasic energy: 200 J (or manufacturer's recommended dose); monophasic 360 J
4. Paddle/pad placement: right upper chest below clavicle and apex at left anterior axillary line below nipple
5. Apply firm pressure (25 lbs) with paddles or ensure complete pad contact
6. Charge while continuing compressions; hold compressions only for shock delivery
7. Clear team: verbal and visual confirmation no one touching patient or bed
8. Deliver shock; resume CPR immediately for 2 minutes before rhythm check
9. Continue ACLS algorithm with epinephrine 1 mg IV/IO every 3-5 minutes and amiodarone 300 mg IV/IO for refractory VF/VT

Thoracostomy (Chest Tube/Small Bore Catheter)

Large Bore Chest Tube

Indications:

- Traumatic hemothorax or hemopneumothorax
- Tension pneumothorax after needle or finger decompression
- Large or symptomatic pneumothorax in a ventilated patient
- Empyema or large effusion requiring drainage when a small catheter is inadequate

Contraindications:

- No absolute contraindications in the unstable patient
- Relative: coagulopathy (correct in parallel, not before, in emergencies), pleural adhesions or prior thoracotomy on that side, and overlying infection — choose an alternative site

Steps:

1. Indication: hemothorax, pneumothorax requiring suction, empyema
2. Position: lateral decubitus with arm abducted or supine with arm behind head
3. Identify triangle of safety: apex at axilla, base at 5th intercostal space, anterior border is lateral edge of pectoralis major, posterior border is anterior edge of latissimus dorsi
4. Insert at 4th or 5th intercostal space at mid-axillary line
5. Sterile prep; local anesthetic along proposed tract including periosteum of rib above
6. Make 3-4 cm incision parallel to rib; blunt dissect with curved clamp over top of rib (avoid neurovascular bundle inferior to rib)

7. Puncture parietal pleura with clamp; spread to create tract; insert finger to confirm intrapleural and sweep adhesions
8. Clamp chest tube (28-36 Fr for adults) with hemostat; insert tube superiorly and posteriorly for air, inferiorly and posteriorly for fluid
9. Advance until last hole is 2-3 cm inside chest wall
10. Connect to chest drainage system with water seal; ensure tidaling
11. Secure with silk suture (horizontal mattress or purse string); apply petroleum gauze, 4x4s, and tape
12. Order chest X-ray to confirm position and resolution of pneumothorax/hemothorax

Small Bore Catheter (Pigtail/Arrow)

Indications:

- Simple or spontaneous pneumothorax
- Free-flowing pleural effusion requiring drainage
- Increasingly acceptable for stable traumatic pneumothorax and select hemothorax

Contraindications:

- Large or clotted hemothorax where the catheter will occlude (use a large bore tube)
- Loculated collections may require imaging-guided placement
- Relative: coagulopathy and overlying infection, as with any thoracostomy

Steps:

1. Indication: simple pneumothorax, small effusions
2. Seldinger technique: insert needle into pleural space; aspirate air/fluid
3. Advance guidewire; remove needle
4. Make small skin incision; dilate if necessary
5. Advance catheter over wire; remove wire and dilator
6. Secure with suture; attach to Heimlich valve or water seal
7. Consider Heimlich valve for outpatient management of spontaneous pneumothorax

Cutaneous

Wound Closure

Indications:

- Lacerations amenable to primary closure to improve healing time, function, and cosmesis, generally within 12–18 hours of injury (up to about 24 hours on the face)

Contraindications:

- Do not close primarily: significantly contaminated or infected wounds, most bites to the hand or delayed bites (face is the exception after thorough irrigation), wounds older than the acceptable window, and deep puncture wounds that cannot be irrigated adequately — use delayed primary closure or secondary intention
- Do not suture over an unreduced fracture or unexplored deep injury to tendon, nerve, or vessel — address the deep injury first
- Retained foreign body until removed or excluded

Steps:

1. Hemostasis: direct pressure, topical hemostatics, or ligation of bleeding vessels
2. Irrigation: high-pressure irrigation (35-70 psi) with 500-1000 mL sterile saline; remove visible contamination
3. Debridement: remove devitalized tissue, foreign bodies, and debris
4. Anesthesia: local infiltration or regional block; avoid epinephrine in digits, nose, ears, penis
5. Layered closure:
6. Deep: absorbable suture (Vicryl 3-0 or 4-0) in dermis, buried knots
7. Superficial: non-absorbable (Ethilon, Prolene) or absorbable (fast-absorbing gut) for skin
8. Suture selection: face 5-0 or 6-0, scalp 3-0 or 4-0, trunk/extremities 4-0 or 5-0
9. Technique: simple interrupted (most common), vertical mattress (eversion), horizontal mattress (tension), running subcuticular (cosmetic)
10. Remove sutures: face 3-5 days, scalp 7-10 days, trunk 10-14 days, extremities 10-14 days, over joints 14 days
11. Alternative: tissue adhesive (Dermabond) for low-tension linear wounds; steri-strips with benzoin for superficial closure
12. Tetanus prophylaxis: Tdap if >10 years since last tetanus or unknown status; tetanus immune globulin if dirty wound and incomplete series

Head, Ear, Eye, Nose, and Throat

Control of Epistaxis

Indications:

- Active anterior or posterior epistaxis unresponsive to direct pressure — stepwise: topical vasoconstrictor and anesthetic, cautery, anterior packing, posterior balloon for posterior sources

Contraindications:

- Cautery: do not cauterize both sides of the septum in the same session (perforation risk); avoid cautery over infected or traumatized mucosa
- Packing in the setting of significant midface or skull base fracture is a relative contraindication — direct visualization and caution with any instrumentation
- Posterior packing mandates admission with monitoring; use caution in patients with tenuous respiratory status

Steps:

1. Identify anterior vs. posterior bleed; locate bleeding point (Kiesselbach's plexus most common)
2. First line: topical vasoconstrictor (oxymetazoline or phenylephrine) and pressure (pinch soft part of nose for 10-15 minutes)
3. Chemical cautery: silver nitrate stick to bleeding vessel and surrounding 2-3 mm; avoid bilateral cautery (septal perforation risk)
4. Electrical cautery: bipolar only; avoid monopolar near pacemaker
5. Anterior packing: petroleum gauze layered from nasal floor toward roof, extending to posterior choana; or Merocel/Rhino Rocket expanded with saline
6. Posterior packing: Foley catheter (12 Fr) inserted to nasopharynx, inflated with 10 mL, pulled anteriorly and clamped; or commercial balloons (Epistat)
7. Prophylactic antibiotics (amoxicillin-clavulanate) for packs left >24 hours to prevent toxic shock syndrome
8. Admit for posterior bleeds, coagulopathy, or failed anterior packing

Flexible Nasopharyngolaryngoscopy

Indications

- Evaluation of the upper airway: suspected supraglottic infection (epiglottitis), foreign body sensation, stridor, voice change, airway assessment before intubation, and nasopharyngeal or laryngeal trauma

Contraindications

- Do not instrument the airway of a child with suspected epiglottitis outside a controlled setting with airway backup
- Severe midface or skull base trauma is a relative contraindication to nasal passage
- Epistaxis obscuring the view and uncooperative patients are practical limitations

Steps:

1. Select appropriate flexible fiberoptic scope: Diagnostic (3.1—4.0 mm outer diameter) vs. Intubating (3.5—4.2 mm outer diameter with suction port).
2. Check white balance and focus on gauze or tongue; confirm fiberoptic light source brightness and battery charge.
3. Test suction channel patency with sterile saline; ensure compatible suction tubing and pressure (100—150 mmHg).

4. Prepare anti-fog solution or warm the scope tip in warm sterile saline (40°C) to prevent fogging; apply surgical lubricant to the distal 15 cm of the scope (avoid lens).
5. Position video monitor at eye level for the operator; ensure two-person team available (operator + assistant to manage medications/suction/tube advancement).
6. Apply topical vasoconstrictor to both nares: Oxymetazoline 0.05 (2 sprays per nare) or phenylephrine 0.5 (soaked pledgets); wait 3—5 minutes for mucosal shrinkage.
7. Administer topical anesthesia: Atomized 4% lidocaine via MAD device (3—5 mL per nare) or nebulized 4% lidocaine (5 mL via nebulizer); for awake intubation, consider bilateral superior laryngeal nerve blocks (1% lidocaine 2 mL each side) and transtracheal injection (3 mL 4% lidocaine through cricothyroid membrane).
8. Optional antisialogogue: Glycopyrrolate 0.2—0.4 mg IV 5—10 minutes prior (reduces secretions that obscure view).
9. Select the more patent nare (wider opening, less septal deviation); if equal, choose the right nare.
10. Orient the scope: The direction of the bending section (controlled by thumb lever) should initially face the nasal floor (medially and inferiorly).
11. Insert gently along the inferior meatus (floor of nasal cavity), directing the scope parallel to the hard palate toward the ear (not upward toward cribriform plate); avoid the middle turbinate.
12. Advance slowly under direct vision; if resistance occurs, apply gentle pressure or switch nares; never force against the turbinates (risk bleeding).
13. Once past the posterior nasal cavity, visualize the nasopharynx: Identify the torus tubarius and soft palate; avoid triggering the gag reflex by minimizing soft palate contact.
14. Request the patient phonate "eeeee" or pant (rapid shallow breathing) to visualize vocal cord mobility; request swallow to observe epiglottic movement.
15. Assess: Symmetry of movement (abduction on inspiration, adduction on phonation), lesions, edema, hematoma, foreign bodies, or secretions; document findings.

Slit Lamp Examination

Indications:

- Evaluation of eye pain, red eye, foreign body sensation, trauma, or vision change: corneal injury and ulcer, anterior chamber cell and flare, hyphema, foreign body identification and removal, and Seidel testing for globe leak

Contraindications:

- No contraindications to the examination itself. If globe rupture is obvious, defer all pressure on the globe (including tonometry and lid manipulation), shield the eye, and involve ophthalmology.

Steps:

1. Position patient with chin on rest, forehead against bar
2. Set magnification (10x or 16x); adjust illumination angle (30-60 degrees)
3. Systematic examination: lids/lashes, conjunctiva, sclera, cornea, anterior chamber, iris, lens
4. Use cobalt blue filter with fluorescein stain to identify abrasions, ulcers, and Seidel test (aqueous leak)
5. Check anterior chamber depth and cell/flare (Tyndall effect)
6. Tonometry if indicated (applanation): anesthetize with proparacaine, fluorescein strip, gently touch cornea with tonometer
7. Evert upper lid to examine for foreign body

Musculoskeletal

Arthrocentesis

Indications:

- Suspected septic arthritis (diagnostic tap is mandatory and urgent)
- New monoarthritis — crystal versus infection
- Symptomatic relief of a tense effusion or hemarthrosis
- Confirmation of traumatic arthrotomy (saline load test)

Contraindications:

- Infection of the overlying skin and soft tissue (cellulitis or abscess in the needle path) — do not pass through infected tissue; if septic joint is still suspected, use an alternative approach or orthopedic consultation
- Joint prosthesis (relative — strongly prefer orthopedics to perform the tap)
- Coagulopathy and anticoagulation are relative; the diagnostic need for a suspected septic joint nearly always outweighs bleeding risk

Steps:

1. Identify joint and approach:
    - Knee: lateral approach, superior and lateral to patella; or medial approach
    - Shoulder: posterior approach 2 cm inferior and medial to posterolateral acromion
    - Ankle: anteromedial or anterolateral
    - Wrist: dorsal approach between extensor tendon compartments
2. Sterile prep; local anesthetic
3. Insert 18-20 gauge needle with 10-60 mL syringe; advance until joint space entered (loss of resistance)
4. Aspirate fluid completely; if dry, inject 1 mL sterile saline and re-aspirate
5. Analyze fluid: gross inspection, cell count, crystal analysis (polarized light), gram stain, culture, glucose, protein
6. Interpretation: non-inflammatory (<2000 WBC), inflammatory (2000-50,000), septic (>50,000 with >90% PMNs), crystal (negatively birefringent gout vs. positively birefringent pseudogout)
7. Post-procedure: compression dressing, rest, ice, elevation

Fracture/Dislocation Immobilization

Indications

- Any fracture or reduced dislocation requiring stabilization for pain control, protection from further injury, and healing; splint (not circumferential cast) in the ED to accommodate swelling

Contraindications

- No contraindications to appropriate immobilization. Document neurovascular status before and after; avoid circumferential casting in the acute phase; do not immobilize before reducing a dislocation with vascular compromise.

Steps:

1. Reduction: confirm neurovascular status pre-reduction; provide analgesia (hematoma block, systemic, or regional)
2. Traction-countertraction technique appropriate for specific dislocation
3. Post-reduction neurovascular check and X-ray confirmation

4. Splint selection: sugar tong (forearm), posterior mold (wrist), coaptation (humerus), posterior ankle stirrup, knee immobilizer, shoulder immobilizer
5. Apply stockinette; padding over bony prominences
6. Wet plaster (10-15 sheets) or fiberglass; mold to position of function
7. Secure with elastic bandage; elevate extremity
8. Return precautions: increased pain, numbness, tingling, cyanosis, loss of pulses

Spine Immobilization

Indications:

- Suspected unstable spinal injury based on mechanism and examination, pending clinical or radiographic clearance (apply validated decision rules — NEXUS or Canadian C-Spine — to avoid unnecessary immobilization)

Contraindications:

- Penetrating trauma without neurologic deficit (immobilization increases mortality — do not backboard these patients)
- Do not force a patient with ankylosing spondylitis or fixed deformity into a neutral position — splint in their position of comfort
- Combative patients where forced immobilization worsens spinal motion (relative — sedate or immobilize as tolerated)
- Prolonged rigid backboard use causes pressure injury and pain; remove the board at the earliest opportunity

Steps:

1. Manual inline stabilization (MILS) until collar applied
2. C-collar sizing: measure from chin to shoulder; ensure front and back plates fit without jaw compression or neck hyperextension
3. Log-roll technique: one person at head maintaining neutral alignment, three people on same side of patient, roll as unit
4. Pediatric considerations: pad under torso to account for occiput, preventing cervical flexion
5. Clear immobilization only after clinical clearance (NEXUS or Canadian C-spine rules) or imaging negative for injury

Nervous System

Lumbar Puncture

Indications:

- Suspected CNS infection (meningitis, encephalitis) — do not let the LP delay antibiotics
- Suspected subarachnoid hemorrhage with a nondiagnostic CT
- Suspected idiopathic intracranial hypertension (diagnostic and therapeutic) and select neurologic diagnostics (e.g., Guillain-Barré)

Contraindications:

- Signs of elevated intracranial pressure from a mass lesion or impending herniation — obtain CT first when risk factors are present (focal deficit, papilledema, immunocompromise, new seizure, depressed mental status)
- Infection over the puncture site
- Coagulopathy: platelets below approximately 50,000, INR above approximately 1.5, or therapeutic anticoagulation — correct or defer
- Suspected spinal epidural abscess at the level of puncture (image instead — do not pass the needle through it)

Steps:

1. Contraindications: increased intracranial pressure (papilledema, focal deficits), coagulopathy, infection at site, spinal epidural abscess risk
2. Position: lateral decubitus with knees flexed toward chest, or sitting leaning forward; maximize interspinous distance
3. Identify landmarks: line between iliac crests (L4 spinous process or L4-L5 interspace); select L3-L4, L4-L5, or L5-S1
4. Sterile prep; local anesthetic
5. Insert spinal needle (22 gauge) with stylet; angle 10-15 degrees cephalad toward umbilicus
6. Resistance encountered at ligamentum flavum, then dura; "pop" sensation when entered
7. Remove stylet; observe CSF return; collect 1-2 mL in each of 4 tubes
8. Opening pressure: manometer attached to needle in lateral decubitus (normal <20 cm H_2O)
9. Replace stylet before withdrawing needle (theoretical prevention of epidermoid tumor)
10. Send for: cell count and differential (tubes 1 and 4), glucose and protein, gram stain, culture, xanthochromia (centrifuge tube 1), cryptococcal antigen, VDRL if indicated
11. Post-procedure: supine position 30-60 minutes, hydration, caffeine; warn of post-dural puncture headache

Obstetrics and Gynecology

Delivery of Newborn

Indications:

- Precipitous delivery: crowning or an irresistible urge to push with imminent delivery — delivery in the ED is managed, not deferred

Contraindications:

- No contraindications to assisting an imminent vaginal delivery
- Do not encourage pushing and prepare for emergent obstetric intervention when a contraindication to vaginal delivery is evident: umbilical cord prolapse (elevate the presenting part, position, emergent cesarean), transverse lie, or known complete placenta previa with hemorrhage

Skills:

1. Prepare sterile field; don sterile gloves if time permits
2. Controlled delivery: support perineum with dominant hand; guide fetal head out with gentle pressure to prevent rapid expulsion
3. Check for nuchal cord: if loose, slip over head; if tight, clamp and cut cord before delivering shoulders
4. Delivery of shoulders: downward traction until anterior shoulder visible under symphysis, then upward traction for posterior shoulder
5. Suction mouth then nose with bulb syringe (mouth first to prevent aspiration when baby gasps)
6. Delayed cord clamping: wait 30-60 seconds if infant vigorous; clamp with two Kelly clamps 3 cm from abdomen, cut between
7. Dry, warm, stimulate; APGAR score at 1 and 5 minutes
8. Manage shoulder dystocia if encountered: McRoberts maneuver (hyperflexion of maternal thighs), suprapubic pressure, Rubin maneuver, Wood's screw maneuver, delivery of posterior arm
9. Third stage management: await placental separation (signs: cord lengthening, gush of blood, uterine firming); gentle traction on cord with suprapubic counterpressure
10. Administer uterotonic: oxytocin 10 units IM or IV after anterior shoulder delivered; methylergonovine 0.2 mg IM or carboprost 250 mcg IM if hemorrhage
11. Inspect perineum for lacerations; repair if necessary

Medical Resuscitation

Pre-Arrival Preparation and Resuscitation Bay Setup

1. Assign roles (airway, procedures, medications, documentation, family liaison)
2. Prepare resuscitation cart: verify defibrillator functionality, pacing capability, and monitor connections
3. Prepare vasopressor infusion pumps with primed tubing (norepinephrine, epinephrine, phenylephrine); calculate weight-based dosing if patient weight known or estimate using Broselow tape or (age + 4) × 2 for pediatrics, or 70 kg standard adult dosing
4. Prepare resuscitation fluids: warmed crystalloid (normal saline or Lactated Ringer's), 4 units O-negative blood (female) or O-positive (male) if hemorrhage suspected, albumin 5 or 25 if available
5. Positioning: elevate head of bed 30 degrees if respiratory distress, supine with legs elevated if suspected hypovolemic shock (unless contraindicated by spinal precautions)
6. Ensure available: arterial line kit, central line kit (triple lumen or introducer), IO drill, ultrasound with cardiac and vascular probes, cooling blankets if hyperthermia suspected, point-of-care ultrasound device

Immediate Primary Survey and Stabilization

1. Airway: Assess patency; GCS <8 or inability to protect airway mandates intubation; prepare rapid sequence intubation with etomidate 0.3 mg/kg or ketamine 1-2 mg/kg plus rocuronium 1.2 mg/kg or succinylcholine 1.5 mg/kg
2. Breathing: Apply supplemental O_2 15L via non-rebreather; if SpO_2 <90% despite 100% FiO_2, escalate to BIPAP (IPAP 10-15, EPAP 5) or intubation; listen for bilateral breath sounds, tension pneumothorax, or flail chest
3. Circulation: Assess pulse quality, capillary refill, skin temperature, mentation; if no pulse, initiate CPR and ACLS algorithm immediately
4. Disability: Rapid glucose check (treat <70 with D50 25-50 mL or D10 2 mL/kg); assess pupils (size, reactivity, asymmetry); GCS calculation
5. Exposure: Remove clothing completely; assess for rashes (meningococcemia, anaphylaxis), track marks, surgical scars, medical alert jewelry; prevent hypothermia (active warming if temp <35°C)

Vascular Access and Hemodynamic Monitoring

1. Establish two large-bore peripheral IVs (14-16 gauge) antecubital or external jugular; if unsuccessful after 2 attempts or if access inadequate, proceed to intraosseous (EZ-IO humeral head or proximal tibia) or central line
2. Central Line Indications: Need for vasopressors, inability to obtain peripheral access, invasive hemodynamic monitoring, hypertonic saline or concentrated potassium administration
3. Arterial Line Indications: Expected hemodynamic instability requiring frequent pressures, need for arterial blood gas monitoring, titration of vasoactive medications (place within 30 minutes of vasopressor initiation if feasible)
4. Attach continuous monitoring: 5-lead ECG, pulse oximetry, non-invasive blood pressure cycling every 2-5 minutes initially, capnography if intubated
5. Obtain point-of-care labs: ABG, lactate, hemoglobin/hematocrit, electrolytes (including magnesium, calcium, phosphate), creatinine, BUN, glucose, coagulation studies, type and screen/crossmatch

Shock Classification and Initial Management

Septic Shock

1. Recognition: Suspected infection + lactate ≥4 or MAP <65 mmHg requiring vasopressors
2. Antibiotics: Administer within 1 hour of recognition; empirical coverage based on source:
3. Community-acquired pneumonia: Ceftriaxone 1 g IV + Azithromycin 500 mg IV or Ceftriaxone + Levofloxacin 750 mg IV
4. Intra-abdominal: Piperacillin-tazobactam 3.375 g IV + Vancomycin loading dose 25 mg/kg (max 2 g) + Metronidazole 500 mg IV
5. Urinary source: Ceftriaxone 1 g IV or Piperacillin-tazobactam if resistant organisms suspected
6. Meningitis: Vancomycin 15-20 mg/kg q8-12h + Ceftriaxone 2 g q12h + Ampicillin 2 g q4h (if Listeria risk >50 years, immunocompromised, or pregnant) + Dexamethasone 0.15 mg/kg (before or with first antibiotic dose)
7. Fluid Resuscitation: 30 mL/kg crystalloid (NS or LR) within first 3 hours; reassess after each 10 mL/kg bolus for signs of fluid overload (JVD, crackles, S3 gallop, rising BNP)
8. Source Control: Drain abscesses, remove infected lines, obtain surgical consultation for necrotizing fasciitis, cholangitis, or intestinal ischemia within 6 hours

Cardiogenic Shock

1. Recognition: SBP <90 mmHg or MAP <65 mmHg with CI <2.2 L/min/m^2, PCWP >15 mmHg, or clinical signs of hypoperfusion with elevated JVP and pulmonary edema
2. Inotropic Support: Dobutamine 2-20 mcg/kg/min (start at 2.5-5 mcg/kg/min) or Milrinone 0.375-0.75 mcg/kg/min (load with 50 mcg/kg over 10 minutes if not hypotensive)
3. Vasopressor Support: Norepinephrine 0.05-0.5 mcg/kg/min if MAP <65 despite dobutamine; avoid pure alpha-agonists (phenylephrine) which increase afterload
4. Diuretics: Furosemide 40-80 mg IV if volume overloaded; consider bumetanide 1-2 mg IV if furosemide refractory
5. Nitrates: Nitroglycerin 0.4 mg SL or infusion 5-10 mcg/min if SBP >100 and no RV infarct; avoid if RV infarct, severe AS, or preload-dependent state and if hypotensive. Nitrates for preload reduction and improvement of respiratory distress
6. Emergent Interventions: Cardiac catheterization lab activation for STEMI, consider ECMO if refractory, pericardiocentesis if tamponade

Hypovolemic Shock (Hemorrhagic)

1. Recognition: Tachycardia, hypotension, narrow pulse pressure, cool extremities, delayed capillary refill >3 seconds, elevated shock index (HR/SBP >0.9)
2. Hemorrhage Control: Direct pressure, tourniquet for extremity hemorrhage, pelvic binder if suspected pelvic fracture, TXA 1 g IV over 10 minutes (within 3 hours of injury) followed by 1 g over 8 hours
3. Blood Products: Initiate Massive Transfusion Protocol (MTP) if >4 units PRBC anticipated:
4. Ratio: 1:1:1 (PRBC:FFP:Platelets) or 6:4:1
5. Target: Hgb >7 (>8 if CAD), INR <1.5, Plt >50,000, fibrinogen >100 (give cryoprecipitate if <150)
6. Calcium: Replete if ionized calcium <1.0 (give 1 g calcium chloride IV or 3 g calcium gluconate per 4-6 units PRBC)
7. Permissive Hypotension: Maintain SBP 80-90 mmHg (MAP 50-60) until hemorrhage controlled (except TBI, maintain SBP >110)

Anaphylactic Shock

1. Recognition: Hypotension plus mucocutaneous involvement (urticaria, flushing) or respiratory compromise (bronchospasm, stridor, hypoxia) after antigen exposure

2. Epinephrine: 0.3-0.5 mg IM (1:1000 concentration, 0.3-0.5 mL) lateral thigh; repeat every 5-15 minutes if no improvement; if impending arrest, give 0.1 mg IV (1:10,000) over 5 minutes or 0.1-0.5 mcg/kg/min infusion
3. Adjuncts:
4. H1-blocker: Diphenhydramine 50 mg IV (adults) or 1 mg/kg (peds)
5. H2-blocker: Famotidine 20 mg IV
6. Corticosteroids: Methylprednisolone 125 mg IV or Hydrocortisone 500 mg IV (delayed effect, prevents biphasic reaction)
7. Beta-agonists: Albuterol 2.5 mg nebulized for bronchospasm
8. Glucagon 1-5 mg IV over 5 minutes if on beta-blockers (unopposed alpha stimulation)
9. Fluid Resuscitation: 1-2 L crystalloid rapidly (distributive shock causes massive vasodilation and relative hypovolemia)

Adrenal Crisis

1. Recognition: Hypotension refractory to fluids and vasopressors, hyponatremia, hyperkalemia, hypoglycemia, history of steroid use or autoimmune disease
2. Hydrocortisone: 100 mg IV bolus immediately, then 200 mg/day continuous infusion or 50 mg IV q6h (do not wait for ACTH stimulation test if suspected)
3. Fluids: D5NS or NS; correct hypoglycemia with D50 if needed
4. Mineralocorticoid: Fludrocortisone 0.1 mg daily (only if continued deficiency expected)

Vasopressor Selection, Preparation, and Dosing

Norepinephrine (Levophed) - First Line for Septic Shock

1. Preparation: 4 mg in 250 mL D5W or NS (16 mcg/mL) or 8 mg in 250 mL (32 mcg/mL) for central access
2. Dosing: Start at 0.05 mcg/kg/min (3.5 mcg/min in 70 kg adult), titrate by 0.05 mcg/kg/min every 3-5 minutes to MAP >65; usual range 0.05-0.5 mcg/kg/min (up to 35 mcg/min or higher in refractory cases)
3. Indications: Septic shock, cardiogenic shock (with inotrope), anaphylaxis (after epinephrine), spinal shock
4. Adverse Effects: Arrhythmias, digital ischemia, extravasation necrosis (treat with phentolamine 5-10 mg local infiltration)
5. Access: Central line preferred; can run peripherally temporarily through proximal vein with frequent monitoring (risk of extravasation)

Epinephrine

1. Preparation: 1 mg in 250 mL NS or D5W (4 mcg/mL) for infusion; 1:10,000 (0.1 mg/mL) for cardiac arrest
2. Dosing:
   - Cardiac arrest: 1 mg IV/IO every 3-5 minutes (10 mL of 1:10,000)
   - Anaphylaxis: 0.1 mg IV over 5 minutes or 0.1-1 mcg/min infusion (start 0.1 mcg/min, titrate to effect)
   - Shock: 0.01-0.1 mcg/kg/min (0.7-7 mcg/min in 70 kg adult)
3. Indications: Anaphylaxis, cardiac arrest, severe bradycardia unresponsive to atropine, beta-blocker overdose, anaphylactic shock refractory to IM epinephrine
4. Adverse Effects: Tachycardia, ventricular arrhythmias, hyperglycemia, lactic acidosis, renal vasoconstriction

Phenylephrine (Neo-Synephrine)

1. Preparation: 10 mg in 250 mL NS (40 mcg/mL) or 20 mg in 250 mL (80 mcg/mL)

2. Dosing: Start 0.5 mcg/kg/min (35 mcg/min in 70 kg adult), titrate to MAP >65; usual range 0.5-9 mcg/kg/min
3. Indications: Neurogenic shock (spinal cord injury), intraoperative hypotension, atrial fibrillation with RVR (increases BP without increasing heart rate), aortic stenosis (maintains coronary perfusion without increasing contractility)
4. Contraindications: Cardiogenic shock, septic shock (increases afterload without inotropic support), reflex bradycardia risk
5. Pure Alpha-agonist: No beta-1 activity; increases SVR and BP, may decrease cardiac output

Vasopressin (Pitressin)

1. Preparation: 20 units in 100 mL NS (0.2 units/mL) or 40 units in 100 mL (0.4 units/mL)
2. Dosing: Fixed dose 0.03 units/min (1.8 units/hour) OR weight-based 0.01-0.04 units/min; do not titrate (on/off medication)
3. Indications: Septic shock as adjunct to norepinephrine (Vasopressin and Septic Shock Trial - VASST), anaphylaxis refractory to epinephrine, hepatorenal syndrome, variceal bleeding (off-label for shock), diabetes insipidus
4. Physiology: V1 receptor agonist (vascular smooth muscle), not dependent on catecholamine receptors (useful in acidosis or beta-blockade)
5. Caution: Mesenteric ischemia, digital ischemia, hyponatremia (SIADH), myocardial ischemia

Dobutamine

1. Preparation: 250 mg in 250 mL D5W or NS (1000 mcg/mL)
2. Dosing: 2.5-20 mcg/kg/min; start at 2.5-5 mcg/kg/min and titrate every few minutes based on cardiac output or clinical response
3. Indications: Cardiogenic shock with low output, acute decompensated heart failure, inotropic support without significant vasoconstriction, cardiac stress testing
4. Physiology: Beta-1 agonist (primary), mild beta-2 agonist (vasodilation), minimal alpha activity; increases contractility and heart rate, decreases SVR
5. Contraindications: Hypertrophic obstructive cardiomyopathy (HOCM), severe aortic stenosis (may worsen gradient), atrial fibrillation with rapid ventricular response (may accelerate AV conduction)

Resuscitation Fluids

Crystalloid Solutions

1. Normal Saline (0.9%):
   - Composition: 154 Na, 154 Cl, pH 5.0-5.5
   - Indications: Initial resuscitation, head injury (isotonic), hyperkalemia, metabolic alkalosis
   - Caution: Hyperchloremic metabolic acidosis with large volumes (>30 mL/kg), potential renal vasoconstriction
2. Lactated Ringer's (Hartmann's):
   - Composition: 130 Na, 109 Cl, 28 lactate, 4 K, 3 Ca
   - Indications: Burns, sepsis, trauma (reduces acidosis compared to NS), diabetic ketoacidosis
   - Contraindications: Hyperkalemia (contains 4 K), severe metabolic alkalosis, concurrent blood transfusion (calcium chelates citrate in PRBC)
3. Plasma-Lyte A:
   - Composition: 140 Na, 98 Cl, 50 acetate/gluconate, 5 K, 3 Mg
   - Most physiologically balanced; minimal effect on acid-base status

Colloid Solutions

1. Albumin 5%: Iso-oncotic; expands plasma volume similar to crystalloid but stays intravascular longer; indications: large volume paracentesis, spontaneous bacterial peritonitis, hepatorenal syndrome, burn resuscitation if crystalloid requirements excessive (>30 mL/kg in first 8 hours)
2. Albumin 25%: Hyperoncotic; draws fluid from interstitial to intravascular; indications: nephrotic syndrome, cirrhosis with ascites, cerebral edema (controversial)

Blood Products

1. Packed Red Blood Cells (PRBC):
   - Dose: 1 unit raises Hgb by 1 or Hct by 3% in stable adults
   - Indications: Hgb <7 (restrictive strategy), <8 if CAD or active bleeding with hemodynamic instability
   - Type and crossmatch requires 45 minutes; type-specific 15 minutes; O-negative immediate
2. Fresh Frozen Plasma (FFP):
   - Dose: 15-20 mL/kg (typically 4 units in adults)
   - Indications: INR >1.5 with active bleeding, massive transfusion protocol, warfarin reversal (with PCC preferred if available), TTP plasmapheresis replacement
3. Platelets:
   - Dose: 1 apheresis unit (equivalent to 6 pooled units) or 6-10 pooled units
   - Indications: Plt <10,000 (prophylaxis), <50,000 with active bleeding or invasive procedure, <100,000 with CNS bleeding
4. Cryoprecipitate:
   - Dose: 10 units (1 unit per 10 kg)
   - Indications: Fibrinogen <100-150, DIC with bleeding, hemophilia A (when factor VIII concentrate unavailable)

Fluid Resuscitation Endpoints

1. Dynamic Assessment: Passive leg raise (PLR) with stroke volume measurement or pulse pressure variation (PPV) <13% suggests fluid non-responsiveness
2. Static Markers: MAP >65 mmHg (or >80 if chronic hypertension), urine output >0.5 mL/kg/hr, lactate clearance >10 at 2 hours, normalization of base deficit
3. IVC Ultrasound
   - Greater than ~50% collapsibility suggests the patient is likely volume-responsive (hypovolemic or preload-dependent). These patients are more likely to benefit from a fluid bolus.
   - Less than ~50% collapsibility suggests adequate or elevated volume status, where fluids may not improve cardiac output and could cause harm
4. Tissue Perfusion: Capillary refill <3 seconds, warm extremities, decreasing mentation abnormalities

Critical Medical Conditions

Acute Coronary Syndrome with Cardiogenic Shock

1. Aspirin 325 mg chew (if not given), Clopidogrel 600 mg loading or Ticagrelor 180 mg, Heparin bolus 60 units/kg (max 4000) then 12 units/kg/hr
2. Emergent PCI within 90 minutes (door-to-balloon); fibrinolysis only if PCI unavailable within 120 minutes and <12 hours symptoms
3. IABP or Impella for mechanical support if medical therapy fails
4. Avoid nitrates if SBP <90 mmHg or RV infarct (inferior MI with right-sided leads showing ST elevation)

Acute Pulmonary Embolism with Massive/Submassive

1. Massive PE (sustained hypotension SBP <90 or shock): Systemic thrombolysis unless absolute contraindication (Alteplase 100 mg IV over 2 hours or 0.6 mg/kg bolus over 15 minutes for PE <50 kg)
2. Submassive (RV dysfunction, elevated troponin/BNP, normotensive): Consider thrombolysis if clinical deterioration; heparin drip otherwise
3. Surgical embolectomy or catheter-directed thrombolysis if thrombolysis contraindicated or failed
4. Fluids: cautious 500 mL bolus only if clear hypovolemia; avoid aggressive fluids (RV failure is pressure overloaded, not volume depleted)

Status Epilepticus

1. First line: Benzodiazepines - Lorazepam 4 mg IV (repeat x2) or Diazepam 10 mg IV (repeat x2) or Midazolam 10 mg IM if no IV access
2. Second line: Levetiracetam 60 mg/kg IV (max 4500 mg) or Fosphenytoin 20 mg PE/kg IV (max 1500 mg PE) or Valproic acid 40 mg/kg IV (max 3000 mg)
3. Refractory: Propofol 2 mg/kg bolus then 50-200 mcg/kg/min or Midazolam 0.2 mg/kg bolus then 0.1-0.4 mg/kg/hr; intubate and continuous EEG
4. Pyrexia management (for febrile seizures)

Severe Hyperkalemia (>6.5 or ECG changes)

1. Stabilize Myocardium: Calcium chloride 1 g IV over 5-10 minutes (or calcium gluconate 3 g); repeat if ECG changes persist; onset 1-3 minutes, duration 30-60 minutes
2. Shift K Intracellularly:
    - Regular insulin 10 units IV + D50 25 g IV (onset 15-30 min, duration 4-6 hours)
    - Albuterol 10-20 mg nebulized over 15 minutes (beta-2 agonist)
    - Sodium bicarbonate 50-100 mEq IV if metabolic acidosis present (pH <7.2)
3. Eliminate K:
    - Kayexalate 15-30 g PO/PR (onset hours, risk of intestinal necrosis)
    - Loop diuretics: Furosemide 40-80 mg IV if renal function adequate
    - Hemodialysis: definitive treatment if refractory or renal failure
4. Monitor: Continuous ECG, serial K every 30-60 minutes, treat underlying cause

Thyroid Storm

1. Block Synthesis: Propylthiouracil (PTU) 600-1000 mg loading dose then 200 mg q4-6h OR Methimazole 60-80 mg/day (PTU preferred if pregnant)
2. Block Release: Iodine (SSKI 5 drops q6h or Lugol's solution) given 1 hour AFTER thionamide (to prevent new hormone synthesis)
3. Block Conversion (T4 to T3): Hydrocortisone 300 mg IV load then 100 mg q8h (also treats possible adrenal insufficiency)
4. Supportive: Propranolol 1-2 mg IV (or 60-80 mg PO q4h) to control adrenergic symptoms, aggressive cooling (acetaminophen only, avoid aspirin), fluids, treat precipitating cause

Serotonin Syndrome

1. Recognition: Mental status change + autonomic instability + neuromuscular abnormalities (clonus, hyperreflexia, hyperthermia) in context of serotonergic drug use
2. Cyproheptadine (serotonin antagonist): 12 mg PO/NGT initially, then 2 mg q2h until response (max 32 mg/day)
3. Benzodiazepines: Lorazepam 2-4 mg IV for agitation, tremor, seizures
4. Cooling: External cooling blankets, ice packs, evaporative cooling if temp >40°C; consider dantrolene if hyperthermia refractory (controversial)

5. Supportive: IV fluids, discontinuation of offending agents, intubation if airway compromise from muscle rigidity

Malignant Hyperthermia

1. Dantrolene: 2.5 mg/kg IV bolus immediately, repeat until symptoms abate (may require 10 mg/kg total); then 1 mg/kg q4-6h x 24-48 hours to prevent recurrence
2. Cooling: Stop triggering agents (volatile anesthetics, succinylcholine), hyperventilate with 100% O_2, ice packs to groin/axilla, cooled IV fluids, bladder/gastric lavage with iced saline
3. Labs: ABG (metabolic acidosis, hypercapnia), CK, lactate, electrolytes (hyperkalemia), coagulation studies (DIC risk)
4. Support: Treat hyperkalemia with calcium, insulin/glucose, bicarbonate; maintenance fluids; ICU admission

Beta-Blocker Overdose

1. Glucagon: 5-10 mg IV bolus over 2-5 minutes (causes hyperglycemia, nausea/vomiting), then 1-5 mg/hour infusion
2. High-Dose Insulin (HIE): Regular insulin 1 unit/kg IV bolus then 1-10 units/kg/hour infusion with dextrose support (euglycemic clamp)
3. Lipid Emulsion: 20 Intralipid 1.5 mL/kg bolus over 2-3 minutes, then 0.25 mL/kg/min for 30-60 minutes
4. Epinephrine: High-dose infusion (0.1-1 mcg/kg/min) often required; norepinephrine adjunct
5. Calcium: Calcium chloride 1-2 g IV for myocardial contractility support

Calcium Channel Blocker Overdose

1. Calcium: Calcium chloride 1 g IV every 10-20 minutes (up to 3 g) or calcium gluconate 3 g IV; monitor ionized calcium (target high normal)
2. High-Dose Insulin: Same protocol as beta-blocker overdose (insulin 1 unit/kg bolus, then 0.5-2 units/kg/hr)
3. Vasopressors: Norepinephrine first line; epinephrine if bradycardic; glucagon as adjunct
4. Lipid Emulsion: Same dosing as beta-blocker overdose
5. Transcutaneous or Transvenous Pacing: For bradycardia refractory to medications

Trauma Resuscitation

Pre-Arrival Activation and Resuscitation Bay Preparation

1. Activate Level I Trauma Response; notify trauma surgeon, anesthesiologist, OR, blood bank, and interventional radiology if hemodynamically unstable
2. Prepare hemorrhage control station: commercial tourniquets (CAT or SOF-T), hemostatic gauze (Combat Gauze, ChitoGauze), pelvic binder (T-POD or SAM), traction splints, temporary intravascular shunt kit
3. Prime massive transfusion cooler: 4 units O-negative packed red blood cells (PRBCs), 4 units fresh frozen plasma (FFP), 1 apheresis platelet unit; request thawed plasma (AB or type-specific) immediately available
4. Prepare TXA: 1 g in 100 mL NS (infuse over 10 minutes), followed by second dose 1 g in 250 mL NS over 8 hours if within 3 hours of injury
5. Set up rapid infusers (Level 1 or Belmont) with warming capability; ensure calcium chloride 1 g vials readily available (administer 1 g per 4-6 units PRBC anticipated)
6. Positioning: trauma stretcher with ability for Trendelenburg and reverse Trendelenburg; ensure C-collar sizes (small, medium, large) at head of bed; prepare log-roll equipment (spinal board if indicated)
7. Assign roles explicitly: Team Leader (maintains global oversight, does not perform procedures), Airway Physician, Procedure/Access Physician, Documentation Nurse, Medication Nurse, Radiology Technician

Primary Survey: ABCDE with Cervical Spine Protection

A - Airway with C-Spine Protection

1. Manual inline stabilization (MILS) immediately; immobilize cervical spine with rigid collar simultaneously with airway assessment
2. Assess patency: inspect for facial fractures (Le Fort I-III), mandibular instability, airway edema, expanding neck hematoma, stridor, soot in oropharynx (inhalation injury)
3. Immediate airway indication: GCS ≤8, severe maxillofacial trauma, copious vomiting/bleeding, respiratory distress with hypoxia (SpO_2 <90% on high-flow O_2), expanding neck hematoma, airway burn
4. Rapid Sequence Intubation (Trauma Modifications):
5. Induction: Etomidate 0.3 mg/kg IV (hemodynamically neutral) or Ketamine 1-2 mg/kg IV (preferred if hypotensive, preserves sympathetic tone)
6. Paralysis: Rocuronium 1.2 mg/kg IV (avoid succinylcholine if >48 hours since burns, crush injury, denervation, or hyperkalemia risk)
7. Cricoid pressure during rapid sequence if no contraindication (C-spine fracture with risk of displacement)
8. Video laryngoscopy - preferred for all airway mangment - c-spine can be manually stabilized so collar does not interfere with airway managment, minimize neck movement during intubation
9. Surgical airway standby: scalpel-bougie-tube technique ready if failed intubation; perform cricothyrotomy (needle cricothyrotomy only as bridge in pediatric patients <12 years)
10. Post-intubation: verify ETT position (waveform capnography, auscultation, chest X-ray at teeth/lip level), secure with tube holder, always order post intubation sedation

B - Breathing and Ventilation

1. Inspect chest wall: paradoxical movement (flail chest), open chest wounds (sucking chest wound), tracheal deviation, JVD (tension pneumothorax or cardiac tamponade), subcutaneous emphysema
2. Auscultate bilaterally; if absent breath sounds or tympanic percussion:

3. Immediate needle decompression: 14-gauge 3.25-inch angiocath, 2nd intercostal space midclavicular line OR 4th/5th intercostal space anterior axillary line (preferred to avoid cardiac vessels)
4. Follow immediately with tube thoracostomy: 28-36 Fr for hemothorax, 20-28 Fr for pneumothorax; insert at 5th intercostal space mid-axillary line (triangle of safety)
5. Open pneumothorax: Cover with three-sided occlusive dressing (Asherman valve or improvised); if tension develops, remove dressing temporarily
6. Massive hemothorax (>1500 mL initial output or >200 mL/hr for 2-4 hours): Chest tube placement, prepare autotransfusion if available, emergent thoracotomy if exsanguinating
7. Ventilation strategy: Lung-protective tidal volumes 6 mL/kg predicted body weight; avoid hyperventilation ($PaCO_2$ 35-40 mmHg) unless signs of cerebral herniation (see TBI section); PEEP 5 cm H_2O if hypotension resolved

C - Circulation and Hemorrhage Control

1. Assess pulse quality, skin color, capillary refill (>2 seconds abnormal), mentation; calculate Shock Index (HR/SBP >0.9 indicates significant shock)
2. Immediate Hemorrhage Control:
3. Extremity hemorrhage: Apply tourniquet 2-3 inches proximal to wound (not over joint), tighten until bleeding stops and pulse eliminated; mark time on tourniquet; maximum 2 hours before neurovascular compromise (temporary release only in OR)
4. Junctional hemorrhage (groin/axilla): Combat Gauze or Celox packing with 3-5 minutes firm pressure; wound clamp if amputation
5. Pelvic fracture: Apply pelvic binder at level of greater trochanters (not waist); tighten until symphysis compressed to 1 cm or until stability achieved; leaves on until OR or angiography
6. Vascular Access:
7. Two large-bore peripheral IVs (14-16 gauge) or 18-gauge IO (intraosseous) in proximal humerus (preferred for rapid flow) or proximal tibia if peripheral access fails after 2 attempts or 90 seconds
8. Central line (9 Fr introducer catheter) only if peripheral/IO unsuccessful or if vasoactive medications required; femoral vein preferred in trauma (avoid IJ/subclavian if coagulopathic or thoracic trauma)
9. Blood Products: Initiate Massive Transfusion Protocol (MTP) if:
10. SBP <90 mmHg with suspected torso hemorrhage
11. HR >120 with suspected active bleeding
12. Known PRBC requirement >4 units in 4 hours
13. Initial Hgb <10 with ongoing bleeding
14. Resuscitation Strategy:
    - Permissive Hypotension: SBP 80-90 mmHg (MAP 50-60) until hemorrhage controlled, EXCEPT in Traumatic Brain Injury (TBI) - maintain SBP >110-120 mmHg (cerebral perfusion pressure >60)
    - Initial fluid: Warmed blood products preferred; if delayed, limited crystalloid (250 mL boluses) to maintain radial pulse or mentation
15. TXA: 1 g IV over 10 minutes immediately if within 3 hours of injury (CRASH-2 criteria); second 1 g over 8 hours; contraindicated if isolated TBI without extracranial bleeding (CRASH-3 nuance)
16. Calcium: 1 g Calcium Chloride (or 3 g Calcium Gluconate) IV with first 4 units PRBC, then every 4-6 units or if ionized calcium <1.0

D - Disability (Neurologic Evaluation)

1. Rapid neurologic assessment: GCS (verbal component assumed if intubated), pupillary size/reactivity (asymmetry suggests uncal herniation or direct ocular trauma), lateralizing signs
2. TBI Management Prior to OR:

- o Sedation: Propofol 25-50 mcg/kg/min or Etomidate infusion if hypotensive; avoid hypotension (single most important factor for secondary brain injury)
- o Hyperosmolar Therapy if signs of herniation (unilateral dilated pupil, Cushing's triad, asymmetric posturing):
- o Mannitol 0.25-1 g/kg IV (keep serum osmolarity <320 mOsm/L or hypertonic saline 3 250 mL over 30 minutes (preferred if hypotensive, also expands intravascular volume)
- o Hyperventilation: Only as bridge to OR if herniation signs present ($PaCO_2$ target 30-35 mmHg); otherwise maintain normocapnia
- o Head of Bed: 30 degrees once spinal precautions cleared or if cervical collar applied with reverse Trendelenburg

3. Spinal Cord Injury:
    - o Neurogenic Shock: Hypotension with bradycardia (loss of sympathetic tone); treat with fluids PLUS Phenylephrine (pure alpha) or Norepinephrine to maintain MAP >85-90 (preserve spinal cord perfusion)
    - o High-dose Methylprednisolone: NOT recommended (NASCIS III showed no benefit, increased infection risk); do not administer
4. Maintain mean arterial pressure >85 for first 7 days if spinal cord injury confirmed

E - Exposure and Environmental Control

1. Remove all clothing; inspect posterior surfaces during log-roll maintaining spinal alignment
2. Identify entry/exit wounds (circle with marker, cover with sterile dressing); do not remove impaled objects (stabilize in place)
3. Prevent hypothermia: Warm resuscitation bay to 75-80°F (24-27°C); use forced-air warming blankets (Bair Hugger) on torso (not over extremity IV sites); infuse warmed fluids and blood; consider warmed humidified oxygen
4. Advanced Rewarming strategies if temperature <35°C: Warmed bladder irrigation, warmed peritoneal lavage, extracorporeal rewarming for severe hypothermia with cardiac arrest

Adjuncts to Primary Survey

FAST Examination

1. Perform during primary survey (C phase) if patient unstable; do NOT delay transport to OR for CT if positive FAST in unstable patient
2. Views: Pericardial (subxiphoid or parasternal), hepatorenal (Morison's pouch), splenorenal, suprapubic (bladder with retroperitoneal view), thoracic (pleural sliding for pneumothorax, effusions)
3. Positive FAST (hemoperitoneum or pericardial fluid) + Hemodynamic instability = Immediate OR (laparotomy or sternotomy/pericardial window)
4. Negative FAST + Unstable + No obvious thoracic/abdominal source = Consider pelvic fracture (binder applied), retroperitoneal hemorrhage, or long bone fractures

X-Rays

1. Chest X-ray (portable AP supine): Verify ETT, OGT, central line positions; evaluate for hemothorax, pneumothorax, widened mediastinum (aortic injury), rib fractures, pulmonary contusions
2. Pelvis X-ray: If hemodynamically unstable, single AP view to identify pelvic fracture pattern (open book, vertical shear, lateral compression) to guide binder placement and angiography vs OR decision
3. C-Spine X-ray: Only if patient stable and CT unavailable; otherwise CT C-spine is imaging of choice for clearance

Secondary Survey (Head-to-Toe Examination)

1. Head: Scalp lacerations (bleeding control with Raney clips or staples), depressed skull fractures, Battle's sign, raccoon eyes, CSF otorrhea/rhinorrhea (gauze loosely placed, do not pack), hemotympanum, facial stability (Le Fort fractures)
2. Maxillofacial/C-spine: Mandible instability, tracheal deviation, cervical step-offs; maintain collar until cleared
3. Chest: Clavicle tenderness, flail segments (paradoxical motion), subcutaneous emphysema; re-evaluate breath sounds after patient repositioning
4. Abdomen: Seat belt sign (intestinal injury risk), Grey-Turner's sign (retroperitoneal hemorrhage), Kehr's sign (referred shoulder pain from splenic injury), peritoneal signs; DRE for sphincter tone, blood (spinal injury), prostate position (urethral injury)
5. Pelvis/Perineum: Stability testing (gentle compression of iliac wings - only once to avoid displacing clot), blood at urethral meatus, scrotal hematoma (butterfly sign), open book deformity
6. Extremities: Tenderness, deformity, compartments (tense, painful with passive stretch), pulses (ABI <0.9 suggests vascular injury), motor/sensory function
7. Back/Spine: Log-roll maintaining alignment; inspect for step-offs, ecchymosis, exit wounds

Critical Injury-Specific Management Prior to OR

Traumatic Brain Injury (Severe - GCS ≤8)

1. Sedation/Analgesia: Fentanyl 25-50 mcg IV (prevents coughing/straining) + Propofol 25-75 mcg/kg/min; avoid hypotension (maintain SBP >110)
2. ICP Management: Head midline, 30 degrees elevation, avoid jugular compression (loose collar); Mannitol 0.25-1 g/kg or 3 saline 250 mL for signs of herniation
3. Seizure Prophylaxis: Levetiracetam 1000-1500 mg IV if severe TBI (GCS <8) or penetrating head wound; load immediately
4. Coagulopathy Reversal: If on anticoagulants:
   - Warfarin: PCC 25-50 units/kg + Vitamin K 10 mg IV
   - DOACs: PCC 50 units/kg (consider andexanet alfa for rivaroxaban/apixaban if available)
   - Platelet dysfunction (aspirin/clopidogrel): Platelet transfusion if active ICH and going to OR
5. Hyperventilation: Only for acute herniation (blowing pupil); otherwise $PaCO_2$ 35-40

Thoracic Trauma

1. Tension Pneumothorax: Immediate decompression followed by chest tube; do NOT await X-ray confirmation in unstable patient
2. Massive Hemothorax: Chest tube placement (large bore 36 Fr), autotransfusion if available; OR if >1500 mL immediate return or >200 mL/hr for 4 hours
3. Cardiac Tamponade: Pericardiocentesis only if patient decompensating and OR not immediately available; otherwise immediate thoracotomy/sternotomy; volume loading to maintain preload
4. Traumatic Aortic Injury (suspected widened mediastinum): Beta-blockade (Esmolol 50-100 mcg/kg/min or Labetalol 10-20 mg IV) to maintain HR <100 and SBP 90-100 (permissive hypotension to prevent rupture); emergent vascular surgery consultation

Abdominal Trauma

1. Unstable with Positive FAST: Direct to OR; no CT; pre-operative antibiotics (Cefazolin 2 g IV or Ampicillin/Sulbactam 3 g IV if penetrating)
2. Stable with Questionable FAST: CT abdomen/pelvis with IV contrast (oral contrast not needed in acute trauma); look for active extravasation (requires angiography or OR), grade of solid organ injury

3. Retroperitoneal Hematoma: Do NOT explore if stable and non-expanding; if expanding or pulsatile = vascular injury, requires OR or angiography
4. Open Abdomen: If bowel eviscerated, cover with sterile saline-moistened gauze and impermeable dressing; do not attempt reduction in ED if contaminated or edematous

Pelvic Fracture

1. Mechanism: High-energy (MVC, fall >10 feet, crush)
2. Hemorrhage Control: Mechanical stabilization with pelvic binder or sheet tied at greater trochanters (reduces pelvic volume, stabilizes fracture, limits venous bleeding)
3. Decision Tree:
    - Hemodynamically unstable + Pelvic fracture on X-ray + FAST negative = Angiography (embolization) vs Pre-peritoneal packing vs External fixation
    - Hemodynamically unstable + Positive FAST = OR first (laparotomy), then address pelvis
4. Contraindications to Binder: Open pelvic fracture with perineal wound (apply carefully to avoid contaminating wound), lateral compression fracture (may worsen internally rotated hemipelvis - check X-ray pattern first)
5. Urethral Injury Signs: Blood at meatus, high-riding prostate, scrotal hematoma, butterfly bruising → Do NOT place Foley; perform retrograde urethrogram first or place suprapubic catheter

Extremity Trauma

1. Vascular Injury Hard Signs: Active bleeding, expanding hematoma, bruit/thrill, pulseless limb, audible "wound blowout" → Immediate operative exploration or temporary intravascular shunt
2. Compartment Syndrome: Pain out of proportion, pain with passive stretch, paresthesias, pallor, pulselessness (late sign), tenseness → Fasciotomy in ED if delayed OR; measure compartment pressures if equivocal (>30 mmHg or within 30 mmHg of diastolic pressure)
3. Amputation: Preserve amputated part in moist gauze, placed in plastic bag, then on ice (never directly on ice); tourniquet control of stump; tetanus prophylaxis
4. Open Fractures: Splint in position of function; cover with sterile saline dressing; antibiotics within 3 hours (Cefazolin 2 g IV + Gentamicin 5 mg/kg if Gustilo grade III, add Penicillin 2-4 million units if soil contamination/clostridium risk)

Burns

1. Airway: Intubate if inhalation injury suspected (soot in oropharynx, singed nasal hairs, hoarseness, stridor, closed space fire, carboxyhemoglobin >10); early intubation before edema develops
2. Fluid Resuscitation (Parkland Formula): 4 mL × weight (kg) × %TBSA burned (2nd and 3rd degree only); half in first 8 hours from time of injury (not ED arrival), quarter next 8 hours, quarter final 8 hours; use LR; titrate to urine output 0.5-1 mL/kg/hr
3. Escharotomy: If circumferential full-thickness burns restricting ventilation (chest) or perfusion (extremities); perform in ED if compartment syndrome developing
4. Carbon Monoxide: 100% O_2 until carboxyhemoglobin <10%; hyperbaric if CO >25%, pregnant with CO >15%, or neurological deficits

Damage Control Resuscitation Principles (Pre-OR)

1. Blood Product Strategy: Maintain ratio approaching 1:1:1 (PRBC:FFP:Platelets); utilize whole blood if available (military/remote settings)
2. Minimize Crystalloid: Goal <2 L crystalloid prior to blood products to prevent dilutional coagulopathy and edema
3. Arterial Blood Gas Monitoring: Track base deficit, lactate, hemoglobin, ionized calcium every 30 minutes; pH <7.2 indicates need for bicarbonate (1 mEq/kg) if hemodynamically unstable with arrhythmias

4. Rewarming: Core temperature <34°C impairs coagulation cascade; target >35°C prior to OR if possible using all measures available
5. Reversal of Anticoagulation: As detailed in TBI section; have 4-factor PCC immediately available for trauma patients on warfarin

Special Populations

Pregnancy (>20 weeks)

1. Positioning: Left lateral displacement of uterus (tilt board or manual displacement) to relieve IVC compression; if CPR required, perform manual left uterine displacement or 15-degree left tilt
2. Physiologic Changes: Increased blood volume (tolerate 1000-1500 mL blood loss before decompensation), hemodilution (Hgb normally 10-11), supine hypotension syndrome
3. Fetal Monitoring: If viable fetus (>24 weeks) and mother hemodynamically stable, apply fetal monitor; if unstable, maternal stabilization takes precedence
4. Perimortem Cesarean Section: If mother in arrest >4 minutes with no ROSC and fetus viable (>24 weeks), perform resuscitative hysterotomy at bedside to improve maternal cardiac output and potentially save fetus

Pediatric Trauma

1. Airway: Uncuffed ETT size = (Age/4) + 4; depth = (Age/2) + 12; cuffed = (Age/4) + 3.5
2. Fluid: 20 mL/kg boluses (warm LR or NS); blood 10-15 mL/kg; avoid permissive hypotension (maintain age-appropriate BP)
3. Chest Tube: 16-24 Fr depending on size; insert at 4th intercostal space
4. Hypothermia: Higher risk; aggressive warming essential

Neonatal Resuscitation

Pre-Arrival Preparation and Resuscitation Environment

1. Activate neonatal resuscitation team; notify NICU, neonatology, and respiratory therapy; prepare for precipitous delivery if maternal peripartum
2. Temperature control (critical priority): Warm resuscitation room to 74°F-77°F (23°C-25°C); preheat radiant warmer; prepare polyethylene plastic wrap (1-liter bag or wrapping sheet) and pre-warmed towels for very low birth weight (<1500 g) or preterm (<32 weeks)
3. Prepare oxygen blender with ability to titrate from 21% (room air) to 100%; avoid 100% oxygen initially for term infants (room air or 21-30 preferred initially)
4. Airway equipment:
5. Face masks: newborn size (cup covers nose and mouth but not eyes), premature size
6. Self-inflating bag (240-500 mL) with pressure manometer and 21% oxygen inlet (do not use anesthesia bags that require compressed gas)
7. T-piece resuscitator (Neopuff) with pressure limiting device (30-40 cm H_2O PIP max)
8. Laryngoscope: Miller 0 (preterm) and Miller 1 (term) straight blades; suction catheter (10 F or 12 F), meconium aspirator adapter
9. ETT: 2.5 mm (ID) for <1000 g or <28 weeks, 3.0 mm for 1000-2000 g or 28-34 weeks, 3.5 mm for >2000 g or >34 weeks; 3.5 mm for term infants; stylet optional
10. Depth marking: 5.5-6 cm at lip for 3.0 mm tube, 7 cm for 3.5 mm tube (calculate: 6 + weight in kg for nasal depth, 7 + weight for oral depth approximation)
11. Vascular access: Umbilical catheterization tray (3.5 Fr single-lumen for >28 weeks, 5 Fr for term), umbilical tape, sterile scissors, sterile drapes, hemostats, 3-0 silk suture, 3-way stopcock, 5-10 mL syringes, normal saline flushes; intraosseous needle (EZ-IO 15 mm) as backup
12. Medication preparation (calculate for 3 kg term infant unless known otherwise):
    - Epinephrine 1:10,000 (0.1 mg/mL): draw 3 mL (0.3 mg total) in 1 mL aliquots
    - Normal saline 10 mL in syringe for volume expansion
    - Dextrose 10 (D10): 2-4 mL/kg (6-12 mL for 3 kg infant)
    - Naloxone (rarely indicated): 0.1 mg/kg (0.3 mg max)
    - Sodium bicarbonate 4.2 (0.5 mEq/mL): 2 mEq/kg (6 mEq for 3 kg)
13. Pulse oximeter with neonatal probe (pre-ductal: right hand or wrist; post-ductal: foot) and pre-ductal cardiac monitor leads (leads I, II, III)

Initial Actions

1. Warm, dry, stimulate, position:
2. Place infant on preheated radiant warmer with head toward provider
3. Remove wet linen immediately; dry vigorously with warm towel (stimulation + temperature preservation)
4. Position: Sniffing position with slight extension; 2 cm shoulder roll may be needed for exaggerated occiput of neonate
5. Clear airway: Bulb suction mouth then nose only if obvious obstruction or meconium present with poor muscle tone; routine suctioning not recommended (causes bradycardia and apnea)
6. Assessment of 3 questions (within first 5-10 seconds):
    1. Is the infant term gestation (>37 weeks)?
    2. Does the infant have good muscle tone (flexed extremities, active movement)?

    3. Is the infant breathing or crying?
    4. If all 3 answers "Yes": Skin-to-skin contact with mother; delay cord clamping >60 seconds if stable; observe for breathing; no resuscitation needed
7. If any answer "No": Proceed to initial steps under radiant warmer
8. Cord management: Delayed cord clamping (60 seconds minimum) for vigorous term and preterm infants; if immediate resuscitation needed, clamp and cut cord within 30 seconds to allow movement to warmer

Initial Steps and Positive Pressure Ventilation (PPV)

1. Open airway: Jaw thrust if nasal obstruction suspected (neonates are obligate nasal breathers); suction only if airway obstructed
2. Tactile stimulation: If not breathing, flick soles or rub back vigorously
3. Assess heart rate: Auscultate apical pulse or palpate umbilical stump at base; if HR <100 bpm or gasping/apnea after 10-15 seconds stimulation, initiate PPV immediately
4. Pulse oximetry: Apply to right hand/wrist (pre-ductal) within 60 seconds of birth; target pre-ductal SpO_2:
    - 1 min: 60-65%
    - 2 min: 65-70%
    - 3 min: 70-75%
    - 4 min: 75-80%
    - 5 min: 80-85%
    - 10 min: 85-95%
5. FiO_2: Start 21% (room air) for term infants ≥35 weeks; 21-30% for 32-35 weeks; increase to 60% if SpO_2 below target after 90 seconds; 100% only if HR not responding
6. Technique: Two-person technique preferred—one holds mask with "C-E" configuration (thumb and index finger form "C" over mask, remaining fingers form "E" under jaw for jaw thrust), second squeezes bag or adjusts T-piece
7. Initial breaths: May require 30-40 cm H_2O to expand lungs (functional residual capacity), then decrease to 20-25
8. Assess effectiveness of PPV (within 15 seconds):
9. Rising heart rate (HR >100 bpm is primary indicator of adequate ventilation)
10. Improving SpO_2
11. Bilateral breath sounds and chest rise (visible but not excessive; overventilation causes pneumothorax)
12. If inadequate chest rise or HR not improving:
13. MR. SOPA mnemonic (correct in order):
    - Mask adjustment: Reapply, ensure seal over nose and mouth (not eyes)
    - Reposition airway: Sniffing position; check for secretions (suction if obstructed)
    - Suction mouth and nose (if secretions present)
    - Open mouth: Slightly open jaw/mouth to reduce obstruction from large tongue
    - Pressure increase: Increase PIP to 30-40 cm H_2O
14. Alternative airway: Endotracheal intubation or laryngeal mask (size 1 for >1500 g or >34 weeks)

Chest Compressions (Cardiac Resuscitation)

1. Indication: Heart rate <60 bpm after 30 seconds of adequate PPV (with 100% FiO_2 and reassessment of airway/ventilation)

2. Ratio: 3:1 compression to ventilation (90 compressions and 30 breaths per minute = 120 events/minute)
3. Technique:
    - Two-thumb technique preferred (encircling hands around chest, thumbs on sternum)
    - Landmarks: Lower third of sternum (just below nipple line), one finger-breadth below xiphoid process
    - Depth: One-third of AP diameter of chest (≈1.5 cm in term infant, 1 cm in preterm)
    - Allow full recoil; thumbs should not lift off chest
    - Alternative: Two-finger technique (single rescuer): Index and middle fingers perpendicular to sternum; less effective, reserve for single rescuer or if access needed
4. Reassessment: Check HR every 60 seconds; if HR >60 bpm, discontinue compressions but continue PPV; if HR remains <60 bpm after 60 seconds of compressions + PPV, proceed to medications

Vascular Access and Medication Administration

1. Umbilical Venous Catheter (UVC) - Preferred Access:
2. Cleanse umbilical stump with antiseptic (iodine or chlorhexidine)
3. Place loose ligature around base of cord (umbilical tape)
4. Cut cord with sterile scalpel 1-2 cm from skin (leave 1-2 cm stump); avoid cutting too close (avoids peritoneal entry)
5. Identify vessels: Two thick-walled arteries (small lumen, spurting blood), one thin-walled vein (large lumen, thin wall, non-pulsatile)
6. Grasp artery with fine forceps to use as traction; identify vein (larger, superior/12 o'clock position in anatomical position)
7. Insert catheter (3.5 Fr for preterm, 5 Fr for term) into vein; advance gently 2-4 cm until blood return; should meet slight resistance at 2-3 cm if in artery (do not advance further)
8. Depth estimation: Shoulder-umbilicus distance plus 2 cm; or (weight in kg × 3) + 9 cm + umbilical stump length; tip should be at T8-T9 (just above diaphragm, below liver)
9. Confirm blood return (venous, darker, non-pulsatile); secure with suture or tape bridge; connect to stopcock
10. UVC tip position verification: X-ray confirms tip at T8-T9 or just above diaphragm; if too low (liver), reposition; if too high (RA), withdraw
11. Intraosseous (IO): Proximal tibia or distal femur if UVC unsuccessful; use manual IO needle or EZ-IO 15 mm needle
12. Medications (via UVC or IO):
    - Epinephrine: 0.1-0.3 mL/kg of 1:10,000 solution (0.01-0.03 mg/kg or 0.1-0.3 mL/kg); repeat every 3-5 minutes as indicated; if no UVC/IO, may give 0.5-1 mL (0.05-0.1 mg) of 1:10,000 via ETT (absorption unpredictable)
    - Volume Expansion: 10 mL/kg Normal Saline 0.9% over 5-10 minutes; indications: suspected blood loss (acute blood loss, fetal-maternal hemorrhage, twin-twin transfusion), poor response to epinephrine, pallor despite oxygenation; reassess after each bolus; avoid if cardiogenic shock suspected
    - Dextrose: D10 2-4 mL/kg (0.2-0.4 g/kg) IV/IO; check glucose immediately in any depressed neonate; treat hypoglycemia (<40 in first 4 hours, <45 thereafter)
    - Naloxone: Generally not recommended in neonatal resuscitation; if maternal opioid effect suspected and infant apneic but has strong pulse, focus on PPV first; naloxone may precipitate withdrawal seizures; if absolutely necessary (rare): 0.1 mg/kg IM/IV/ETT (max 0.4 mg); duration 30-60 minutes (shorter than maternal opioids), observe for rebound apnea

- Sodium HCO_3: 2 mEq/kg (4.2 solution = 0.5 mEq/mL; give 4 mL/kg) slow IV; only after adequate ventilation established (risk of intraventricular hemorrhage, hypernatremia); rarely indicated in initial resuscitation

Specific Neonatal Conditions Requiring Critical ED Management

Meconium-Stained Amniotic Fluid (MSAF)

1. Current Guidelines: No longer routine intubation and tracheal suctioning for all meconium-stained infants
2. Action: If infant is vigorous (strong respiratory effort, good muscle tone, HR >100): Observe, clear mouth/nose with bulb syringe, do not intubate for suctioning
3. If non-vigorous (depressed respirations, poor tone, HR <100): Intubate immediately and suction trachea before initiating PPV; use meconium aspirator attached to ETT (20 cm H_2O suction applied to ETT while withdrawing); repeat intubation/suctioning until no meconium retrieved or HR indicates need for PPV (then proceed with PPV)

Pneumothorax/Tension Pneumothorax

1. Recognition: Asymmetric chest movement, diminished breath sounds, sudden deterioration with bagging, transillumination (bright glow with fiberoptic light)
2. Needle decompression: 4th intercostal space in anterior axillary line or 2nd intercostal space midclavicular; use 23-gauge butterfly needle or 24-gauge angiocath (smaller than adults to avoid lung laceration); attach to three-way stopcock and 20 mL syringe
3. Chest tube: 8-10 Fr for term infants; 5-8 Fr for preemies; insert at 4th ICS mid-axillary

Congenital Heart Disease - Ductal-Dependent Lesions

1. Prostaglandin E1 (Alprostadil):
2. Dose: 0.05-0.1 mcg/kg/min IV via UVC (start at 0.05); may decrease to 0.025 once stable
3. Indications: Suspected ductal-dependent systemic circulation (HLHS, critical coarctation, severe AS) or pulmonary circulation (pulmonary atresia with intact septum, critical PS, tricuspid atresia) presenting with profound cyanosis or shock after 100% FiO_2 and ventilation optimized
4. Preparation: Standard concentration 20 mcg/mL (mix 500 mcg in 25 mL NS). Starting dose 0.05 mcg/kg/min; for a 3 kg infant = 9 mcg/hr = 0.45 mL/hr. Titrate to effect (range 0.01-0.1 mcg/kg/min).
5. Side effects: Apnea (intubate prior to starting if possible), flushing, hypotension, fever, seizure-like activity (jitteriness), diarrhea

Hypoglycemia

1. Definition: <40 in first 4 hours; <45 thereafter
2. Treatment: D10 2-4 mL/kg IV/IO bolus (0.2-0.4 g/kg); recheck in 15 minutes; if persistent, start continuous infusion D10 at 80-100 mL/kg/day (5-8 mg/kg/min glucose)
3. Refractory hypoglycemia: Consider glucagon 0.03 mg/kg IV/IM (max 1 mg) if hyperinsulinemic state; hydrocortisone 2 mg/kg IV if adrenal insufficiency; octreotide for persistent hyperinsulinism

Sepsis/Early-Onset Sepsis

1. Risk factors: Maternal fever >38°C, chorioamnionitis, prolonged rupture of membranes (>18 hours), GBS positive mother without adequate prophylaxis
2. Antibiotics: Ampicillin 50 mg/kg IV + Gentamicin 2.5 mg/kg IV or Cefotaxime 50 mg/kg IV (avoid ceftriaxone in neonates due to bilirubin displacement and calcium precipitation); obtain blood culture prior to antibiotics if stable
3. Acyclovir: If HSV suspected (maternal history, vesicular lesions): 20 mg/kg IV q8h

Gastroschisis/Omphalocele

1. Gastroschisis (bowel outside abdomen, no sac): Cover bowel with sterile saline-moistened gauze, then plastic wrap (Saran wrap) to prevent heat/water loss; position side-lying to prevent kinking of mesentery; NGT to suction; IV fluids 1.5-2x maintenance; immediate surgical consult; avoid prolonged attempts at reduction in ED
2. Omphalocele (sac covering contents): Cover with sterile saline gauze and plastic wrap; avoid rupturing sac; handle gently; similar fluid management

Post-Resuscitation Stabilization Prior to NICU Transfer

1. Temperature: Maintain normothermia (36.5°C-37.5°C) or therapeutic hypothermia per protocol; avoid hyperthermia (>38°C)
2. Ventilation: Wean FiO_2 to maintain SpO_2 90-95% (pre-ductal); avoid hyperoxia; if persistent pulmonary hypertension suspected (pre-post ductal SpO_2 difference >10%, or R>L differential), maintain PaO_2 80-100 and consider iNO (inhaled nitric oxide 20 ppm) if available
3. Circulation:
4. Pressors: Dopamine 5-20 mcg/kg/min (first line for hypotension); Dobutamine 2.5-20 mcg/kg/min if poor contractility; Epinephrine 0.05-0.3 mcg/kg/min for shock unresponsive to fluids/dopamine
5. Fluids: Maintenance 60-80 mL/kg/day for first 24 hours (preterm 60-70, term 60-80), increase 10-20 mL/kg/day daily
6. Glucose: Maintain 80-100; start D10 infusion at 60-80 mL/kg/day (4-6 mg/kg/min) if not already established
7. Laboratory studies: Blood gas (correlate pre-ductal SpO_2 with PaO_2), CBC, glucose, calcium (ionized), electrolytes, blood culture if sepsis suspected
8. Lines: Secure UVC (mark external length); consider arterial line (radial or umbilical) if hemodynamically unstable
9. Neurologic: Assess for seizures (subtle: eye deviation, lip smacking, apnea); consider EEG if available; maintain euglycemia and normothermia

Pediatric Resuscitation

Pre-Arrival Preparation and Resuscitation Bay Setup

1. Calculate estimated weight immediately: Use length-based resuscitation tape (Broselow) or formula (Age + 4) × 2 for children 1—10 years; infant 3—10 kg (median 5 kg at 6 months, 10 kg at 1 year); adolescent use adult dosing
2. Prepare medication cards/tape displaying weight-based dosing for all emergency drugs; pre-calculate epinephrine 0.01 mg/kg (0.1 mL/kg of 1:10,000) and 0.01 mg/kg IM (0.01 mL/kg of 1:1,000 for anaphylaxis)
3. Airway equipment selection (verify against calculated weight):
   - ETT Size (uncuffed): (Age/4) + 4; cuffed: (Age/4) + 3.5 (use cuffed ETTs for infants/children to reduce air leak and aspiration risk)
   - Depth at lips: (Age/2) + 12 (oral); (Age/2) + 15 (nasal)
   - Laryngoscope Blade: Straight (Miller 0—1) for infants <2 years; curved (Macintosh) for >2 years
   - BVM: Neonatal (<3 kg), infant (3—10 kg), child (10—30 kg), adult (>30 kg)
   - Suction: 10—12 Fr catheter for infants, 14 Fr for toddlers, Yankauer for children >3 years
   - Intraosseous (IO) drill: EZ-IO with 15 mm (7—39 kg) and 25 mm (>40 kg) needles; or manual IO needle (Jamshidi) for neonates
   - Defibrillator: Pediatric pads (<8 years or <25 kg); adult pads if pediatric unavailable (anterior-posterior placement); energy 2 J/kg first, 4 J/kg subsequent, maximum 10 J/kg or adult dose
4. Temperature management: Servo-controlled warming mattress, warmed blankets, radiant warmer for infants, warmed IV fluids (set to body temperature 37°C)
5. Family presence: Assign dedicated staff member to explain procedures and offer parental presence during resuscitation (evidence supports reduced PTSD for families and staff)

Primary Survey: Pediatric-Specific ABCDE

A - Airway

1. Positioning: Neutral sniffing position for infants (occiput naturally elevated; do not place roll under shoulders as this causes flexion and obstruction due to prominent occiput)
2. Active airway opening: Jaw thrust (preferred in trauma to maintain C-spine alignment) or chin lift; avoid head tilt-chin lift if cervical spine injury suspected
3. Suction: Aggressive suction of oropharynx; use large-bore catheter for meconium or particulate matter (infants do not tolerate nasal suctioning well—bradycardia risk)
4. Adjuncts:
5. Oropharyngeal airway (OPA): Measure from corner of mouth to angle of jaw; size (Age/2) + 2
6. Nasopharyngeal airway (NPA): Size (Age/2) + 2 to (Age/2) + 3; avoid in head trauma (basilar skull fracture risk) or coagulopathy
7. Intubation indications: GCS ≤ 8, respiratory failure (RR >60 or <20 with fatigue), shock unresponsive to fluids, airway protection (bulging fontanelle, craniofacial trauma), refractory status epilepticus
8. Rapid Sequence Intubation (RSI) - Pediatric Modifications:
   - Pretreatment: Atropine 0.02 mg/kg (minimum 0.1 mg, maximum 0.5 mg) for infants <1 year or any child receiving succinylcholine (prevents bradycardia); lidocaine 1 mg/kg if increased ICP suspected (though evidence limited)
   - Induction: Ketamine 1—2 mg/kg IV (hemodynamic preservation) or Etomidate 0.3 mg/kg IV (avoid in sepsis due to adrenal suppression); avoid Propofol if hypovolemic (hypotension)

- Paralysis: Rocuronium 1.2—1.6 mg/kg IV (preferred if risk of difficult airway—can be reversed with sugammadex if needed) OR Succinylcholine 2 mg/kg IV (contraindicated if hyperkalemia risk: burns >24 hr old, crush injury, denervation, muscular dystrophy)
- Cricoid pressure: Controversial in pediatrics; may distort airway anatomy; apply only if aspiration risk high and release if bag-mask ventilation difficult
- Tube selection: Use cuffed tubes (low pressure, high volume) for all ages; cuff pressure <20—25 cm H_2O; uncuffed only if tube size between available sizes

9. Confirmation: Qualitative and quantitative waveform capnography (mandatory); auscultation in axilla (not just stomach); symmetric chest rise; condensation in tube; 5th vital sign: capnography
10. Post-intubation: Secure with tape (not commercial holders in infants—too heavy) or surgical cotton umbilical tape; sedation: Fentanyl 1—2 mcg/kg/hr + Midazolam 0.05—0.1 mg/kg/hr or Propofol 20—50 mcg/kg/min (avoid hypotension)

B - Breathing

1. Respiratory rates by age: Newborn 30—60, Infant (<1 yr) 25—40, Toddler 20—30, School-age 15—25, Adolescent 12—20
2. Signs of impending respiratory failure: Nasal flaring, suprasternal/intercostal/subcostal retractions, head bobbing, grunting (infants), paradoxical breathing (abdomen sucks in when chest expands), altered mental status, cyanosis
3. Oxygen delivery:
    - Neonates: 100% O_2 (concern for retinopathy of prematurity only in chronic use; emergency resuscitation requires 100%)
4. Children: Titrate to 94—99% SpO_2 (avoid hyperoxia post-resuscitation)
5. Ventilation parameters:
    - Rate: 20—30 breaths/minute for infants, 20 for school-age, 12—20 for adolescents
    - Tidal volume: 6—8 mL/kg predicted body weight
    - PEEP: 5 cm H_2O initially; increase if atelectasis/ARDS
    - I:E ratio: 1:2 to allow complete exhalation (prevent breath stacking)
6. Specific interventions:
    1. Tension pneumothorax: Needle decompression with 18-gauge needle or angiocath, 4th intercostal space anterior axillary line (avoid midclavicular line in infants due to thymus and cardiac proximity)
    2. Chest tube: Size (Age/4) + 4 (French); insert at 4th—5th intercostal space mid-axillary line
    3. Asthma/Croup: Racemic epinephrine 0.5 mL of 2.25 solution in 3 mL NS nebulized for upper airway obstruction; Magnesium sulfate 50 mg/kg (max 2 g) IV for severe asthma

C - Circulation

1. Bradycardia is a pre-arrest sign in children (unlike adults where tachycardia precedes arrest); HR <60 with poor perfusion despite oxygenation/ventilation = CPR
2. Hypotension formula: Systolic BP <70 + (Age × 2) mmHg (or <70 for 1—10 years)
3. Vascular Access (hierarchical approach):
    - Peripheral IV: Two attempts maximum 90 seconds; use scalp veins in infants if extremities failed
    - Intraosseous (IO): First-line access in decompensated shock or cardiac arrest; preferred sites: proximal tibia (flat medial surface 1—2 cm below tibial tuberosity) or distal femur (lateral surface 2—3 cm above lateral condyle) in infants; humeral head in older children; contraindicated if fracture, previous IO attempt in same bone, or infection over site
    - Central Access: Internal jugular or femoral; subclavian higher complication rate in children; ultrasound-guided placement

4. Fluid Resuscitation:
   - Crystalloid: 20 mL/kg NS or LR over 5—20 minutes (warm fluids); reassess after each bolus; maximum typically 60—80 mL/kg before blood products unless ongoing hemorrhage
   - Blood products: 10—15 mL/kg PRBC initially; type-specific preferred; O-negative for females of childbearing age, O-positive acceptable for males/infants (low anti-D risk); FFP 10—15 mL/kg; Plt 5—10 mL/kg (usually 1 apheresis unit or 6—10 pooled units)
5. Glucose: Check immediately; treat <70 with D10 2—4 mL/kg IV (0.2—0.4 g/kg); never use D50 in pediatrics (causes hyperosmolar injury, necrosis if extravasation)
6. Calcium: 10—20 mg/kg Calcium Chloride (0.1—0.2 mL/kg of 10 solution) or 30—60 mg/kg Calcium Gluconate per 10—15 mL/kg PRBC transfused

D - Disability (Neurologic)

1. Pediatric GCS: Modified for children; verbal score adjusted for age (smiles, coos, cries appropriately = 5; inconsolable crying = 4; inappropriate crying = 3; agitated = 2; no response = 1)
2. AVPU: Alert, Voice, Pain, Unresponsive (quicker than GCS for triage)
3. Fontanelles: Bulging anterior fontanelle indicates increased ICP (except crying infant); sunken indicates dehydration
4. Seizure management: See status epilepticus section below
5. Temperature: Hypoglycemia and hypothermia common in septic infants; check rectal temperature (core) in critically ill children

E - Exposure

1. Complete undressing (log-roll maintaining C-spine alignment); measure weight if Broselow tape unavailable
2. Pediatric-specific injury patterns:
   - Non-accidental trauma (NAT): Retinal hemorrhages, bruising in non-mobile infants, patterned burns, multiple fractures in various stages of healing, subdural hematomas of different ages
   - Torus (buckle) fractures vs growth plate injuries (Salter-Harris classification)

Pediatric Cardiac Arrest Algorithm (Asphyxial Arrest)

1. Check pulse: Brachial (infants), Carotid/femoral (children); check for ≤ 10 seconds
2. Pulseless or HR <60 with poor perfusion despite oxygenation/ventilation:
3. Begin CPR: Compression-to-ventilation ratio 30:2 (single rescuer) or 15:2 (two rescuers)
4. Compression depth: 1/3 AP diameter of chest (≈ 4 cm infants, 5 cm children)
5. Rate: 100—120/minute (metronome)
6. Recoil: Allow complete chest recoil; rotate compressors every 2 minutes (fatigue occurs rapidly)
7. Defibrillation:
   - Manual defibrillator preferred (attenuated pediatric dose 2 J/kg first, 4 J/kg subsequent)
   - If AED only (automated): Use pediatric attenuator if <8 years or <25 kg; if unavailable, use adult pads anterior-posterior (do not let pads touch)
8. Epinephrine: 0.01 mg/kg IV/IO (0.1 mL/kg of 1:10,000) every 3—5 minutes; if no IV/IO, endotracheal dose 0.1 mg/kg (0.1 mL/kg of 1:1,000 diluted in 3—5 mL NS)
9. Reversible causes (H's and T's):
   - Hypoxia, Hypovolemia, Hydrogen ion (acidosis), Hypo-/Hyperkalemia, Hypoglycemia, Hypothermia
   - Tension pneumothorax, Tamponade (cardiac), Toxins, Thrombosis (pulmonary/coronary), Trauma

10. Post-ROSC care:
    - Targeted temperature management: 32°C—34°C for 24 hours (or maintain normothermia 36°C —37.5°C); avoid fever >38°C
    - Hemodynamics: Systolic BP >5th percentile for age; MAP >65 (adolescents) or age-appropriate
    - Glucose control: 80—180; avoid hypoglycemia
    - Ventilation: Normocapnia ($PaCO_2$ 35—45); avoid hyperventilation (cerebral vasoconstriction)

Pediatric Bradycardia Algorithm (Pre-Arrest)

1. Identify: Heart rate below age-appropriate normal with signs of poor perfusion (pallor, delayed capillary refill, hypotension, altered LOC)
2. Oxygenate/ventilate: Ensure adequate oxygenation and ventilation first (most pediatric bradycardia is hypoxic)
3. Epinephrine: If HR <60 despite oxygenation/ventilation, begin CPR and give Epinephrine 0.01 mg/kg IV/IO (0.1 mL/kg 1:10,000)
4. Atropine: 0.02 mg/kg IV/IO (minimum 0.1 mg, maximum 0.5 mg for child, 1 mg for adolescent); repeat once; indications: increased vagal tone, AV block, cholinergic toxicity
5. Transcutaneous pacing: If bradycardia unresponsive to medications and CPR; use pediatric pads; start at 20—30 mA above capture threshold (usually 50—100 mA in children)

Pediatric Tachycardia Algorithm

Narrow Complex (SVT)

1. Recognition: HR >220 (infants) or >180 (children) with abrupt onset; P waves absent or abnormal; narrow QRS (<0.08 sec)
2. Vagal maneuvers: Ice to face (diving reflex) in infants; Valsalva in older children (blowing through straw, bearing down)
3. Adenosine: 0.1 mg/kg rapid IV/IO push (maximum 6 mg first dose), followed immediately by 5—10 mL NS flush; second dose 0.2 mg/kg (maximum 12 mg); must be given via proximal IV or IO (delays in circulation time reduce efficacy)
4. Synchronized cardioversion: If unstable (hypotension, altered mental status, signs of shock): 0.5—1 J/kg; increase to 2 J/kg if ineffective; sedate if possible but do not delay if unstable

Wide Complex (VT)

1. Unstable: Synchronized cardioversion 0.5—1 J/kg (increase to 2 J/kg)
2. Stable: Amiodarone 5 mg/kg IV over 20—60 minutes (max 300 mg); OR Procainamide 15 mg/kg IV over 30—60 minutes (avoid if prolonged QT)
3. Pulseless VT/VF: Defibrillation 2 J/kg, then 4 J/kg, then ≥ 4 J/kg (maximum 10 J/kg or adult dose); Epinephrine every 3—5 minutes; consider Amiodarone 5 mg/kg bolus for refractory VF/VT

Critical Conditions and Specific Interventions

Pediatric Septic Shock

1. Recognition: Cold shock (vasoconstricted: delayed capillary refill, thready pulses, cool extremities) vs Warm shock (vasodilated: bounding pulses, flash capillary refill, widened pulse pressure) more common in adults but seen in children
2. Antibiotics: Within 60 minutes; empirical:
    - Neonates (0—28 days): Ampicillin 50 mg/kg + Gentamicin 2.5 mg/kg or Cefotaxime 50 mg/kg (avoid ceftriaxone due to bilirubin displacement)

- Infants/children: Ceftriaxone 50 mg/kg (max 2 g) or Cefotaxime 50 mg/kg + Vancomycin 15 mg/kg if MRSA suspected
- Meningitis coverage: Add Vancomycin 15 mg/kg + Ceftriaxone/Cefotaxime; consider Acyclovir 20 mg/kg if HSV encephalitis suspected

3. Fluid resuscitation: 20 mL/kg NS or LR boluses over 5—10 minutes; up to 60—80 mL/kg in first hour if ongoing shock; reassess perfusion after each bolus
4. Vasopressors (begin if fluid refractory or signs of fluid overload/cardiomegaly on CXR):
   - Cold shock: Epinephrine 0.05—0.3 mcg/kg/min (first line) or Dopamine 5—10 mcg/kg/min (if central access not available—can cause arrhythmias)
   - Warm shock: Norepinephrine 0.05—0.3 mcg/kg/min (first line) or Phenylephrine (pure alpha) if high output with low SVR
5. Hydrocortisone: 2 mg/kg (max 100 mg) if catecholamine-resistant shock and concern for adrenal insufficiency (chronic steroid use, hypopituitarism, congenital adrenal hyperplasia)

Pediatric Anaphylaxis

1. Epinephrine: 0.01 mg/kg IM (0.01 mL/kg of 1:1,000) into lateral thigh (vastus lateralis); maximum 0.5 mg; repeat every 5—15 minutes
2. Adjuncts:
   - H1: Diphenhydramine 1 mg/kg IV (max 50 mg)
   - H2: Famotidine 0.25 mg/kg IV or Famotidine 0.25 mg/kg IV
   - Corticosteroids: Methylprednisolone 1—2 mg/kg IV (max 125 mg) or Prednisolone 1 mg/kg PO
   - Beta-agonists: Albuterol 2.5 mg nebulized (or 0.15 mg/kg with minimum 2.5 mg) for bronchospasm
3. Fluid resuscitation: 20 mL/kg NS bolus for hypotension; repeat as needed (distributive shock)
4. Glucagon: 20—30 mcg/kg (max 1 mg) IV if on beta-blockers (refractory to epinephrine)

Pediatric Status Epilepticus

1. First line: Benzodiazepines
   - Lorazepam 0.1 mg/kg IV/IO (max 4 mg per dose; may repeat once)
   - Diazepam 0.2—0.5 mg/kg IV/IO/PR (max 10 mg)
   - Midazolam 0.2 mg/kg IM or intranasal (0.2 mg/kg spray into nares, max 10 mg) if no IV access
2. Second line:
   - Levetiracetam 60 mg/kg IV (max 4500 mg) over 15 minutes OR
   - Fosphenytoin 20 mg PE/kg IV (max 1500 mg PE) over 10 minutes OR
   - Valproic acid 20—40 mg/kg IV (max 3000 mg) over 10 minutes (avoid if metabolic disorder suspected)
3. Refractory: Intubation with RSI (avoid long-acting paralytics to monitor for seizure activity); continuous EEG monitoring; Midazolam infusion 0.1—0.4 mg/kg/hr or Propofol infusion 1—2 mg/kg/hr (risk of propofol infusion syndrome—limit duration)
4. Metabolic correction: Glucose (treat hypoglycemia), Pyridoxine 100 mg IV if neonatal seizures or isoniazid toxicity

Diabetic Ketoacidosis (DKA)

1. Fluid resuscitation: 10—20 mL/kg NS over 1—2 hours (isotonic resuscitation); then 0.45—0.9 NS with maintenance fluids
2. Insulin: Start 0.05—0.1 units/kg/hr only after fluid resuscitation initiated and no longer in shock; delay if pH <6.9 until after initial fluid bolus

3. HCO_3: Controversial; generally avoid unless pH <6.9 with hemodynamic compromise; give 1—2 mEq/kg over 1 hour if used
4. Cerebral Edema: 1—2 mmol/kg Mannitol (0.25—0.5 g/kg) or 3% Hypertonic Saline 5 mL/kg over 15 minutes for altered mental status, bradycardia, or hypertension; emergent intubation with hyperventilation only if herniation signs ($PaCO_2$ target 30—35)
5. Potassium: Add to fluids once urine output confirmed and K^+ <5.5; typical replacement 20—40 fluid

Hypoglycemia

1. Asymptomatic: Feed oral glucose if alert; D10 2—5 mL/kg IV if NPO
2. Symptomatic/Seizing: D10 2—4 mL/kg (0.2—0.4 g/kg) IV; if no IV, Glucagon 0.5 mg IM (1 mg if >25 kg); recheck glucose in 10 minutes
3. Hyperinsulinemic states: Octreotide 1 mcg/kg SC/IV (max 50 mcg) for sulfonylurea overdose; Hydrocortisone 2 mg/kg IV if adrenal insufficiency suspected

Toxic Ingestions (Specific Antidotes)

1. Naloxone: 2 mg (total dose) IN (atomized into nares) or 0.04—0.1 mg/kg IV every 2 minutes; avoid large boluses in opioid-dependent patients (precipitates withdrawal)
2. N-Acetylcysteine: 150 mg/kg in 3 mL/kg D5W over 60 minutes (loading), then 50 mg/kg in 7 mL/kg over 4 hours, then 100 mg/kg in 14 mL/kg over 16 hours (for acetaminophen toxicity)
3. Physostigmine: 0.02 mg/kg IV (max 0.5 mg) for anticholinergic toxicity with severe delirium (contraindicated in TCA overdose—risk of asystole)
4. Sodium HCO_3: 1—2 mEq/kg IV for wide-complex tachycardia due to TCA or other sodium channel blocker; maintain serum pH 7.45—7.55
5. Calcium: Calcium Cl 10—20 mg/kg (0.1—0.2 mL/kg of 10) for calcium channel blocker overdose or hydrofluoric acid burns

Pediatric Trauma Modifications

1. Blood volume: 80 mL/kg (neonate) to 70 mL/kg (child); loss of 25 blood volume causes shock signs
2. C-spine: Occiput causes natural flexion; pad under torso (not head) to achieve neutral position for intubation
3. FAST: Positive if >10 mL free fluid; ultrasound probe selection based on size
4. Traumatic brain injury: Maintain CPP >50—60 (age dependent); avoid hypotonic fluids (D5W, 0.45 NS); use NS or LR; maintain SBP >90 + (Age × 2)
5. Non-accidental trauma: Skeletal survey for infants <1 year with suspected abuse; ophthalmology for retinal exam

Family Communication and Ethical Considerations

1. Family presence: Offer parents/guardians the option to be present during resuscitation; assign designated support person (nurse/social worker) to explain procedures and provide emotional support
2. Termination of resuscitation: Consider cessation after 20 minutes of high-quality CPR with no reversible cause identified and no ROSC; longer duration may be indicated in hypothermia or toxic ingestions
3. Organ donation: Early notification to organ procurement organization (OPO) if brain death anticipated or imminent; maintain perfusion to organs if possible
4. Documentation: Detailed weight-based dosing calculations, timing of interventions, family discussions regarding prognosis and interventions

Post-Resuscitation Care Prior to PICU Transfer

1. Hemodynamic monitoring: Arterial line if vasopressors required; central venous access for medication administration
2. Temperature control: Actively maintain normothermia (36.5°C—37.5°C) or mild hypothermia (32°C—34°C) per institutional protocol; prevent fever
3. Glucose: Maintain 80—180 with D10—D12.5 maintenance fluids (avoid hypoglycemia)
4. Seizure prophylaxis: Consider if severe TBI or post-hypoxic injury; Levetiracetam 20—30 mg/kg load
5. Ventilation: Lung-protective strategy; avoid excessive PEEP causing barotrauma in children with compliant chest walls
6. Sedation/Analgesia: Fentanyl 1—2 mcg/kg/hr + Midazolam 0.05—0.2 mg/kg/hr or Dexmedetomidine 0.2—0.7 mcg/kg/hr (hemodynamic stability)
7. Gastric protection: PPI or H2-blocker if high risk for stress ulceration; NGT to low intermittent suction
8. DVT prophylaxis: Mechanical (SCDs if size appropriate) only in adolescents; pharmacologic prophylaxis generally not indicated in pre-pubertal children

ULTRASOUNDS

Abscess Incision and Drainage

Indications

- Fluctuant cutaneous abscess confirmed clinically or by ultrasound (ultrasound distinguishes abscess from cellulitis and phlegmon)

Contraindications

- Do not perform simple bedside I&D on: abscesses of the central facial triangle draining to the cavernous sinus (relative — small and superficial may be acceptable), abscesses overlying or involving vessels (mycotic aneurysm, pseudoaneurysm — image first if pulsatile), perirectal abscesses with deep extension, necrotizing infection (needs the OR), and hand deep-space infections (needs surgery)
- Breast abscesses near the areola and large complex collections may warrant surgical or needle drainage instead

Steps:

1. Select linear array probe (high frequency, 5—12 MHz) for superficial collections or curvilinear (2—5 MHz) for deep abscesses >4 cm.
2. Perform non-sterile survey scan to identify hypoechoic or anechoic collection with internal debris, posterior acoustic enhancement, and irregular borders; distinguish from cellulitis (cobblestoning), seroma, or necrotic lymph node.
3. Mark entry site avoiding neurovascular bundles; note depth from skin surface to collection center.
4. Apply sterile probe cover with acoustic gel; maintain sterile field throughout.
5. Administer local anesthetic (lidocaine with epinephrine) via 27—30 gauge needle under ultrasound guidance using in-plane technique to hydrodissect tissue planes.
6. Advance 18-gauge needle into collection under real-time guidance (longitudinal plane preferred) to confirm fluid return; aspirate sample for Gram stain and culture if indicated.
7. Perform incision with #11 blade scalpel at skin entry point; advance to collection depth under ultrasound visualization or using previously marked depth.
8. Insert curved hemostat into cavity under ultrasound guidance to break loculations; confirm disruption of septations via real-time imaging.
9. Place loop drain or packing material; confirm placement within cavity via ultrasound (hyperechoic line within anechoic collection).
10. Post-procedure scan to rule out injury to adjacent structures (vessels, tendon sheaths, bone)

11.

Abscess — Ultrasound Appearance

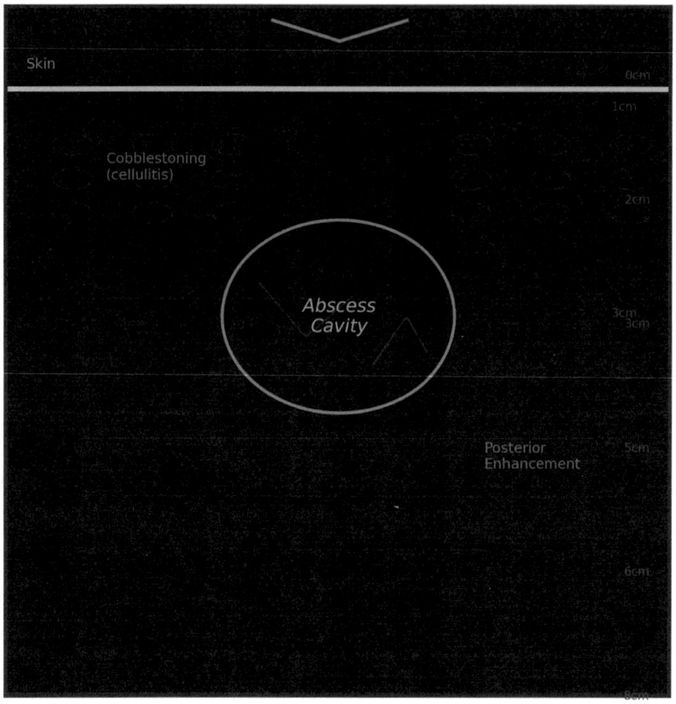

Abscess I&D — Ultrasound-Guided Technique

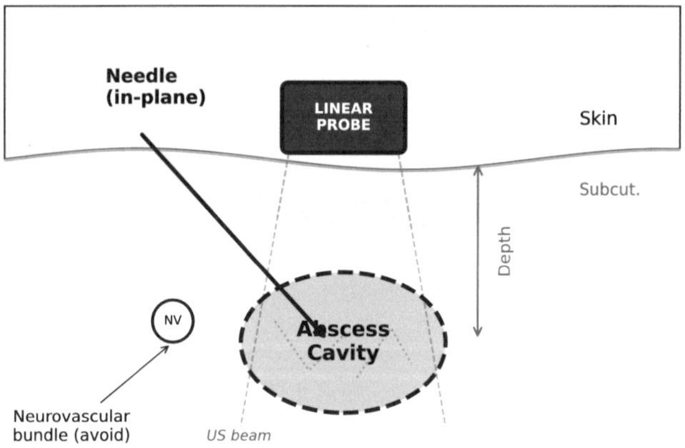

Arthrocentesis

Indications:

- Same indications as landmark arthrocentesis; ultrasound improves success in small effusions, obese patients, and the hip

Contraindications:

- Same as landmark arthrocentesis: overlying infection in the needle path, prosthetic joint (relative — prefer orthopedics), and relative caution with coagulopathy

Steps:

1. Select linear probe for superficial joints (wrist, elbow, ankle) or curvilinear for deep joints (hip, shoulder).
2. Identify joint effusion: anechoic or hypoechoic fluid within joint capsule, distending recesses (suprapatellar, subacromial, radiohumeral).
3. Map neurovascular structures adjacent to target (brachial artery/median nerve at wrist, popliteal vessels at knee); mark safe trajectory.
4. Sterile skin preparation and local anesthetic infiltration.
5. Using in-plane approach, advance 18—22 gauge needle toward fluid collection while visualizing needle tip as hyperechoic dot with comet tail artifact.
6. Aspirate fluid completely; if therapeutic injection, confirm needle tip within joint space before instilling medication (visualize hyperechoic medication microbubbles spreading).
7. For hip arthrocentesis: use anterior approach lateral to femoral neurovascular bundle, targeting femoral head-neck junction; advance under continuous real-time guidance to avoid contact with femoral head cartilage.

Knee Joint Effusion — Suprapatellar Recess

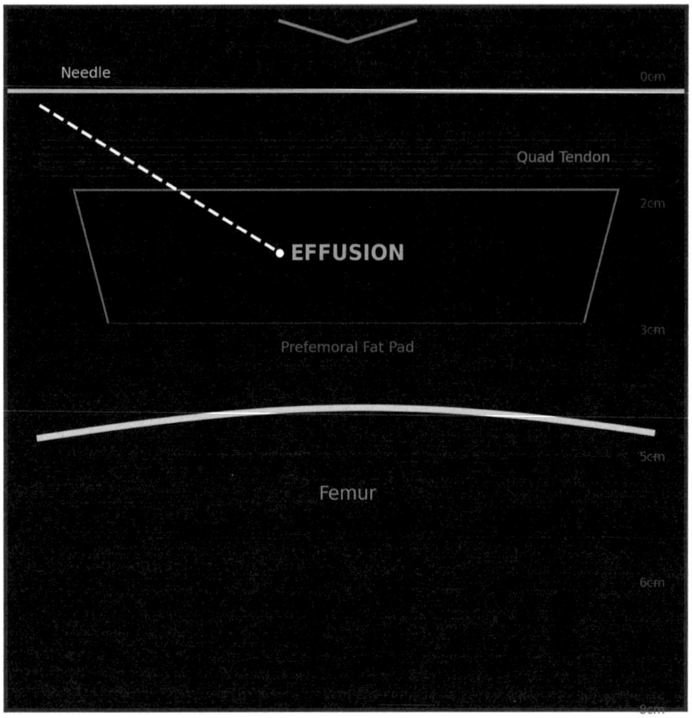

Arthrocentesis — Suprapatellar Approach

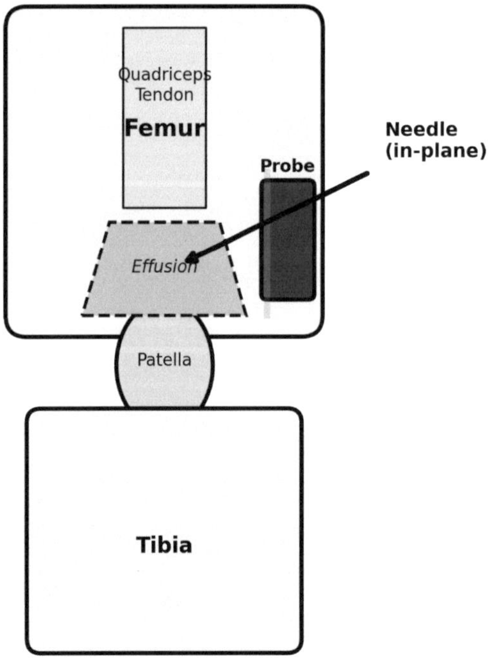

Foreign Body Removal

Indications:

- Radiolucent or palpable soft tissue foreign body (wood, plastic, glass) localized by ultrasound; removal indicated for pain, infection risk, proximity to critical structures, or patient preference

Contraindications:

- Deep foreign bodies adjacent to tendons, nerves, or vessels are better removed in the OR (relative)
- Asymptomatic, small, inert, deeply embedded material may be observed rather than explored
- Do not explore blindly through infected or distorted tissue without imaging localization

Steps:

1. Select high-frequency linear probe (≥10 MHz); optimize depth (2—3 cm) and focus at level of suspected FB.
2. Scan in orthogonal planes to identify hyperechoic focus with specific artifacts: reverberation (comet tail) for metal/glass, variable shadowing or reverberation for wood (depending on hydration and time since implantation), or clean shadowing for bone/glass.
3. Mark skin overlying FB entry point and mark distal extent; measure depth from skin surface.
4. Consider water bath immersion technique for superficial FBs in digits to eliminate near-field clutter.
5. Under sterile conditions, use in-plane needle guidance to advance forceps or hemostat alongside FB; real-time visualization confirms grasping of hyperechoic object.
6. If direct removal impractical, use ultrasound to guide incision down to FB capsule, then extract under direct visualization.
7. Post-removal sweep to confirm complete extraction and evaluate for retained fragments, surrounding abscess formation, or tendon injury

Foreign Body — Linear Probe View

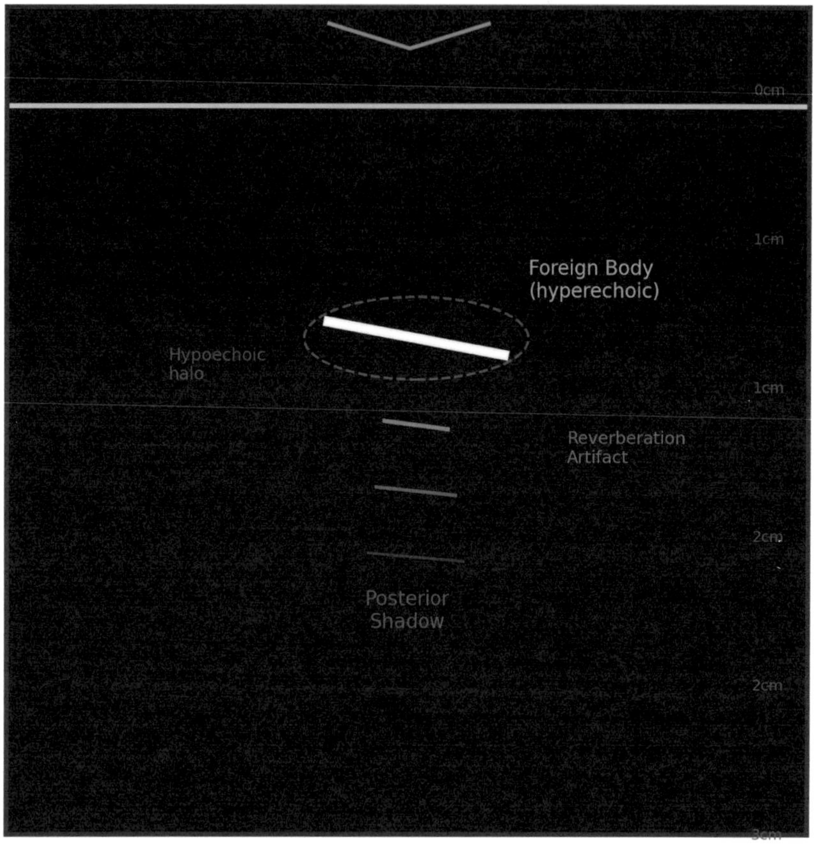

Foreign Body Removal — Ultrasound-Guided

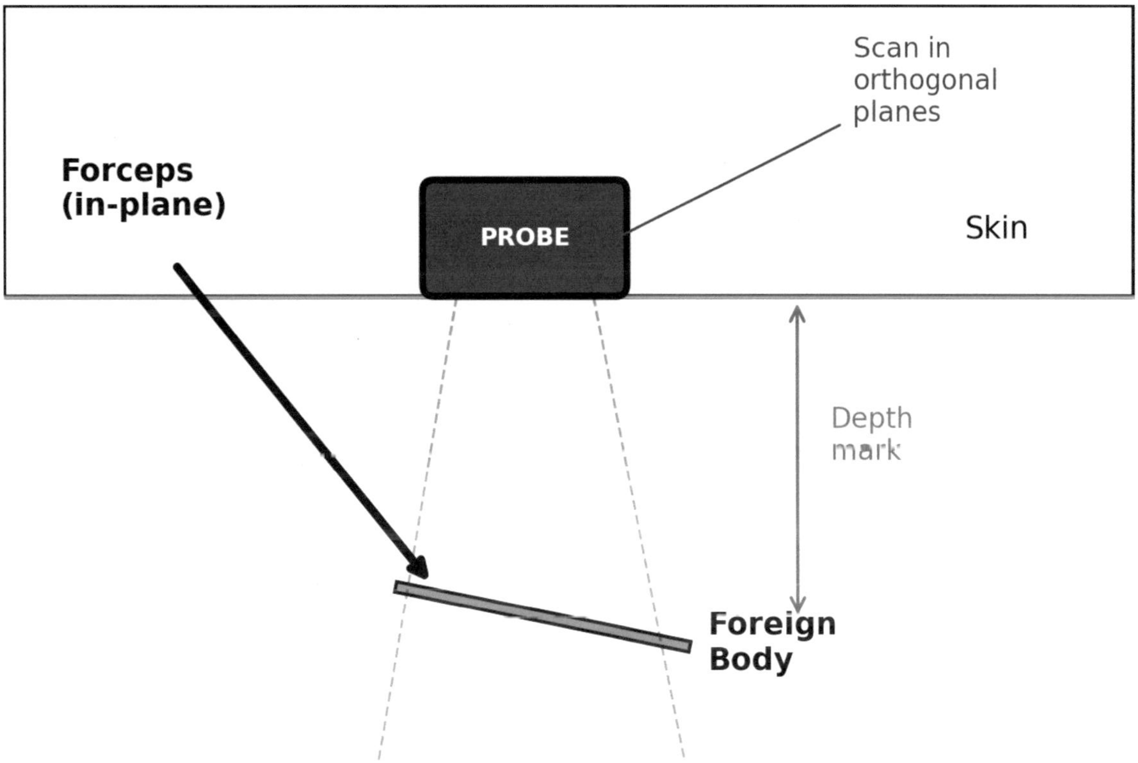

Paracentesis

Indications:

- New-onset ascites requiring diagnostic sampling
- Suspected spontaneous bacterial peritonitis (fever, abdominal pain, encephalopathy, or any deterioration in a cirrhotic with ascites)
- Therapeutic drainage of tense, symptomatic ascites

Contraindications:

- Overlying cellulitis, engorged abdominal wall veins, or surgical scars at the chosen site — move the site under ultrasound
- Bowel obstruction with distension or pregnancy — image-guide carefully and adjust the site
- Coagulopathy from liver disease is NOT a contraindication — routine correction of INR or platelets is not required before paracentesis
- Clinically evident fibrinolysis or DIC is the main hematologic exception

Steps:

1. Select curvilinear or phased array probe (2—5 MHz) for abdominal penetration; patient supine or lateral decubitus.
2. Systematic survey of four quadrants to identify largest fluid pocket; avoid midline (rectus abdominis), scars (adherent bowel), and visible collateral vessels.
3. Identify bowel loops (peristalsis, wall stratification) and measure distance to fluid; target areas with >3 cm fluid depth.
4. Mark entry site at maximal fluid depth with minimal bowel interposition; note depth to peritoneum.
5. Real-time guidance using in-plane technique: advance 18-gauge catheter-over-needle (Angiocath) through abdominal wall layers (skin, subcutaneous, fascia, peritoneum) visualizing tenting of peritoneum and entry into anechoic fluid.
6. Z-track technique (skin displacement 1—2 cm in any direction before peritoneal entry) to prevent leakage.
7. Advance catheter while withdrawing needle; confirm intraperitoneal position by free flow of ascites and ultrasound visualization of catheter within fluid collection.

8. Collect samples (cell count, albumin, culture, cytology); remove catheter and apply pressure.

Paracentesis — Ascites Pocket Identification

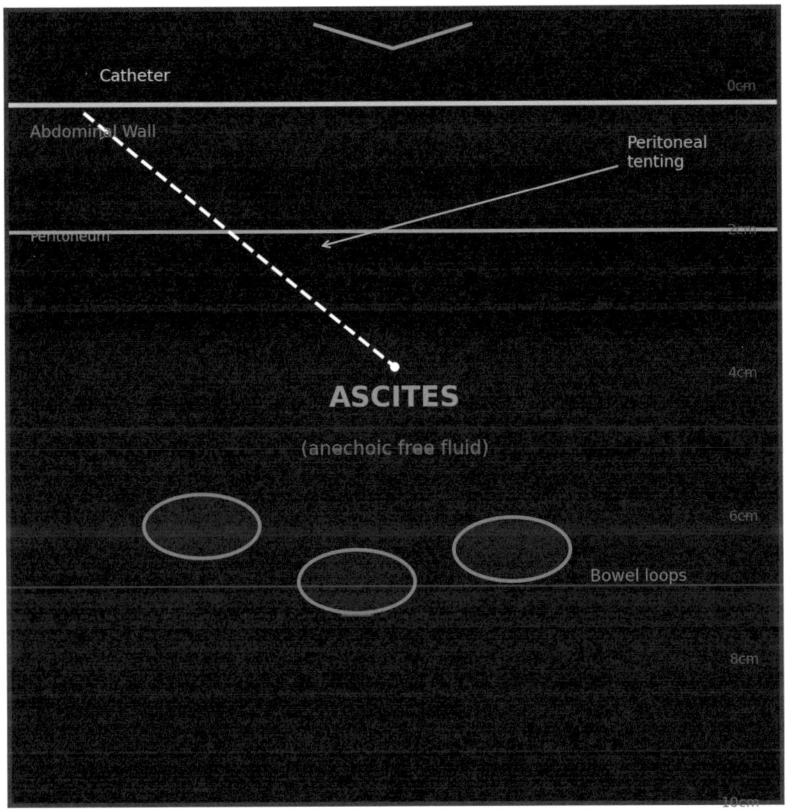

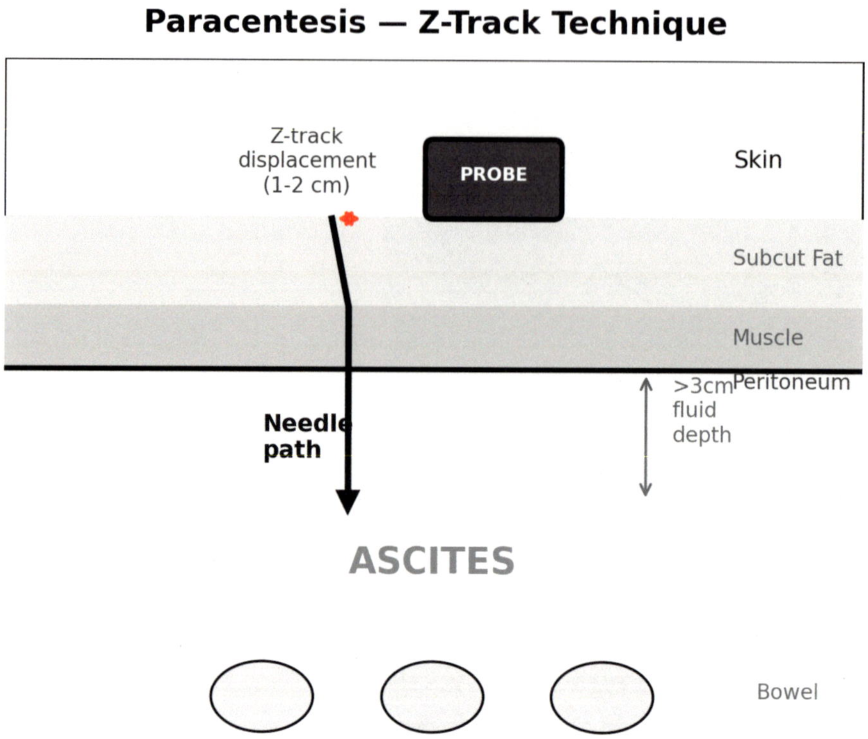
Paracentesis — Z-Track Technique
Z-track displacement (1-2 cm)
PROBE
Skin
Subcut Fat
Muscle
Peritoneum
>3cm fluid depth
Needle path
ASCITES
Bowel

Pericardiocentesis

Indications:

- Cardiac tamponade with hemodynamic compromise (obstructive shock or arrest) — ultrasound-guided at the bedside
- Diagnostic sampling of a large effusion is generally deferred to controlled settings

Contraindications:

- No contraindications in tamponade arrest or peri-arrest
- Traumatic tamponade with cardiac wound: pericardiocentesis is a temporizing measure at most — definitive care is thoracotomy or the OR
- Aortic dissection with hemopericardium (relative — decompression can accelerate the dissection; drain the minimum to restore perfusion en route to surgery)
- Relative in the stable patient: coagulopathy, small or loculated posterior effusions better drained surgically

Steps:

1. Select phased array (2—4 MHz) or curvilinear probe; place patient 30—45 degrees head-up to pool fluid inferiorly.
2. Identify pericardial effusion: anechoic stripe surrounding heart; distinguish from pleural effusion (posterior to descending aorta) and pericardial fat (echogenic, non-mobile).
3. Assess for tamponade: RA/RV diastolic collapse, IVC plethora (distended >2.1 cm with <50 inspiratory collapse).
4. Determine optimal window: subxiphoid (most common, avoids lung/heart), apical (lateral to apex, risk LAD artery), or parasternal (left 5th intercostal, risk internal mammary artery).
5. Measure distance from skin to pericardium; identify and mark rib interspaces to avoid vessel injury.
6. Sterile preparation; local anesthetic with 1% lidocaine.
7. Using subxiphoid approach: insert 18-gauge needle at 30—45 degree angle toward left shoulder under real-time guidance; visualize needle tip entering pericardial space.
8. Advance J-wire (echogenic) through needle; confirm wire position within pericardial sac via ultrasound (avoid RV puncture—wire should not follow cardiac motion into ventricle).
9. Dilate tract and place pigtail catheter; confirm drainage via ultrasound (decreasing effusion size).
10. Monitor for RV/LV puncture (new wall motion abnormality, blood return), coronary laceration, or pneumothorax.

Pericardial Effusion — Subxiphoid View

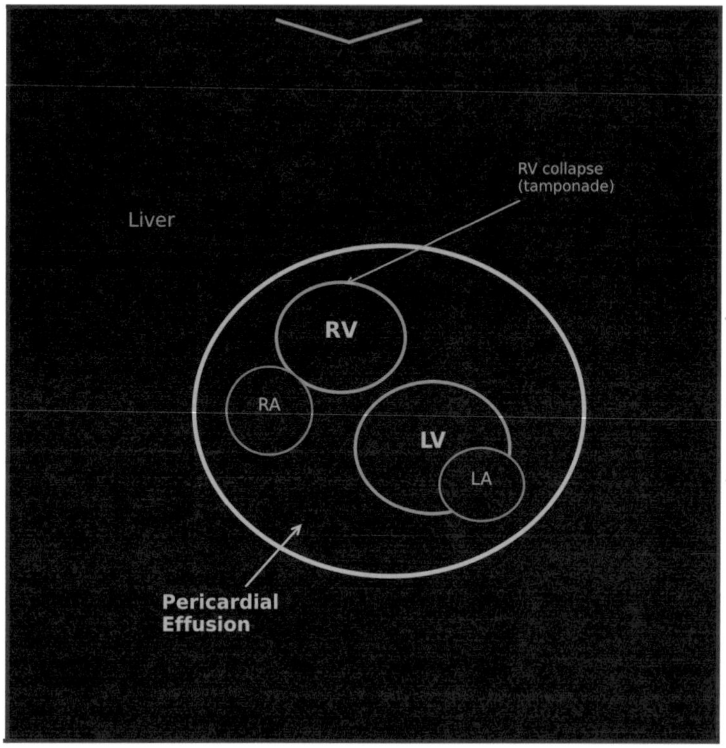

Pericardiocentesis — Subxiphoid Approach

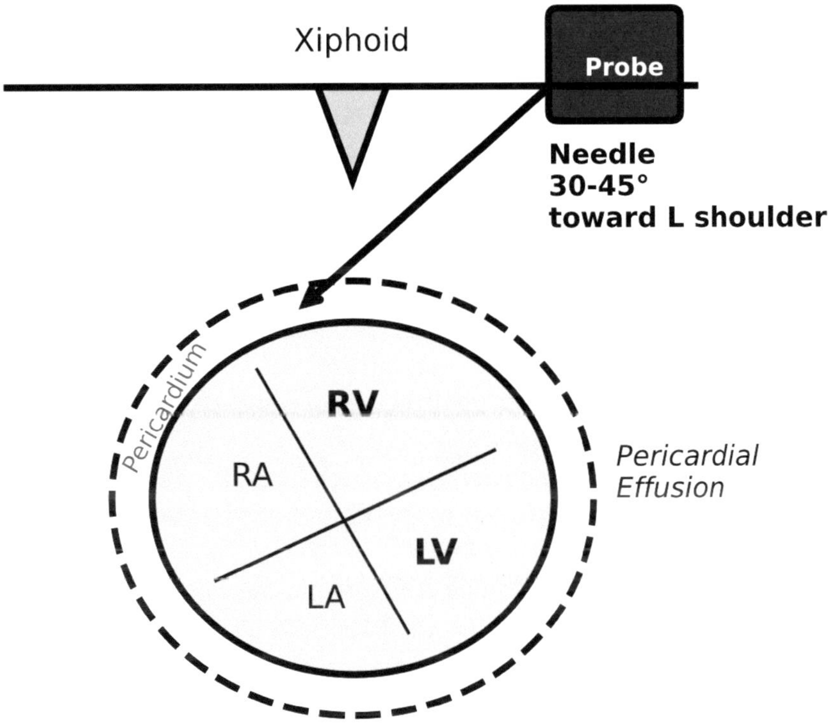

Thoracentesis

Indications:

- Diagnostic sampling of a new or unexplained pleural effusion (infection, malignancy, transudate versus exudate)
- Therapeutic drainage of a large effusion causing dyspnea or hypoxemia

Contraindications:

- Overlying skin infection at the puncture site
- Inability to identify a safe fluid pocket on ultrasound (small or loculated effusion)
- Relative: coagulopathy or anticoagulation (ultrasound guidance makes serious bleeding rare), positive-pressure ventilation (proceed with care), and a single functional lung on the contralateral side

Skills:

1. Select curvilinear or phased array probe; patient seated leaning forward or supine with head elevated 45 degrees.
2. Scan posteriorly using the standard posterior approach (lateral to paraspinal muscles, superior to diaphragm, inferior to scapula) or laterally to identify anechoic pleural fluid; distinguish from consolidated lung (hepatization) or loculated collections.
3. Identify diaphragm (hyperechoic curvilinear structure moving with respiration), liver/spleen, and lung; note depth to fluid and maximal pocket size (>1.5 cm recommended).
4. Avoid intercostal neurovascular bundle (run inferior to ribs); mark site at superior aspect of rib.
5. Real-time guidance: in-plane approach entering above rib, visualizing needle tip enter anechoic fluid collection.
6. Advance catheter-over-needle into pleural space; confirm position with fluid aspiration and ultrasound visualization of catheter within fluid.
7. Attach drainage tubing; monitor for re-expansion pulmonary edema (limit initial drainage to 1—1.5 L).
8. Post-procedure ultrasound to exclude pneumothorax (absence of lung sliding, barcode sign) or hemothorax

Pleural Effusion — Thoracentesis Site

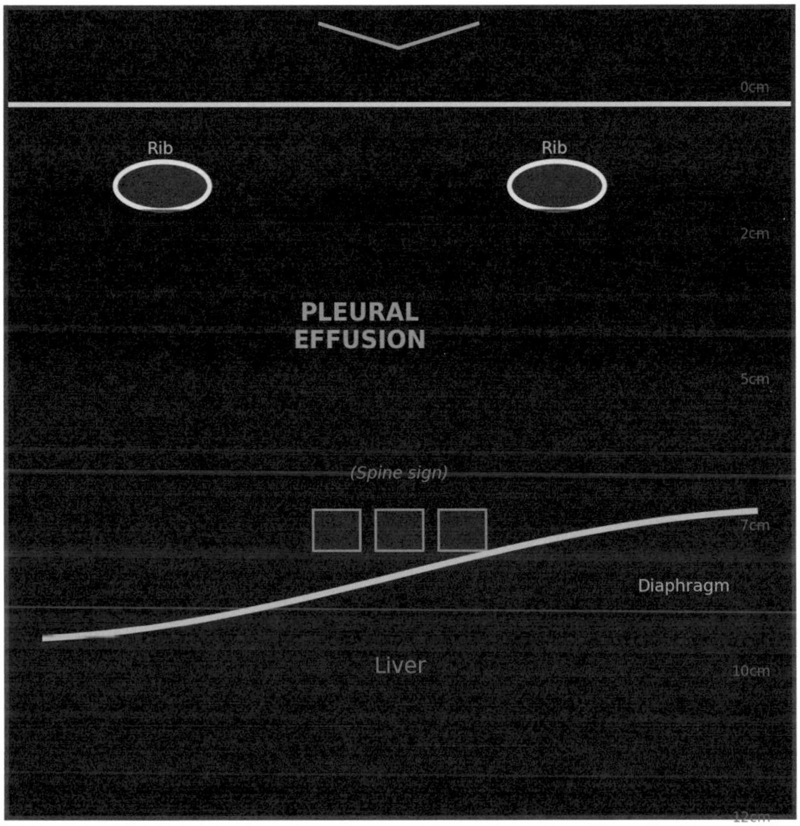

Thoracentesis — Intercostal Approach

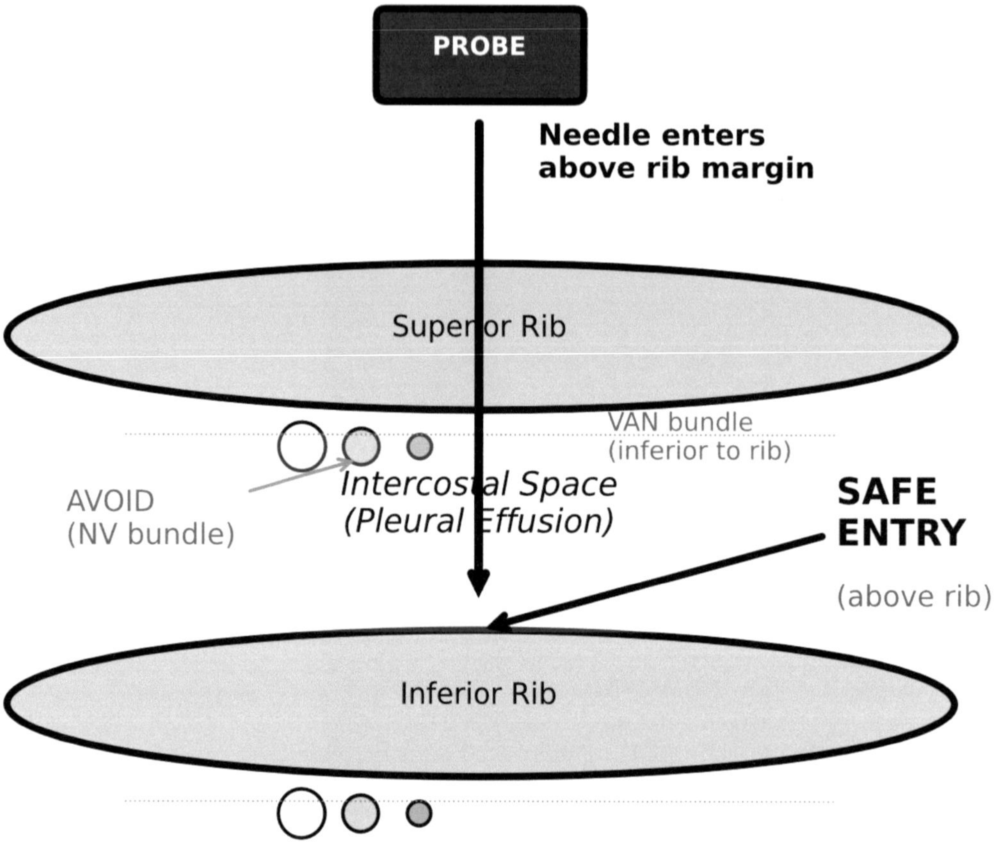

Vascular Access

Central Venous Access (Internal Jugular, Subclavian, Femoral)

1. Select high-frequency linear probe (5—10 MHz); sterile probe cover with gel.
2. Identify vein (compressible, non-pulsatile, venous Doppler phasic with respiration) versus artery (pulsatile, non-compressible, high-velocity Doppler); check for thrombus (intraluminal echogenicity).
3. For IJ: place probe transverse at apex of triangle (clavicular and sternal heads of SCM); target vein lateral to carotid artery.
4. Orient probe to visualize IJ and carotid simultaneously; use in-plane (longitudinal) approach with needle entering at probe edge, visualizing entire shaft, or out-of-plane (transverse) with needle entering at center of probe.
5. Advance needle until tip indenting vein wall; confirm entry by loss of resistance and visualization of tip within lumen (needle tip artifact or "target sign").
6. Confirm guidewire (J-wire) position within vein via ultrasound (hyperechoic line within anechoic lumen); ensure wire does not enter right atrium (visualize SVC/right atrium junction).
7. For subclavian: infraclavicular approach targeting axillary vein (lateral to artery, easily compressible) to avoid pleura and subclavian artery.
8. Post-cannulation: confirm catheter tip position in SVC (right atrial junction) via ultrasound or chest X-ray; rule out pneumothorax (ipsilateral lung sliding assessment).

Internal Jugular Vein — Short Axis View

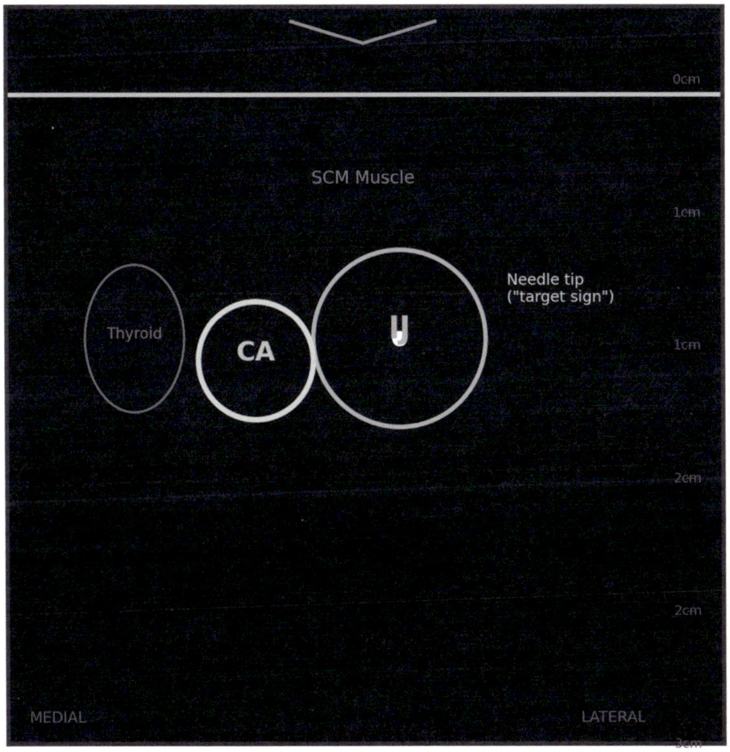

Central Venous Access — Internal Jugular

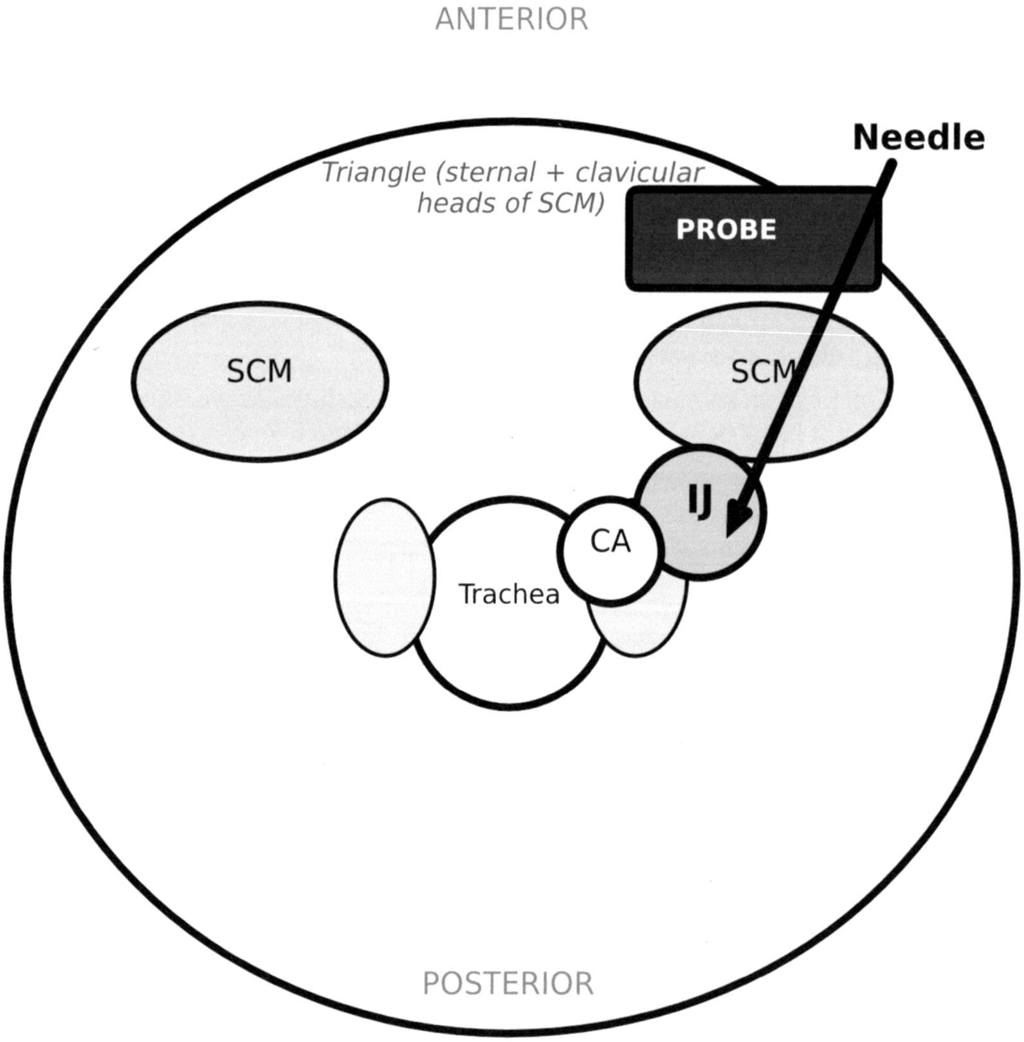

Peripheral Venous Access

1. Select high-frequency linear probe (≥10 MHz); tourniquet placement proximal.
2. Identify superficial veins (cephalic, basilic, median cubital, saphenous): anechoic, compressible, <1 cm depth.
3. Assess vein patency (augmentation with distal compression); avoid veins with thrombosis or significant tortuosity.
4. Static technique: mark vein center; measure depth to guide catheter length selection.
5. Dynamic technique: in-plane approach with 18—20 gauge catheter; visualize needle entering vein anterior wall, confirm flashback, advance catheter while visualizing catheter tip within lumen.
6. Confirm intraluminal position by injecting 5—10 mL normal saline observing turbulence (hyperechoic microbubbles) within vein, not surrounding tissue.

Peripheral IV — Long Axis (In-Plane) View

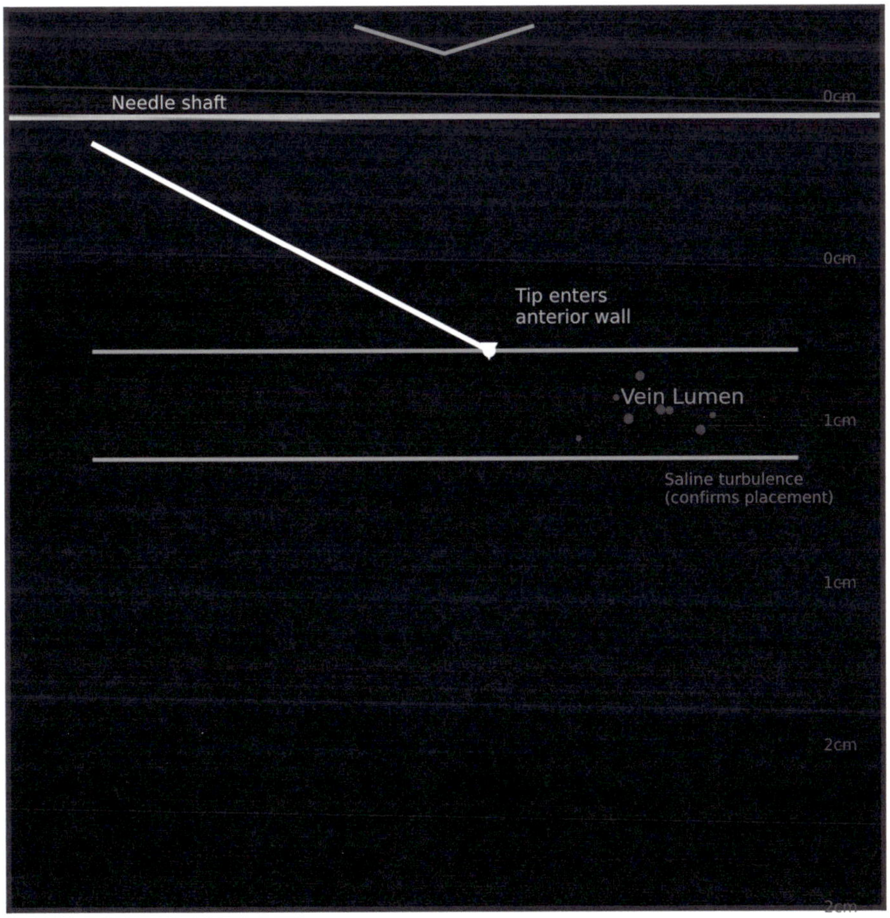

Arterial Access (Radial, Femoral, Brachial)

1. Select high-frequency linear probe; identify artery (non-compressible, pulsatile, circular cross-section with hyperechoic walls).
2. Apply color or spectral Doppler to confirm arterial waveform (high-velocity, triphasic for peripheral arteries).
3. Measure artery diameter to select catheter size (typically 20 gauge for radial, 18 for femoral).
4. Modified Seldinger or direct puncture: in-plane approach at 30—45 degree angle; visualize needle entering anterior wall.
5. Confirm arterial return (pulsatile blood flow); advance guidewire if using Seldinger technique, confirming wire within arterial lumen via ultrasound.
6. Advance catheter; confirm placement by arterial waveform on transducer and ultrasound visualization of catheter within vessel.

Radial Artery — Short Axis View

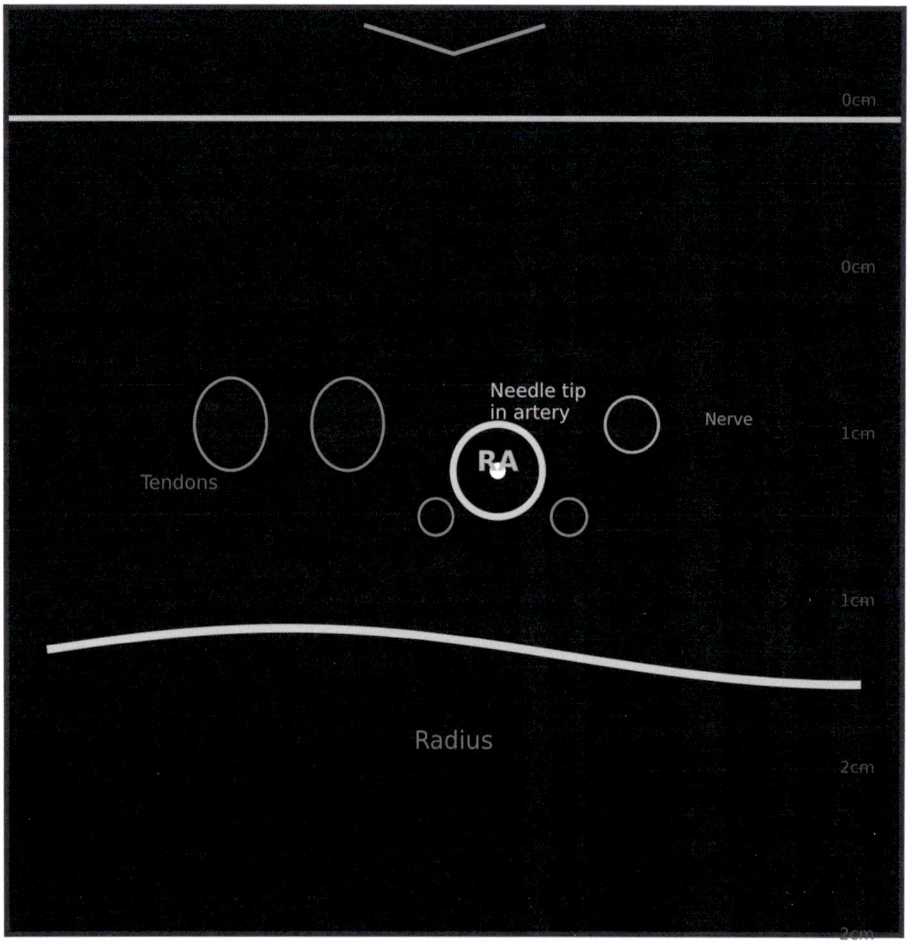

Cardiac Arrest (Medical Etiology Assessment)

1. Select phased array probe (2—4 MHz); place in subxiphoid position for initial view (minimizes CPR interruption).
2. Assess for pericardial effusion: anechoic stripe surrounding heart; if present, assess for RV/RA diastolic collapse indicating tamponade.
3. Evaluate for RV dilation (RV:LV ratio >1:1) suggesting massive pulmonary embolism.
4. Assess cardiac activity: coordinated wall motion vs fibrillatory activity vs standstill (absence of motion).
5. Evaluate IVC: diameter >2.1 cm with <50 collapse suggests volume overload; collapse suggests hypovolemia. Note: IVC assessment is unreliable during active CPR due to positive-pressure ventilation and chest compressions; interpret with caution.
6. If subxiphoid view inadequate, obtain parasternal long-axis during brief CPR pause (≤10 seconds).
7. Consider pulmonary ultrasound for tension pneumothorax (absence of lung sliding, barcode sign) if ultrasound cardiac etiology negative.

Cardiac Arrest — RV Dilation (Massive PE)

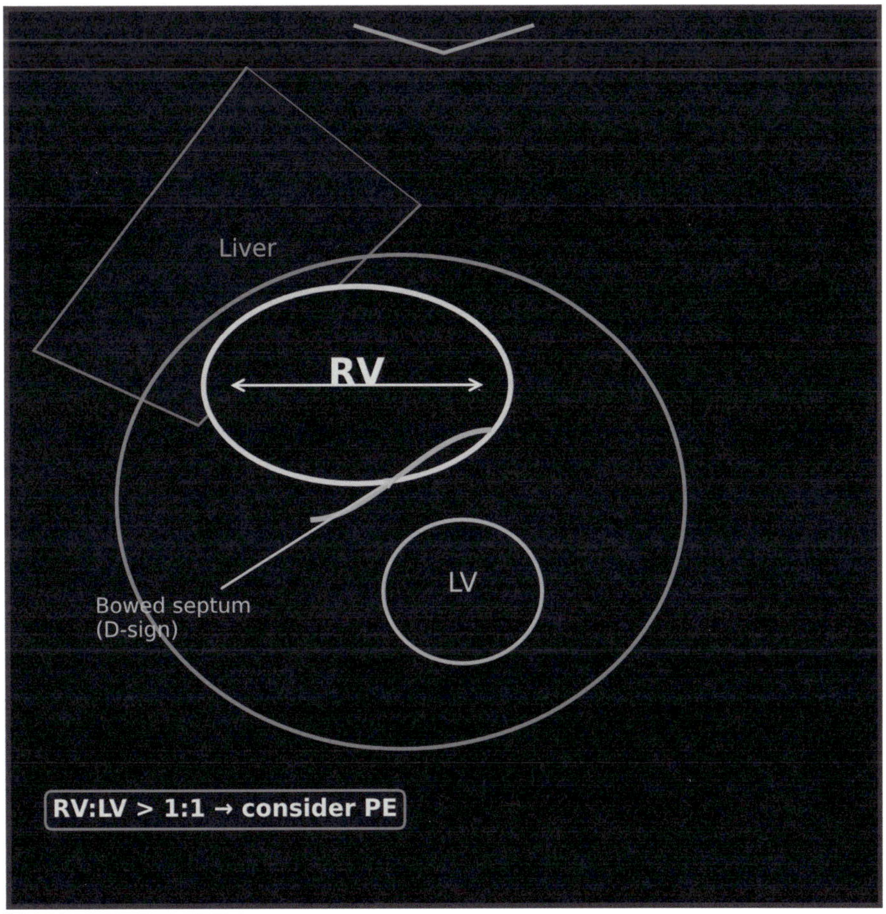

Cardiac Arrest — Subxiphoid View (Normal Chambers)

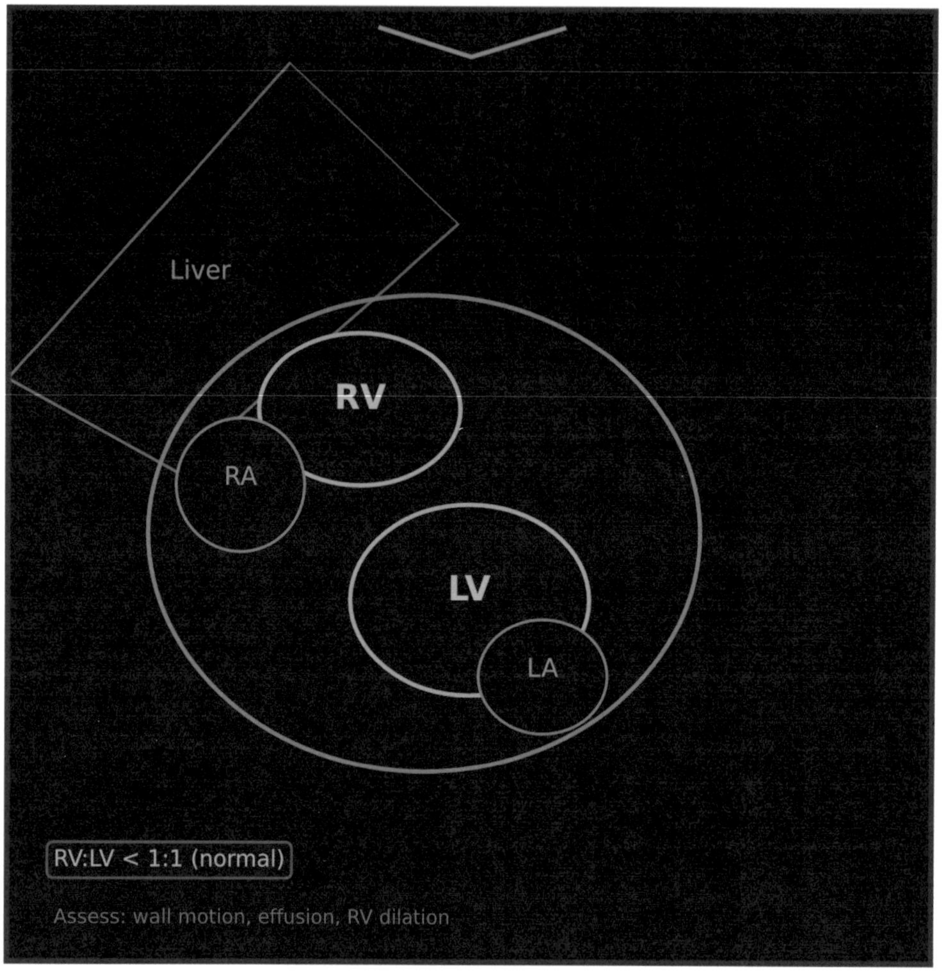

Cardiac Arrest (Traumatic Etiology)

1. Perform FAST exam integration: subxiphoid cardiac view for hemopericardium (hemothorax may mask view), right upper quadrant for hemoperitoneum, left upper quadrant for splenic injury/hemothorax, suprapubic for pelvic hematoma.
2. Assess for pericardial tamponade in penetrating chest trauma: anechoic pericardial collection with RV collapse.
3. Evaluate for massive hemothorax: anechoic fluid above diaphragm in thoracic cavity (>1.5 cm depth indicates need for chest tube).
4. Assess for tension pneumothorax: absence of lung sliding bilaterally, especially in supine trauma patient (anterior chest).
5. Evaluate cardiac activity and chamber size to guide resuscitation efforts.

FAST Exam — Probe Placement Positions

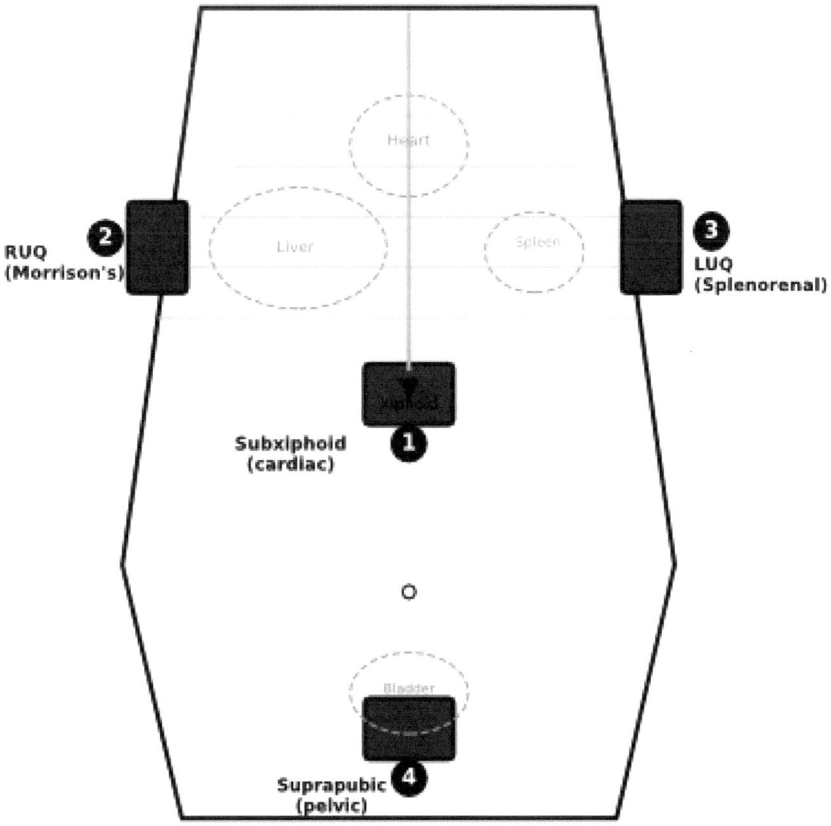

FAST RUQ — Normal (No Free Fluid)

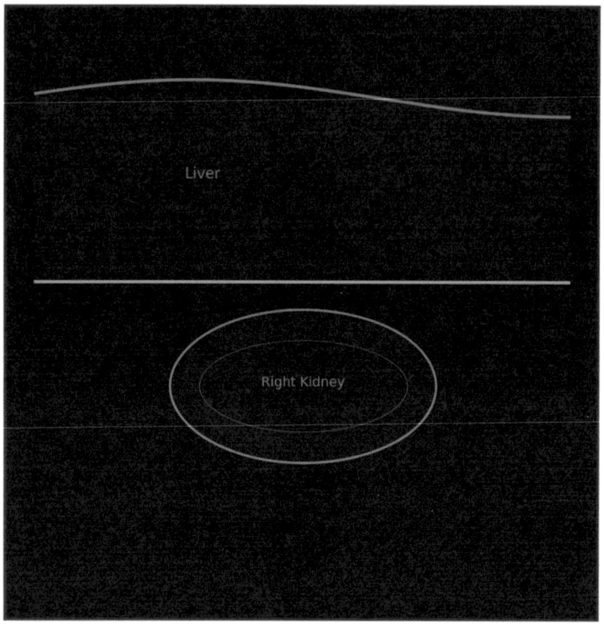

FAST RUQ — Positive (Free Fluid)

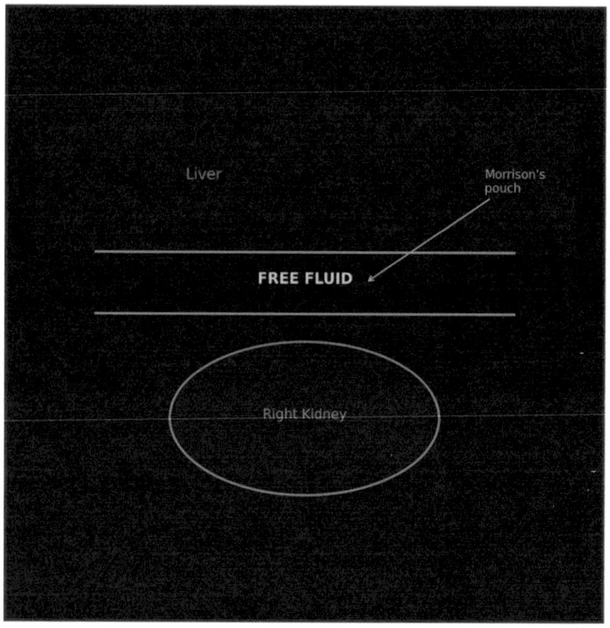

FAST LUQ — Normal

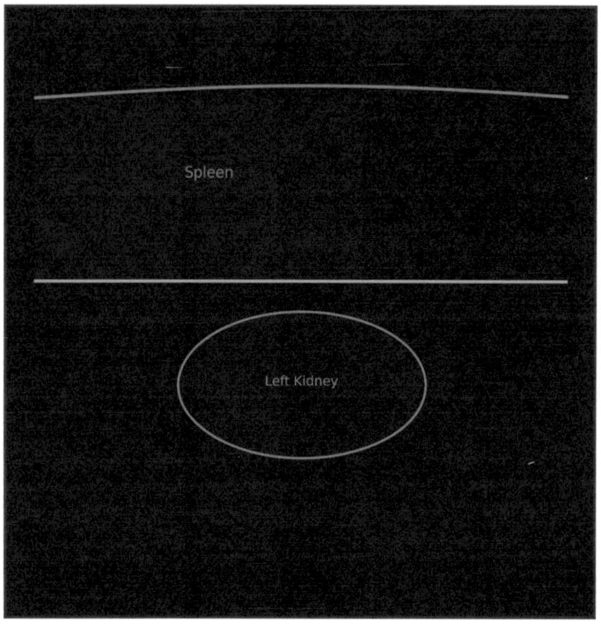

FAST LUQ — Positive (Hemothorax + Hemoperitoneum)

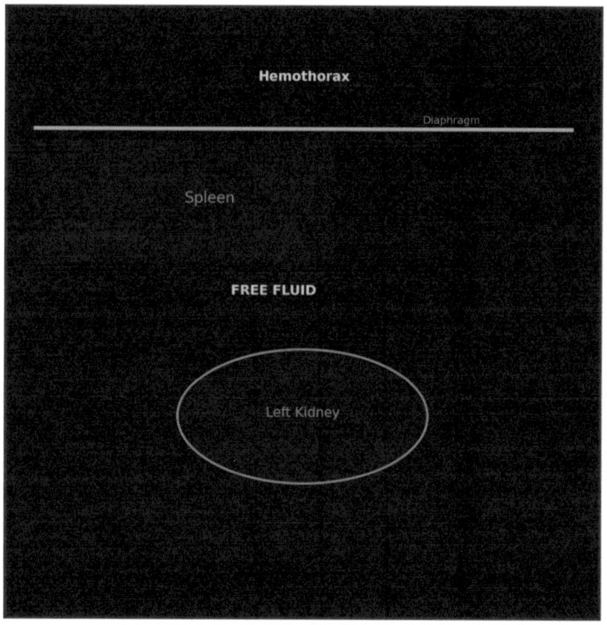

FAST Suprapubic — Normal

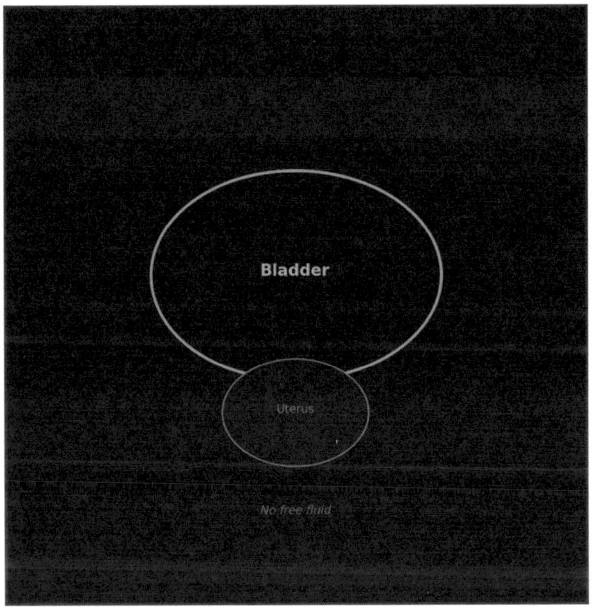

FAST Suprapubic — Positive (Pelvic Free Fluid)

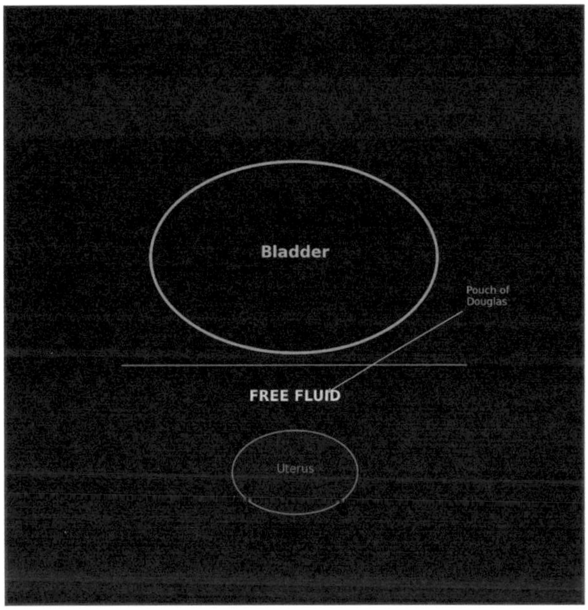

Normal Lung — Seashore Sign (M-mode)

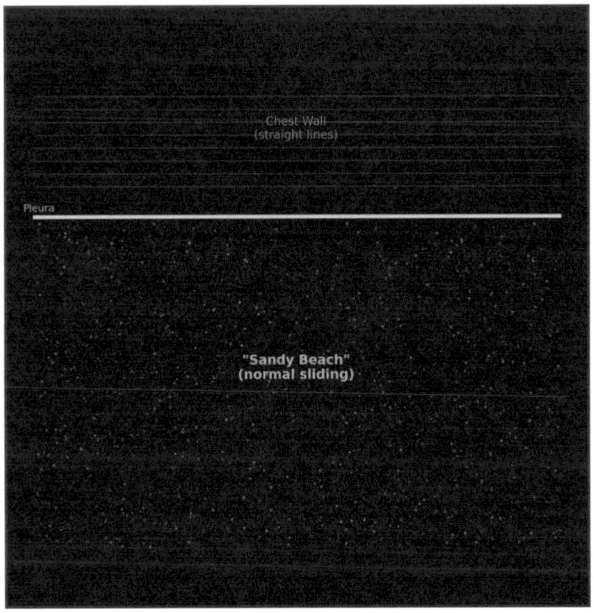

Pneumothorax — Barcode/Stratosphere Sign (M-mode)

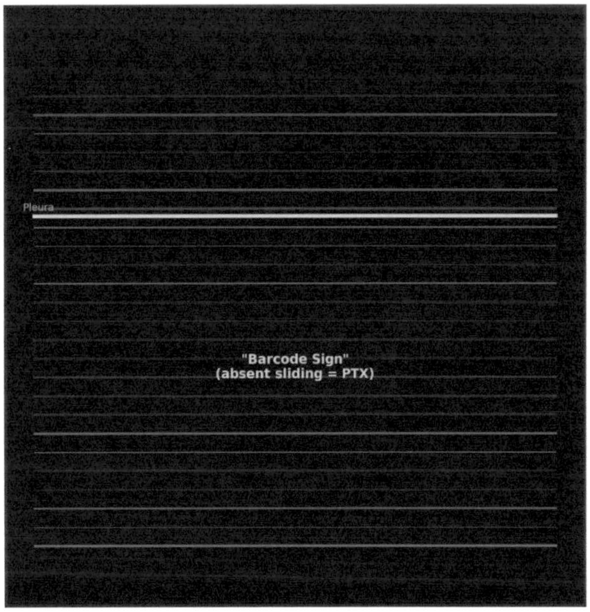

Aorta

1. Select curvilinear (2—5 MHz) for abdominal aorta, phased array for thoracic aortic arch.
2. Transverse and longitudinal scans from xiphoid to umbilicus (proximal, mid, distal segments).
3. Measure outer wall to outer wall: diameter >3.0 cm defines aneurysm; >5.0 cm indicates high risk for rupture.
4. Identify mural thrombus (intraluminal hyperechoic material) and measure residual lumen.
5. Assess for dissection: intimal flap (linear echogenic structure) dividing true (pulsatile, patent) and false lumen (spontaneous echocardiographic contrast, thrombus).
6. Evaluate proximal aorta at diaphragm and distal bifurcation at umbilicus; note iliac artery involvement if aneurysmal.
7. Assess for retroperitoneal hematoma (hypoechoic fluid posterior to aorta, anterior to spine) indicating rupture.

Abdominal Aorta — Transverse (Normal <3cm)

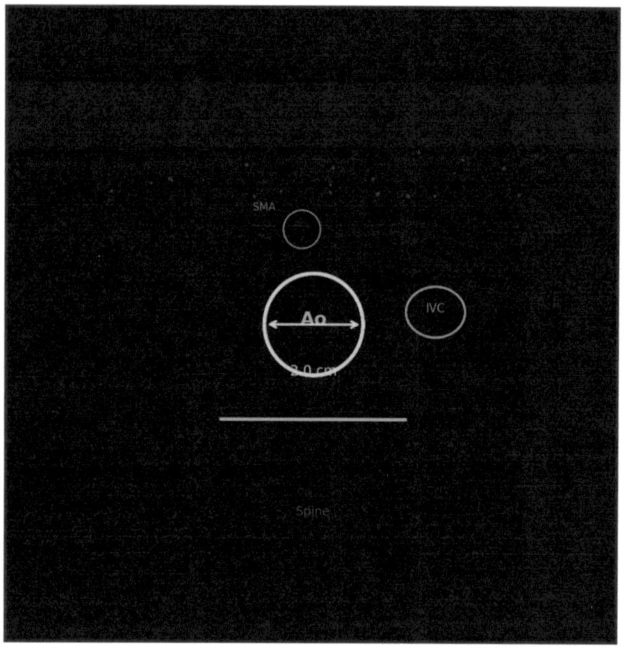

Abdominal Aorta — AAA (>5cm, mural thrombus)

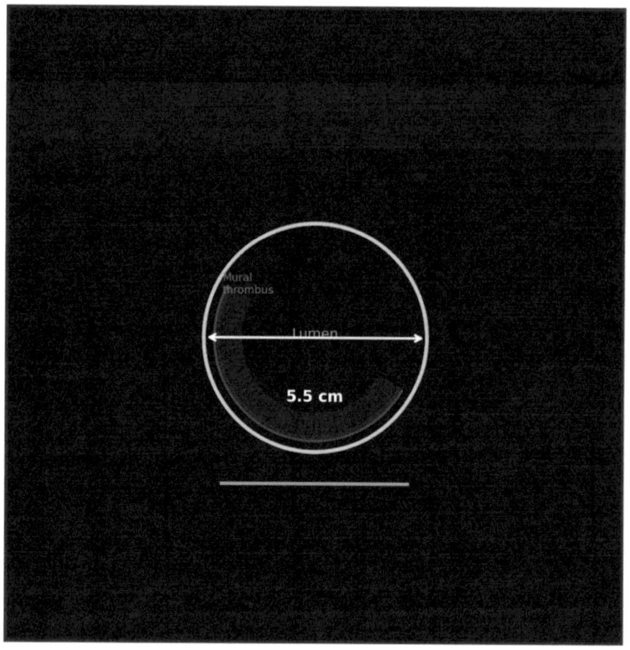

Biliary

1. Select curvilinear probe (2—5 MHz); intercostal or subcostal approach.
2. Identify gallbladder: anechoic pear-shaped structure within gallbladder fossa (interlobar fissure between liver lobes).
3. Assess wall thickness: normal <3 mm; measure anterior wall in sagittal view with perpendicular angle.
4. Evaluate for cholelithiasis: hyperechoic focus with clean posterior acoustic shadowing; assess mobility with patient repositioning (decubitus).
5. Evaluate for cholecystitis: wall thickening, pericholecystic fluid (anechoic stripe surrounding GB), sonographic Murphy's sign (maximal tenderness with probe pressure over GB).
6. Measure common bile duct (CBD) anterior to portal vein: normal <6 mm, <7 mm post-cholecystectomy, increases 1 mm per decade after age 60; assess for choledocholithiasis (shadowing stone within duct).
7. Assess gallbladder size: longitudinal >10 cm or transverse >5 cm suggests hydrops/obstruction.

Gallbladder — Normal Anatomy

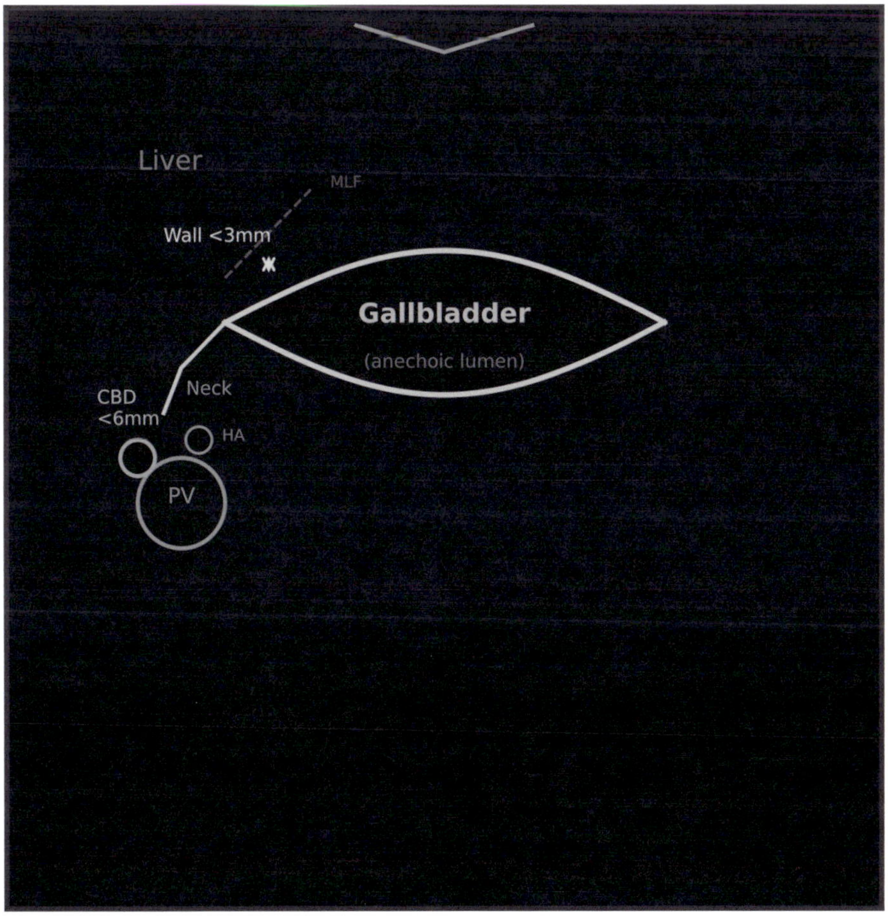

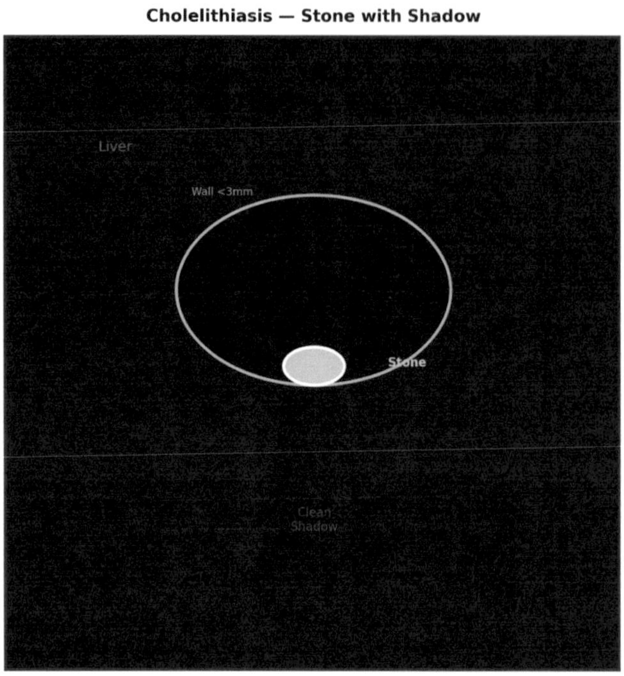
Cholelithiasis — Stone with Shadow
Liver
Wall <3mm
Stone
Clean
Shadow

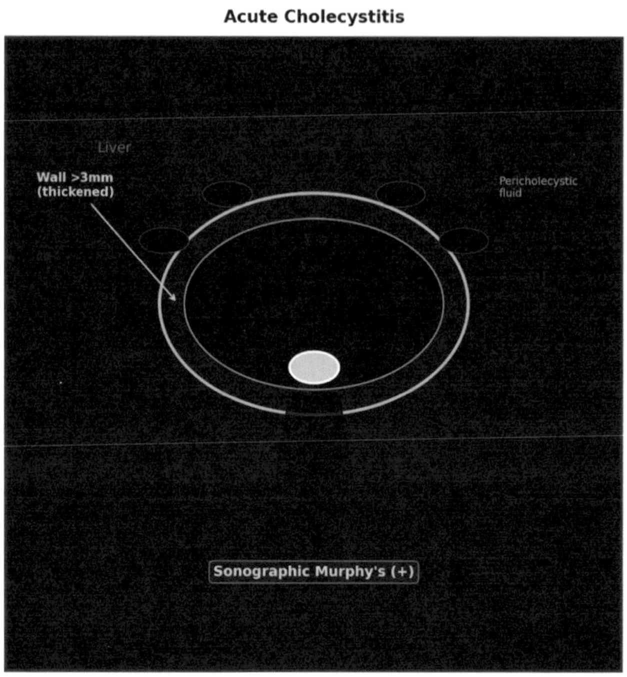
Acute Cholecystitis
Liver
Wall >3mm
(thickened)
Pericholecystic
fluid
Sonographic Murphy's (+)

Bowel

1. Select linear (high frequency) for appendicitis/intussusception or curvilinear for SBO.
2. Appendix: graded compression technique in RLQ; identify blind-ending, non-compressible tubular structure >6 mm outer wall diameter from outer wall to outer wall; assess for appendicolith (hyperechoic with shadowing), periappendiceal fluid, loss of wall layers.
3. Pyloric stenosis: transverse view for "target sign" (mucosa surrounded by hypoechoic muscle); single-wall muscle thickness ≥3 mm (most important criterion), pyloric channel length ≥16 mm, overall pyloric diameter >14 mm. Longitudinal view for "cervix sign" (elongated pylorus).
4. Intussusception: target sign on transverse view (concentric rings of alternating hyperechoic and hypoechoic layers), pseudo-kidney sign on longitudinal view; assess for trapped fluid within intussusceptum (contraindication for reduction).
5. Small bowel obstruction: dilated loops >2.5 cm, increased peristalsis (to-and-fro movement), transition point, free fluid between loops.
6. Hernia: identify fascial defect with bowel loops or fat extending beyond abdominal wall; assess for incarceration (non-compressible, no peristalsis) and strangulation (absent flow on color Doppler).

Appendicitis — Transverse (Target Sign)

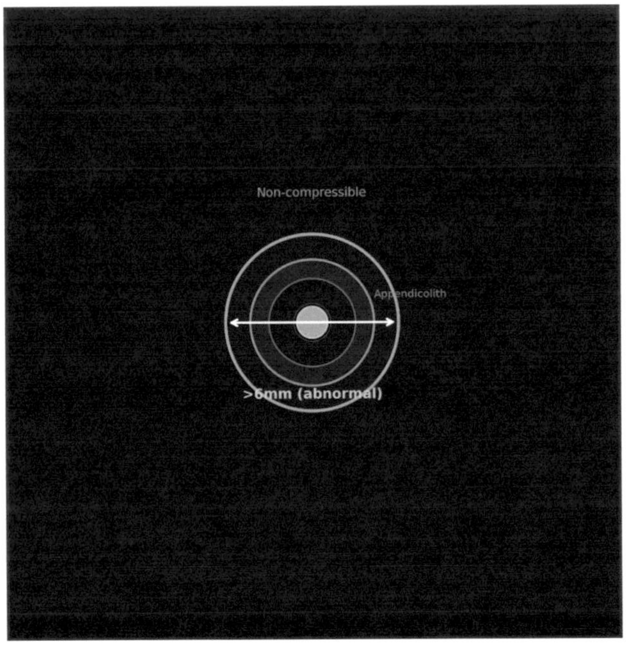

Appendicitis — Longitudinal (Blind-ending)

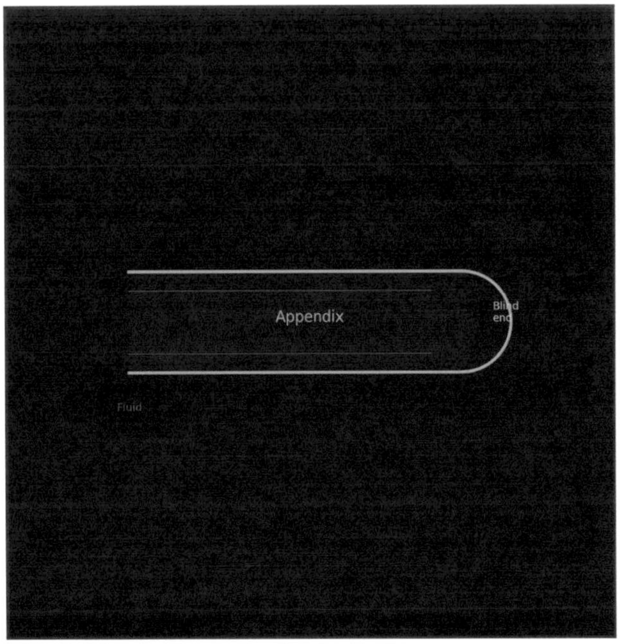

Small Bowel Obstruction — Dilated Loops

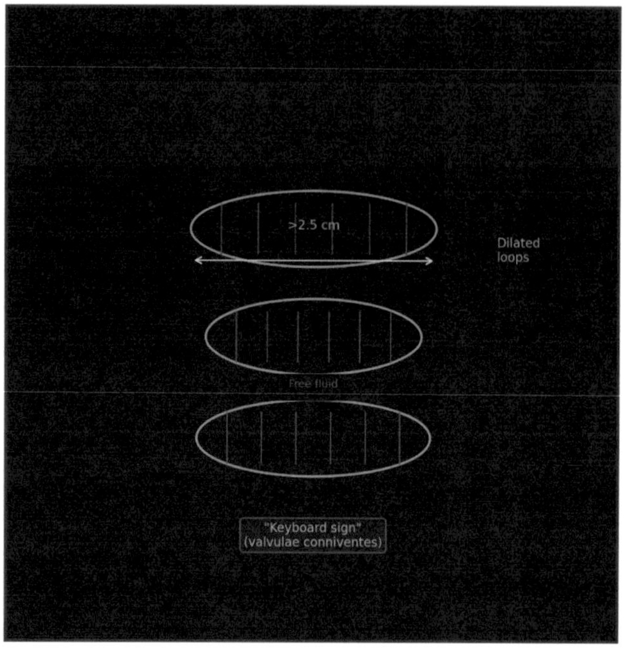

Intussusception — Target Sign (Transverse)

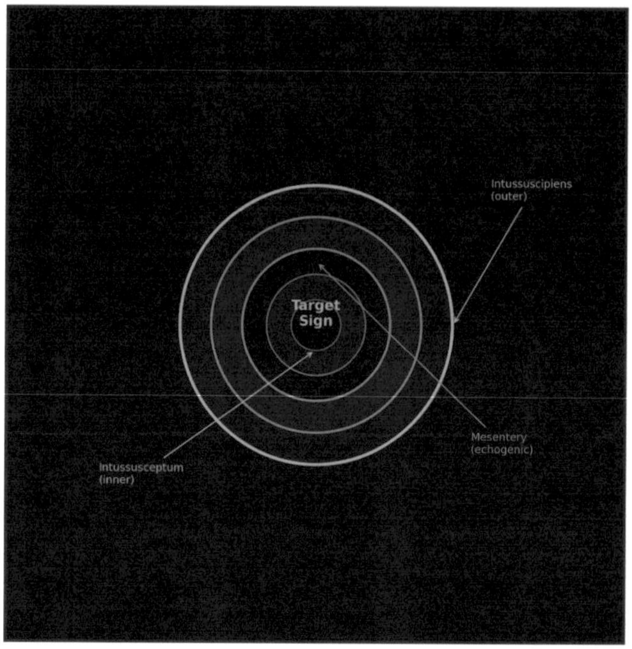

Cardiac

1. Select phased array probe (2—4 MHz).
2. Parasternal long-axis (PLAX): assess LV function (qualitative: hyperdynamic, normal, reduced), pericardial effusion (posterior to LV in systole), RV size, aortic root, mitral valve.
3. Parasternal short-axis (PSAX): assess LV function at papillary muscle level (circular contraction), RV size, pericardial effusion circumferentially.
4. Apical 4-chamber (A4C): assess all four chambers, RV:LV size ratio (normal <0.6:1; ratio >1:1 suggests RV dilation), pericardial effusion (lateral to LV), mitral/tricuspid valves; McConnell's sign (RV free wall akinesis with apical sparing) for PE.
5. Subxiphoid: assess pericardial effusion, RV collapse, IVC size.
6. IVC view (subcostal): assess diameter and collapsibility with sniff (>50% collapse indicates fluid responsiveness).
7. Assess for wall motion abnormalities (WMA): regional hypokinesis/akinesis indicating coronary territory involvement.

Apical 4-Chamber View (A4C)

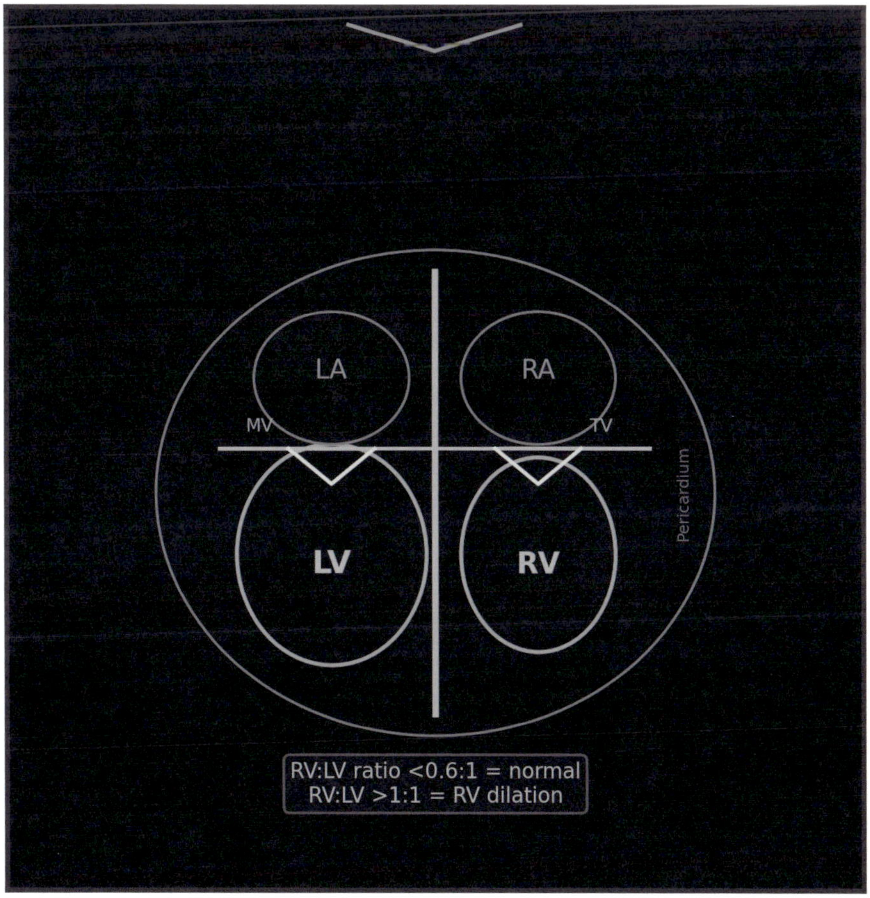

Parasternal Short Axis (PSAX)

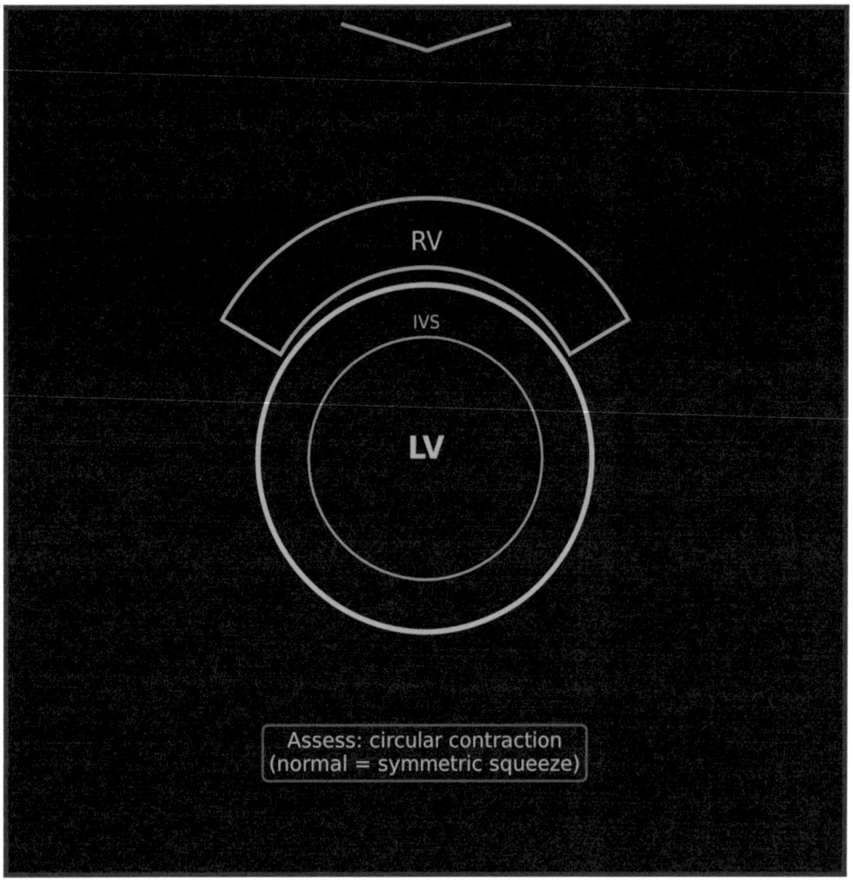

Ocular

1. Select high-frequency linear probe (≥10 MHz); sterile gel on closed eyelid or sterile cover with minimal pressure.
2. Optic nerve sheath diameter (ONSD): measure 3 mm posterior to retina, perpendicular to optic nerve; >5.0 mm suggests elevated ICP (>20 mmHg).
3. Assess for retinal detachment: hyperechoic membrane attached to optic nerve head, mobile with eye movement.
4. Vitreous hemorrhage: swirling echogenic debris within vitreous chamber, gravity-dependent layering.
5. Foreign body: hyperechoic intraocular focus with shadowing or reverberation.
6. Lens dislocation: lens not centered in anterior segment, may be in posterior vitreous.
7. Aqueous/vitreous hemorrhage: anechoic fluid in anterior chamber (hyphema) or vitreous.
8. Posterior vitreous detachment: mobile linear structure not attached to optic nerve.

Ocular — ONSD Measurement

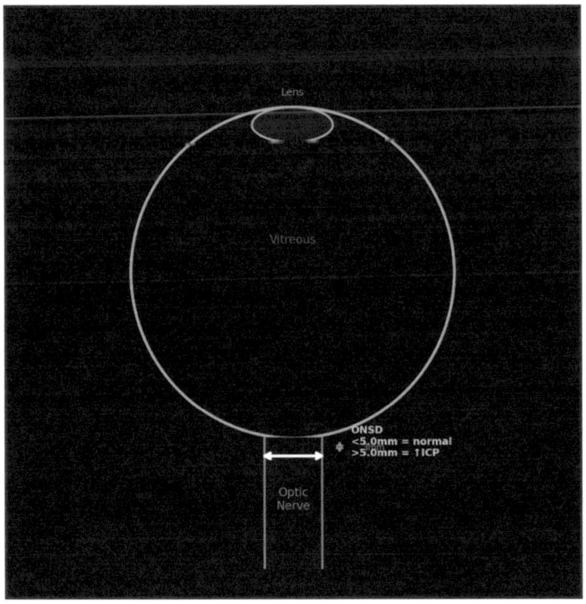

Retinal Detachment

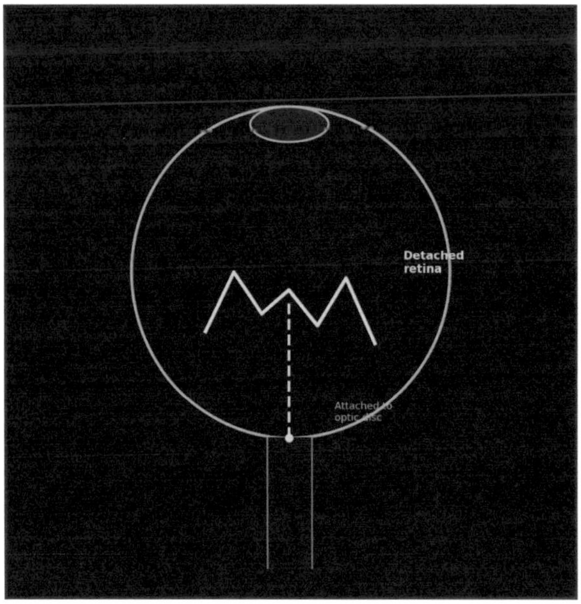

Vitreous Hemorrhage

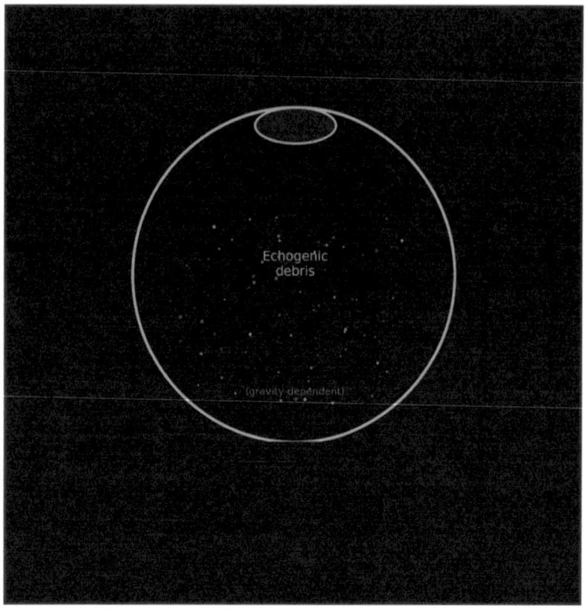

Lens Dislocation

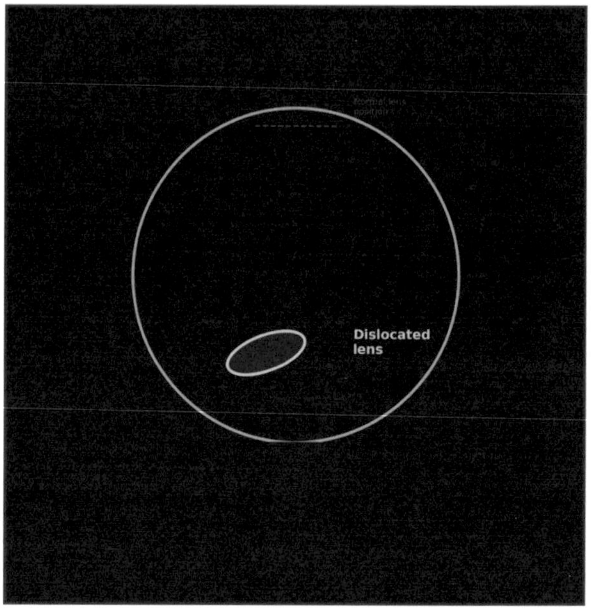

Female Pelvis

1. Select curvilinear (transabdominal) with full bladder or endocavitary (endovaginal) with empty bladder (higher resolution).
2. Transabdominal: identify uterus (midline, pear-shaped, homogeneous myometrium), endometrial stripe (varies by cycle: proliferative 4—8 mm, secretory 7—14 mm, postmenopausal <5 mm unless on HRT).
3. Endovaginal: assess uterus in two planes, measure endometrial thickness (double thickness from anterior to posterior interface).
4. Adnexa: identify ovaries (almond-shaped, follicular cysts), assess for masses (cystic, solid, complex), free fluid in cul-de-sac (anechoic stripe posterior to uterus).
5. Intrauterine pregnancy (IUP): gestational sac (anechoic structure with echogenic rim within endometrium), yolk sac (within sac, confirms IUP), fetal pole, cardiac activity (M-mode documentation).
6. Ectopic pregnancy: empty uterus with decidual reaction, adnexal mass (tubal ring sign—echogenic ring surrounding anechoic gestational sac), moderate free fluid (hemoperitoneum).
7. Assess for ovarian torsion: enlarged ovary (>4 cm), peripheral follicles, absent Doppler flow (not reliable), whirlpool sign (twisted pedicle).

Normal Ovary — Follicular Cysts

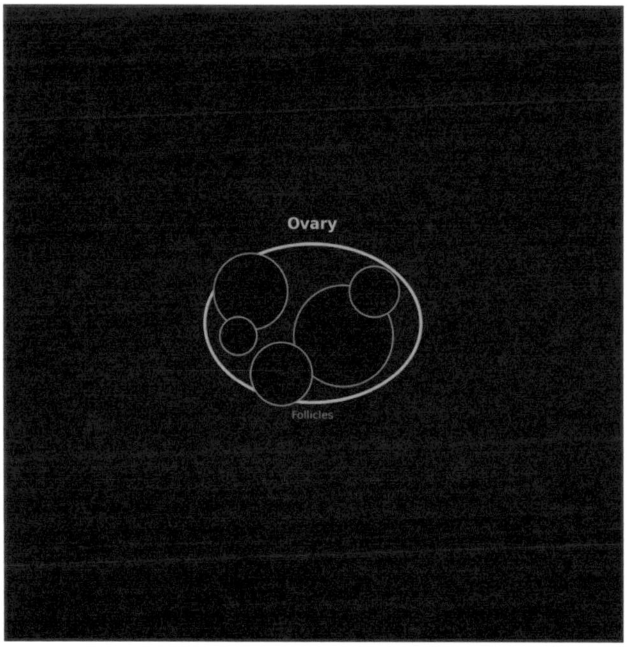

Ovarian Torsion — Enlarged, Peripheral Follicles

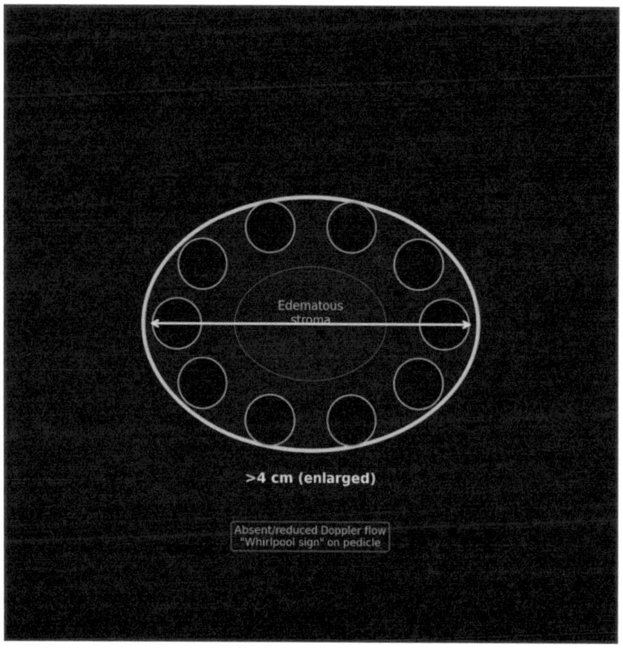

Early IUP — Gestational Sac + Yolk Sac (Endovaginal)

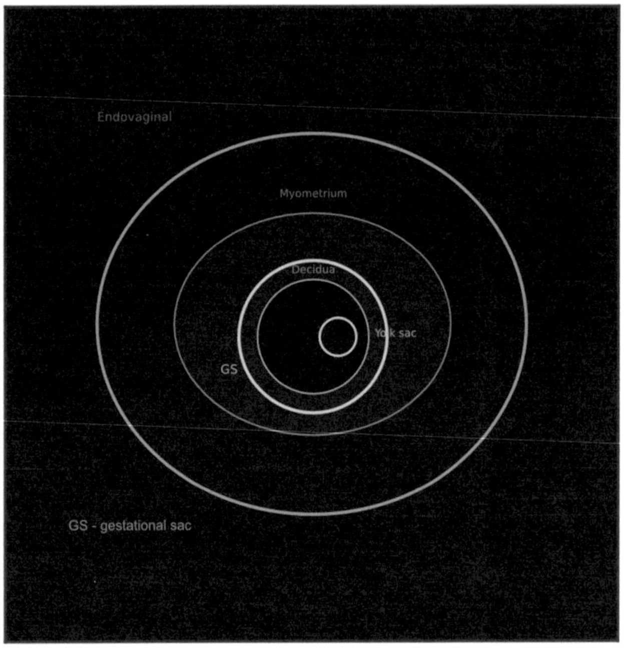

Ectopic Pregnancy — Empty Uterus + Adnexal Mass

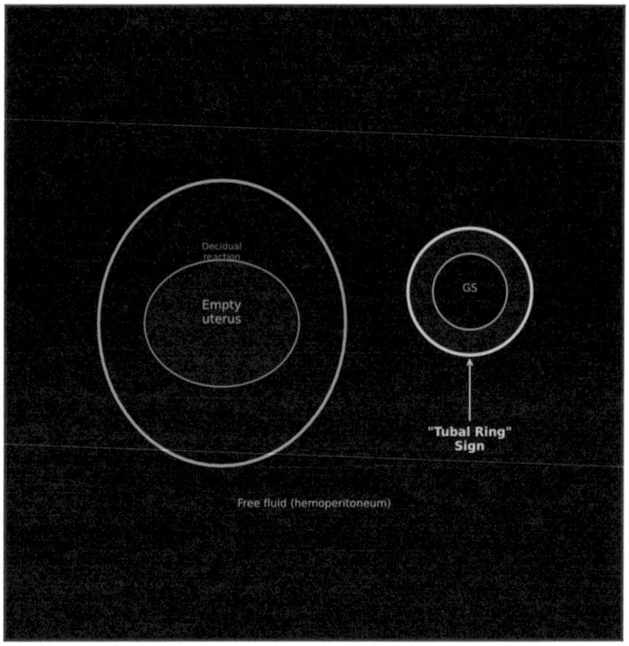

Renal and Bladder

1. Select curvilinear or phased array probe.
2. Right kidney: intercostal or subcostal approach using liver as acoustic window; left kidney: subcostal or posterior approach.
3. Assess cortex, medulla, renal pelvis; grade hydronephrosis: Grade 1 (pelvic splitting), Grade 2 (calyceal dilation without cortical thinning), Grade 3 (cortical thinning, ballooning).
4. Assess for nephrolithiasis: hyperechoic focus with posterior shadowing; assess for ureteral jets (intermittent anechoic stream from ureteral orifice into bladder trigone) to exclude obstruction.
5. Bladder: assess volume (ellipsoid formula: length × width × height × 0.52), wall thickness (<3 mm when distended).
6. Assess for bladder mass, clot (mobile, non-shadowing), or foreign body (catheter balloon appears as hyperechoic ring with clean shadow).

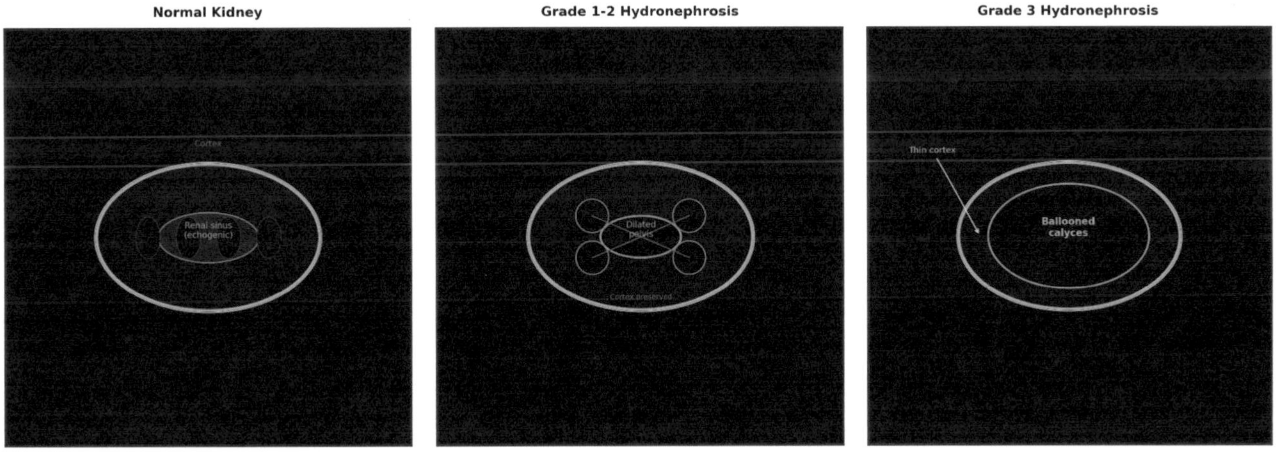

Nephrolithiasis — Stone with Shadow

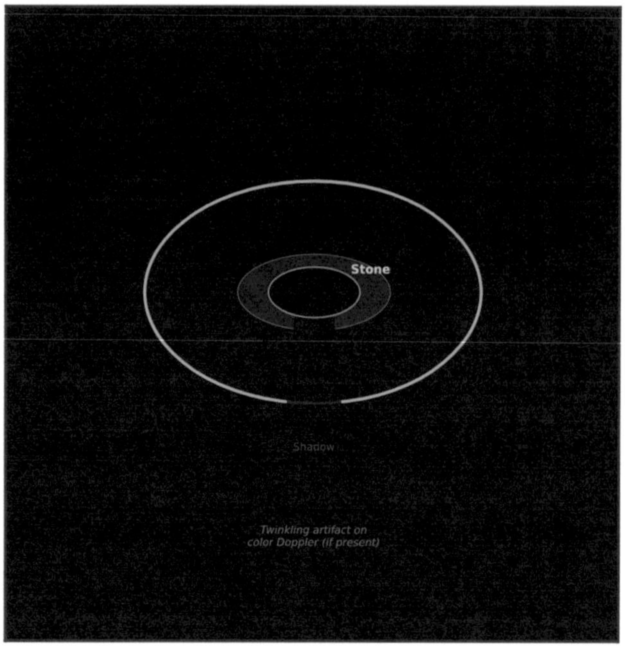

Bladder — Volume Assessment + Ureteral Jets

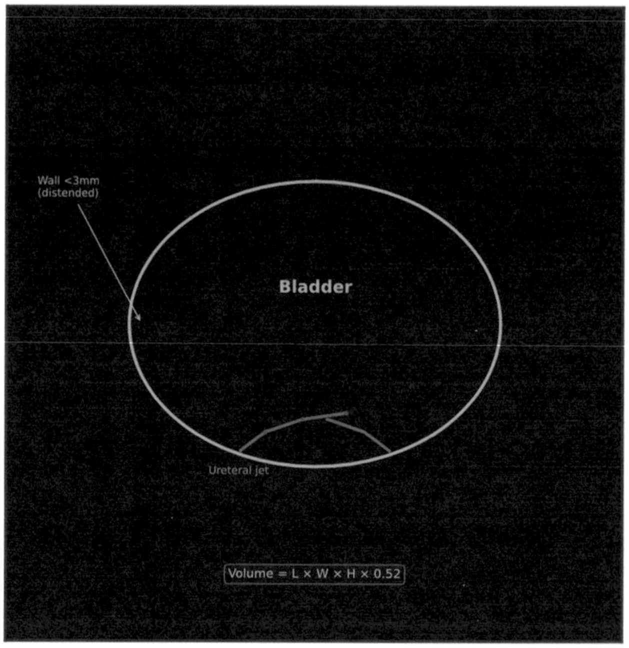

Soft Tissue/Musculoskeletal

1. Select high-frequency linear probe (≥10 MHz).
2. Cellulitis: cobblestoning (hyperechoic fat lobules surrounded by hypoechoic fluid), fluid tracking along fascial planes.
3. Abscess: as detailed in procedural section.
4. Tendon: fibrillar hyperechoic pattern; assess for rupture (hypoechoic gap, loss of fiber continuity), tenosynovitis (anechoic fluid surrounding tendon), anisotropy artifact (change echogenicity with probe tilt).
5. Joint effusion: anechoic/hypoechoic fluid within joint capsule; distinguish from bursitis (subacromial, olecranon, prepatellar).
6. Fracture: cortical step-off, disruption of hyperechoic bone surface, hematoma formation; assess for occult scaphoid or fifth metatarsal fractures.
7. Muscle: assess for tear (hypoechoic collection within muscle belly), hematoma (organized anechoic collection with internal echoes), compartment syndrome (increased echogenicity, thickened fascia, reduced perfusion on Doppler).

Cellulitis — Cobblestoning Pattern

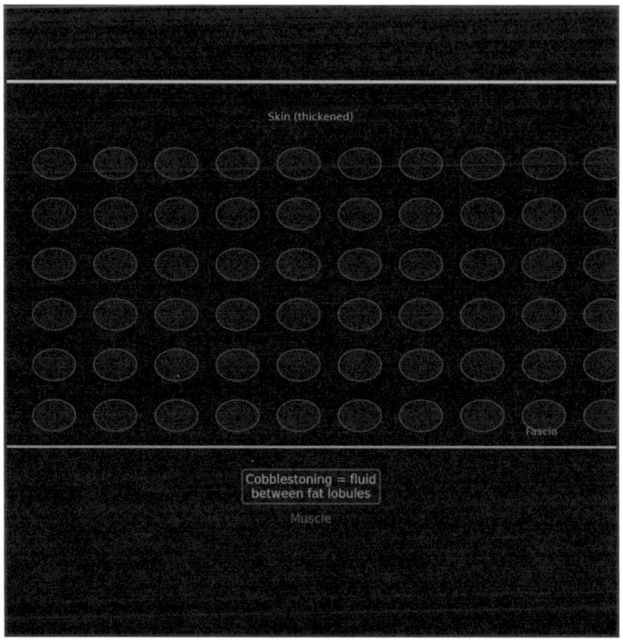

Tendon — Normal vs Tear

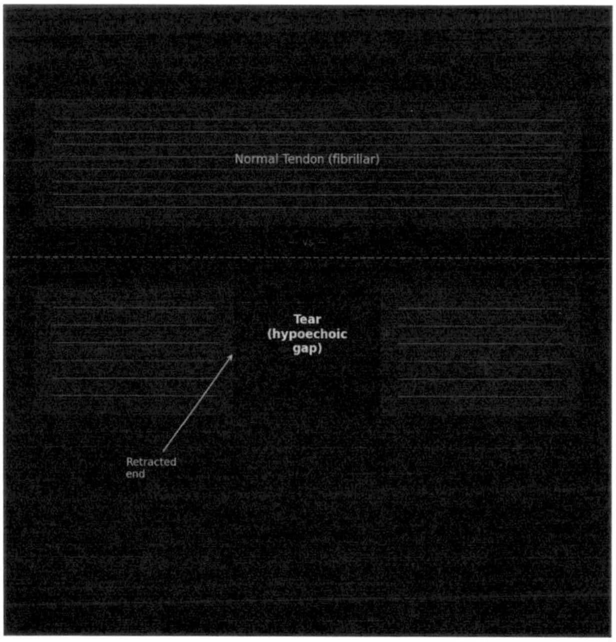

Fracture — Cortical Disruption

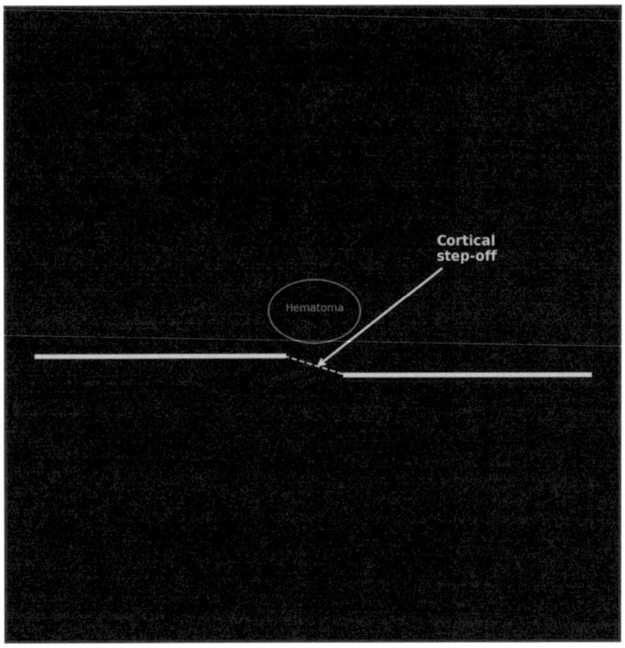

Joint Effusion — Anechoic Fluid in Capsule

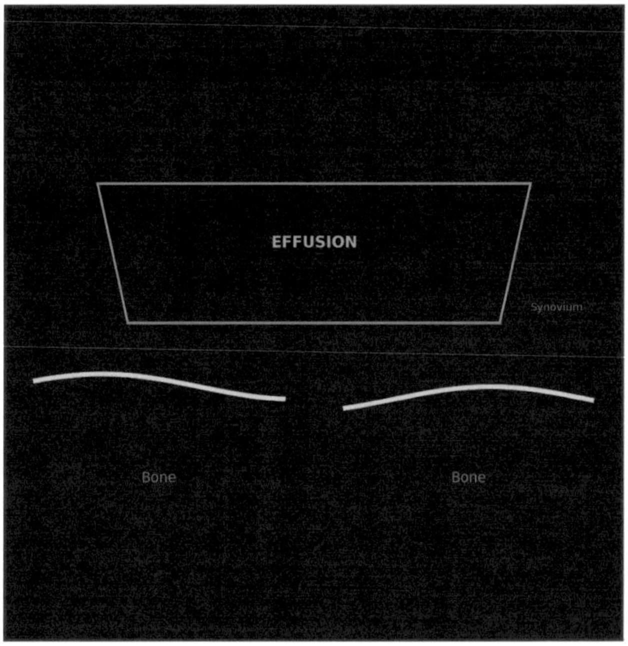

Thoracic

1. Select linear (superficial) or curvilinear (deeper) probe.
2. Pneumothorax: assess for lung sliding (seashore sign on M-mode) at multiple intercostal spaces anteriorly; absence of lung sliding + barcode sign (stratosphere sign on M-mode) indicates pneumothorax; identify lung point (transition zone between sliding and non-sliding).
3. Pleural effusion: anechoic collection above diaphragm, dependent, assess for septations (complex), echogenic debris (hemothorax, empyema), spine sign (vertebral bodies visible above diaphragm indicates effusion).
4. Consolidation: hepatization of lung (tissue-like echogenicity), dynamic air bronchograms (hyperechoic branching structures with movement), shred sign (irregular border between consolidated and aerated lung).
5. Interstitial syndrome: ≥3 B-lines (comet-tail artifacts extending to bottom of screen) in two lung zones bilaterally indicates pulmonary edema; assess for pleural irregularity (thickening, >3 mm).
6. Diaphragm: assess excursion (≥1 cm with deep breath) and thickening fraction (>20 from end-expiration to end-inspiration).

B-lines (Pulmonary Edema)

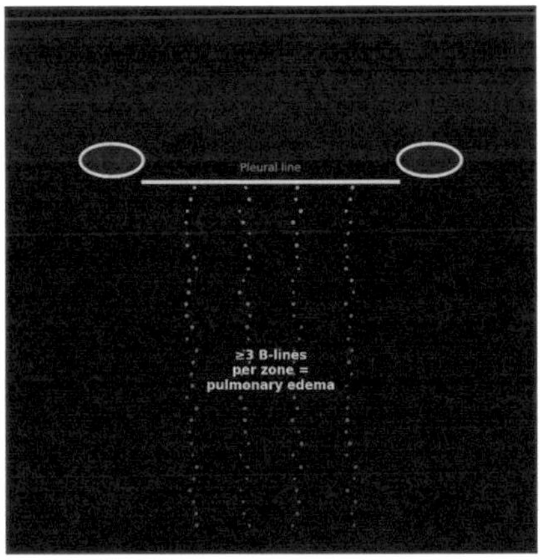

Lung Consolidation (Hepatization)

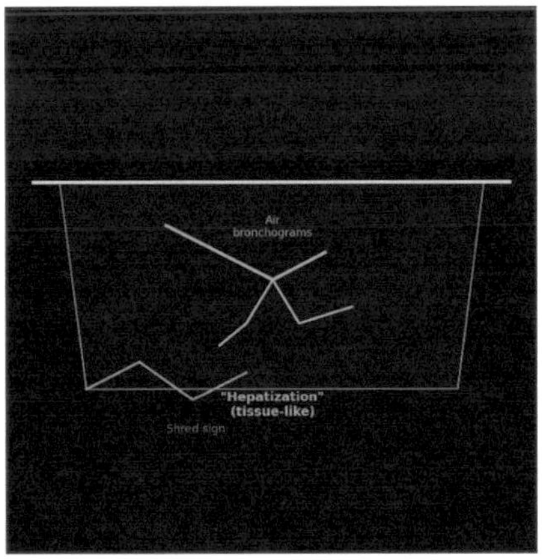

Pleural Effusion + Spine Sign

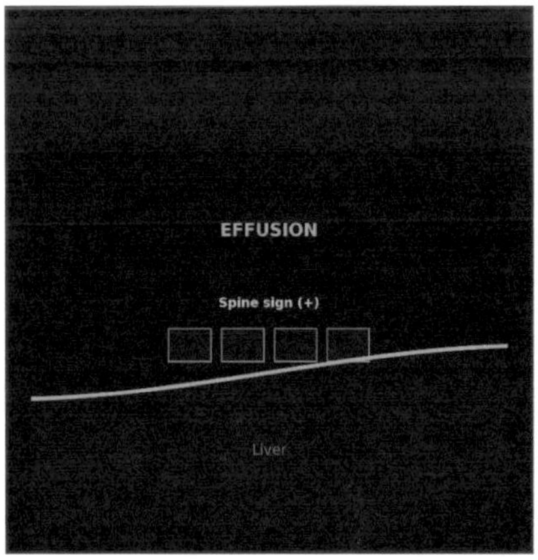

Thoracic US — Probe Placement (8-Zone Protocol)

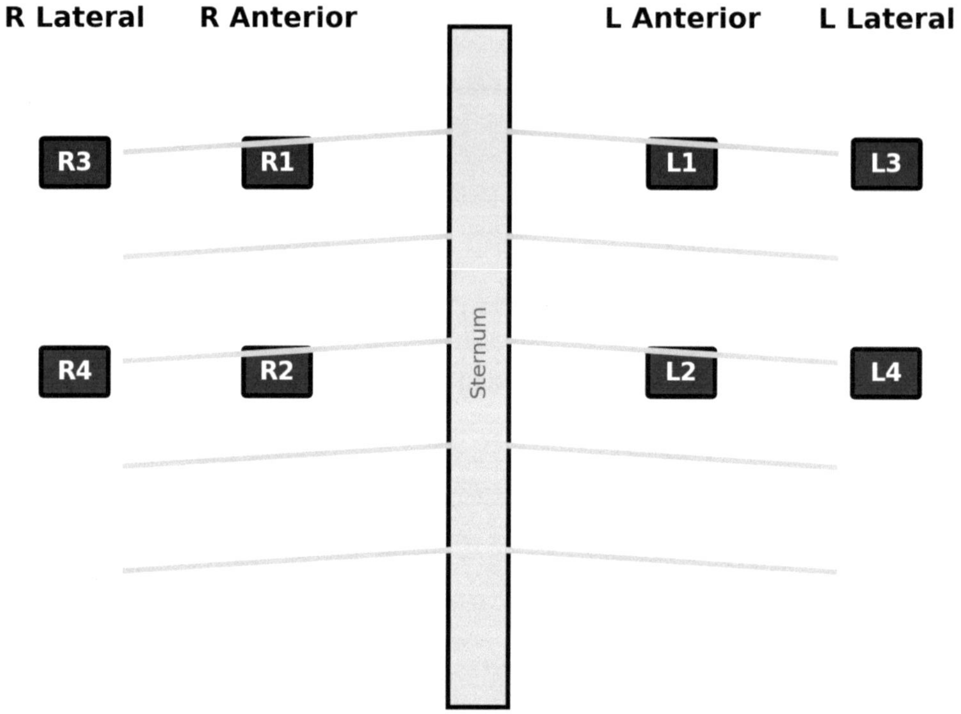

8-Zone Protocol:
• Anterior (2 zones/side)
• Lateral (2 zones/side)
• ≥3 B-lines in 2+ zones = interstitial syndrome

Venous/Arterial Assessment

1. Select linear probe (5—10 MHz).
2. Deep vein thrombosis (DVT): compression technique every 2 cm from groin (common femoral) to popliteal fossa and calf veins (gastrocnemius, soleal); vein should fully collapse with pressure; intraluminal thrombus appears as echogenic material with vein non-compressibility.
3. Augmentation: distal calf squeeze should enhance flow (absence suggests proximal obstruction).
4. Arterial assessment: identify plaque (hyperechoic wall thickening), stenosis (color aliasing, increased velocity on spectral Doppler >200 cm/s), occlusion (absent flow, monophasic waveform proximal).
5. Pseudoaneurysm: anechoic sac communicating with artery via neck; "to-and-fro" waveform on spectral Doppler within sac.
6. Arteriovenous fistula: arterialized venous waveform, high-velocity turbulent flow at communication site.

Compression US — Normal (Vein Collapses)

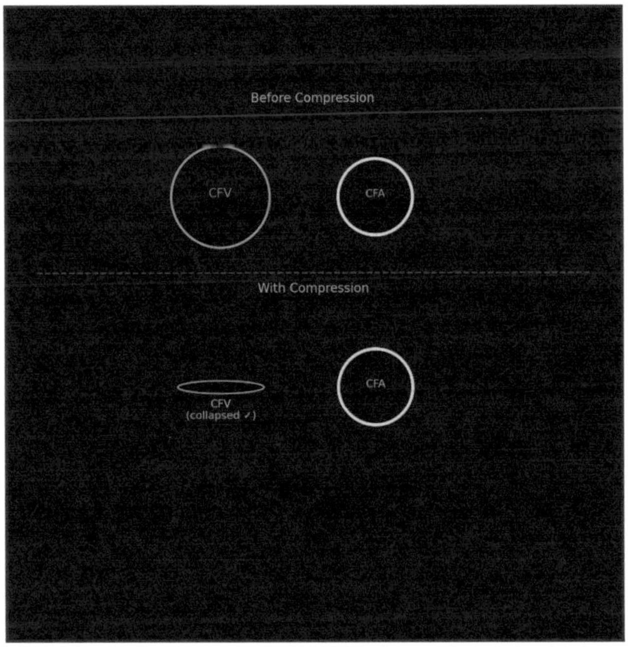

DVT Positive — Vein Non-Compressible

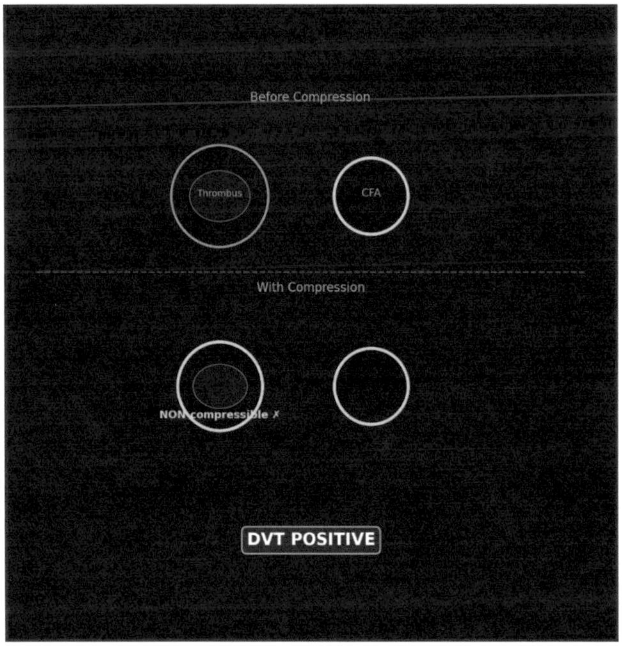

DVT — 2-Point Compression Sites

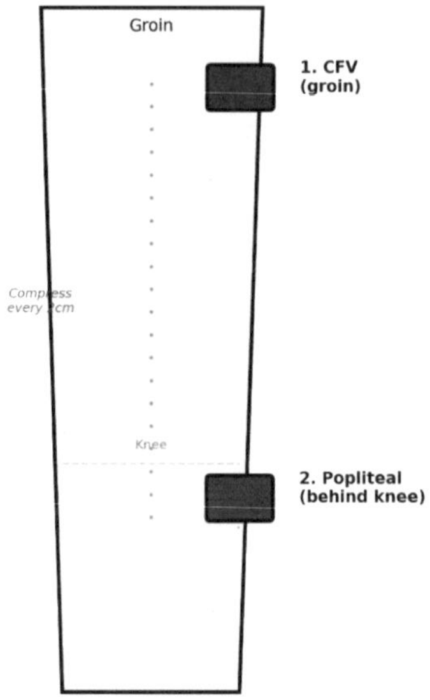

Pseudoaneurysm — "To-and-Fro" Flow

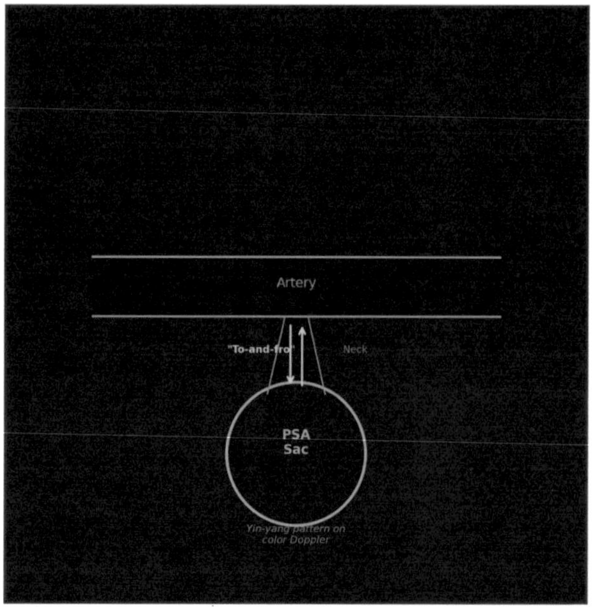

Appendix: Toxidrome Reference

General Approach

- ABC First: Secure airway, support breathing/ventilation, restore circulation; treat abnormal vitals immediately
- Treat the Patient, Not the Poison: Stabilization precedes identification
- Decontamination: Activated charcoal if within 1—2 hours and airway is protected

Anticholinergic Toxidrome

Recognition: "Mad as a Hatter, Blind as a Bat, Dry as a Bone, Red as a Beet, Hot as a Hare"

- Vitals: ↑ HR, ↑ Temperature, ↔ BP, ↓ RR (late)
- Physical Exam: Agitated/delirious, dilated pupils, dry skin, ↓ bowel sounds, urinary retention, flushed
- Common Agents: TCAs, Diphenhydramine, Atropine, Scopolamine, Antipsychotics
- Treatment:
    - Benzodiazepines for agitation and seizures (first line)
    - Active cooling for hyperthermia
    - Physostigmine (0.5—2 mg IV): Reversible cholinesterase inhibitor; diagnostic and therapeutic for severe delirium, dysrhythmias, or intractable seizures. Contraindicated if TCA overdose with QRS prolongation or seizures due to seizure risk.

Cholinergic Toxidrome

Recognition: "Wet as a Hound" — DUMBELS/SLUDGE

- Muscarinic: Bradycardia, miosis, ↑ bowel sounds, salivation, lacrimation, urination, defecation, emesis, diaphoresis
- Nicotinic: Tachycardia, hypertension, muscle fasciculations → weakness/paralysis (stimulation then blockade of nicotinic receptors)
- Common Agents: Organophosphates, Carbamates, Nerve agents (Sarin), Physostigmine
- Treatment:
    - Atropine: Competitive antagonist at muscarinic receptors; titrate to drying of secretions and clearing of bronchoconstriction (may require massive doses)
    - Pralidoxime (2-PAM): Regenerates acetylcholinesterase; effective for organophosphates (not carbamates) — give early before aging
    - Decontamination: Remove clothing; wash skin (Hepatic hydrolysis occurs; don't spread to providers)

Sympathomimetic Toxidrome

Recognition: "Speeding" — Hyperadrenergic State

- Vitals: ↑ BP, ↑ HR, ↑ RR, ↑ Temperature
- Physical Exam: Agitated/combative, dilated pupils, diaphoretic, tremulous, hyperreflexic
- Common Agents: Cocaine, Amphetamines, Bath salts (synthetic cathinones), Ephedrine
- Treatment:
    - Benzodiazepines (first line): For agitation, tachycardia, and hypertension
    - Cooling for hyperthermia (high risk of rhabdomyolysis)

- Avoid pure β-blockers in cocaine toxicity (unopposed α-stimulation worsens hypertension); use Nitroprusside or Phentolamine for severe refractory hypertension

---

Opioid Toxidrome

Recognition: "Code Blue" — Respiratory Depression

- Vitals: ↓ RR (hypoventilation), ↓ HR, ↓ BP, ↓ Temperature
- Physical Exam: Depressed mental status, pinpoint pupils (miosis), ↓ bowel sounds, track marks
- Common Agents: Heroin, Fentanyl, Morphine, Methadone, Oxycodone
- Treatment:
  - Naloxone: Competitive antagonist; start low (0.04—0.4 mg IV) and titrate to respiratory effort (not full arousal) to avoid precipitating withdrawal
  - Airway support: Bag-valve-mask ventilation if apnea; intubation if no response to naloxone
  - Monitor for non-cardiogenic pulmonary edema post-reversal

---

Sedative-Hypnotic Toxidrome

Recognition: "The Coma"

- Vitals: ↓ RR, ↓ HR, ↓ BP, ↓ Temperature
- Physical Exam: Depressed mental status (lethargy to coma), normal or dilated pupils, normal skin turgor
- Common Agents: Benzodiazepines, Barbiturates, Ethanol, Zolpidem, Propofol
- Treatment:
  - Supportive care: Airway protection; mechanical ventilation as needed
  - Flumazenil (Benzo antagonist): 0.2 mg IV — use with extreme caution; only for acute overdose without chronic use or co-ingestion (risk of precipitating withdrawal seizures)

Withdrawal Toxidromes

Alcohol/Benzo Withdrawal:

- Recognition: ↑ Vitals (tachycardia, HTN, hyperthermia), agitation, tremor, seizures
- Treatment: Benzodiazepines (diazepam/lorazepam) — treat with the offending agent or long-acting cross-tolerant agent; Phenobarbital for refractory cases

Opioid Withdrawal:

- Recognition: ↑ Vitals, anxious, dilated pupils, ↑ bowel sounds (hyperactive), yawning, lacrimation, piloerection
- Treatment: Not life-threatening; Clonidine (autonomic symptoms) or Buprenorphine/Methadone for replacement

Oral Board Pearls

- Mixed Overdoses: Common; may see obscured or contradictory signs (e.g., TCA overdose has anticholinergic features plus α-blockade causing hypotension and sodium channel blockade causing QRS widening)
- Hyperthermia: Sympathomimetic and anticholinergic toxidromes; avoid succinylcholine if rhabdomyolysis/hyperkalemia suspected
- Seizures: Benzodiazepines first; consider Pyridoxine (B6) for Isoniazid (INH) toxicity and Physostigmine for anticholinergic-induced seizures

Made in the USA
Las Vegas, NV
03 November 2026

57423148R00276